HUMAN ANATOMY AND PHYSIOLOGY SERIES

SKIN ANATOMY AND PHYSIOLOGY RESEARCH DEVELOPMENTS

HUMAN ANATOMY AND PHYSIOLOGY SERIES

Handbook of Granulocytes:
Classification, Toxic Materials Produced and Pathology
Reuben Hägg and Soren Kohlund (Editors)
2009. ISBN: 978-1-60741-582-4

Skin Anatomy and Physiology Research Developments
Leon F. Bukowskiy (Editor)
2009. ISBN: 978-1-60741-469-8

HUMAN ANATOMY AND PHYSIOLOGY SERIES

SKIN ANATOMY AND PHYSIOLOGY RESEARCH DEVELOPMENTS

LEON F. BUKOWSKY

EDITOR

Nova Biomedical Books

New York

For permission to use material from this book please contact us:
Telephone 631-231-7269; Fax 631-231-8175
Web Site: http://www.novapublishers.com

Library of Congress Cataloging-in-Publication Data

Skin anatomy and physiology research developments / [edited by] Leon F. Bukowskiy.
p. ; cm.
Includes bibliographical references and index.
ISBN 978-1-60741-469-8 (hardcover)
1. Skin. 2. Dermatologic agents. I. Bukowskiy, Leon F.
[DNLM: 1. Skin--anatomy & histology. 2. Skin Diseases. 3. Skin Physiological Phenomena. WR 101 S628 2009]
QP88.5.S554 2009
612.7'9--dc22 2009028882

Published by Nova Science Publishers, Inc. ✦ New York

Contents

Preface

Skin anatomy refers to the structure of the skin, which consists of two principal parts: the outer, thinner portion which is called the epidermis and the inner, thicker portion which is known as the dermis. Alternatively, skin physiology is the subdivision of physiology which concerns the functions of the skin including the regulation of body temperature, protection, sensation, excretion, immunity, blood reservoir and the synthesis of Vitamin D. There are more than a thousand conditions that may affect the skin but some of the most common skin diseases include rashes, bacterial infections, fungal infections, parasitic infections, pigmentation disorders, tumors and cancers and skin diseases that result from trauma. This new book gathers the latest research from around the globe in this field.

Chapter 1 - Lipid-based colloidal delivery systems are an emerging class of health and beauty formulations that combine the benefits of lipid physiological compounds figuring in their composition with the ability to deliver several active pharmaceutical ingredients (APIs) through the skin. Nanoemulsions and lipid nanoparticles have been exploited to increase skin hydration, to maintain and enhance a healthy skin appearance, associated to their unique properties of carrying APIs, such as sunscreens, antioxidants, anti-agings, antifungals and antimicrobials. In comparison to synthetic polymeric colloidal systems, nanoemulsions and lipid nanoparticles are biotolerable, biodegradable, and have low acute and chronic toxicological profile. To to take advantages these properties, research is being done towards the development of newer approaches, which could improve both the aesthetic appeal and performance of a product for topical, dermal and transdermal API delivery. This chapter describes the latest developments in API delivery using nanoemulsions and lipid nanoparticle when formulated in semi-solid vehicles such as gels. These novel formulations provide several advantages over conventional formulations in terms of skin permeation enhancement. Definitions, preparation procedures, characterization and stability of the formulations have been addressed, as well as their applications for topical, dermal and transdermal API delivery.

Chapter 2 - Skin thermal pain is one of the most common problems for humans in everyday life and in thermal therapies, a process in which the thermal behaviour of skin tissue is critical. In spite of its importance, the underlying physical and neural mechanisms of skin thermal pain are not clearly understood, and there are few attempts to model it. Besides, due to the lengthy thermal relaxation time in biological tissue, non-Fourier thermal behaviour has been experimentally observed, attracting increasingly more attention to this phenomenon. In this study, a new thermal-neural model is developed in order to investigate the possible role of non-Fourier thermal behaviour of skin tissue and its role in the transduction process of skin thermal pain sensation. In the model, the non-Fourier thermal behaviour of skin tissue is coupled to the neural response of the nociceptor (special receptor for pain sensation). The results demonstrate that the predicted thermal-neural responses of nociceptors from different bioheat transfer models can deviate substantially under constant surface temperature heating, implying that the non-Fourier thermal feature may play an important role in the nociceptor transduction process of skin thermal pain.

Chapter 3 - Ultraviolet radiation and oxygen together can cause severe damage to biological tissues. The outermost layer of the human skin, the stratum corneum, is of particular interest because of its constant exposure to these irritants. The effects of both noxious factors were examined to learn more about the molecular processes of damage, which may lead to the development of potential protective agents. Furthermore, the mechanisms of action of the molecules already applied to human skin as photoprotectives should be revealed completely. Skin lipid models are introduced as in vitro screening systems for the antioxidative properties of several test substances. Three lipid systems of variable complexity with increasing similarity to human skin were established. Ferrous sulfate, an electron donator and catalyst of the Haber-Weiss reaction, was added to the samples to trigger the formation of reactive oxygen species via a Fenton-like reaction. The amount of lipid peroxidation was quantified by the thiobarbituric acid assay detecting malondialdehyde. Investigations on a molecular level were carried out by use of the instrumental analytical methods mass spectrometry and electron paramagnetic resonance spectroscopy. The findings show that lipid model systems represent a useful approach in drug screening for powerful UV protectors. Hyaluronic acid was found to act antioxidatively in the skin lipid models, ascorbic acid acted as a prooxidant in all lipid model systems. Further investigations of both substances revealed the molecular mechanisms of the observed effects. The topical administration of ascorbic acid, therefore, needs critical re-consideration. Human skin has constant exposure to UV light and oxygen. Therefore, the administration of protectors in pharmaceutical formulations or sunscreens, as found in this study, may be helpful for the protection of the human skin against UV induced damage. In vivo experiments with hyaluronan and its fragments should follow to allow in vitro-in vivo correlation and clinical interpretation of the data.

Chapter 4 - The concealed information test (CIT) is a method of psychophysiological detection that identifies information a knowledgeable (guilty) person does not wish to reveal (Lykken, 1974, 1998). The rationale behind the use of CIT is based on theory and research on orienting responses (ORs) and habituation processes in humans.

Most experimental CIT studies have used electrodermal responses (e.g., skin conductance, skin resistance) as the single autonomic measure to examine various aspects of the CIT. In these studies, electrodermal measures were identified as an efficient means for detecting concealed information and for distinguishing between individuals who do or do not possess this knowledge.

Field research, however, produced large rates of false-negative outcomes and lower skin resistance detection efficiency than experimental studies. These discrepancies might have resulted from factors affecting perception and memory and from the use of a small number of

CIT questions. Other explanations concern the manner in which the test was applied and possible use of countermeasures to which electrodermal responses are particularly vulnerable.

The present review describes findings from experimental and applied research studies using electrodermal measures reported in the CIT literature from a somewhat different perspective. This review highlights several concerns of CIT testing and suggests solutions based on the most recent CIT research.

Chapter 5 - The use of vesicles as skin drug delivery system was introduced in the early eighties by Mezei & Gulasekharam. They reported that standard vesicles (liposomes) of dipalmitoylphosphatidylcholine (DPPC) and cholesterol (CH) increased the concentration of triamcinolone acetonide in the epidermis and dermis by 4-5 times and reduced percutaneous absorption compared with a standard ointment. This effect is known as localized effect. After this report researchers applied standard vesicles and recorded mainly localized effects and rarely targeted delivery to skin appendages or improved transdermal drug delivery. Suddenly, Cevc and coworkers introduced a new type of vesicles, *Transfersomes* in which phospholipids are the major components as liposomes but included an edge activator (surfactant) which provides the ultradeformability and flexibility of the vesicular membrane. These *Transfersomes* were reported to penetrate intact skin delivering therapeutic amounts of drugs such as insulin in efficiency similar to subcutaneous administration of the same formulation. It was difficult to conceive that large lipid vesicles could penetrate the densely packed stratum corneum in great numbers. Accordingly many workers have tested this hypothesis with controversial findings being reported regarding the mechanism of action, with the ultradeformable vesicles being better than standard liposomes. Other researchers included ethanol in liposomes to impart membrane flexibility. These vesicles were termed ethosomes. However, it is important to emphasize that, the higher the membrane flexibility and deformability of the vesicles the lower is their physical stability. Accordingly, the more stable vesicles, niosomes were studied. These vesicles comprise surfactant as the major component with cholesterol and may contain minute amounts of phospholipids. Niosomes are now considered as promising transdermal delivery systems with some surfactants producing highly flexible formulations.

This chapter will critically evaluate different types of vesicles as skin drug delivery systems with respect to their functions from surface to dermal and transdermal effects. The assessment will extend to highlight the possible mechanisms of actions of vesicles before finally reporting on the feasibility of these vesicles for scaling up.

Chapter 6 - Skin contains a network of extracellular matrix (ECM) proteins, including collagen and elastin. Collagen provides structure whereas elastin gives skin firmness and elasticity. The ECM proteins can be degraded or remodelled by the matrixmetalloproteinases (MMPs) and elastase. The MMPs are inhibited by tissue inhibitors of matrixmetalloproteinases (TIMPs). The dermal fibroblasts are primarily responsible for the ECM maintenance. However, there is cross talk between the epidermis and dermis via growth factors and cytokines; which regulate signaling pathways, transcription factors and gene expression. Transforming growth factor (TGF-β) released by epidermal keratinocytes stimulates ECM expression in fibroblasts.

With chronological aging there is fine wrinkling and loss/atrophy of collagen and elastin/fibrillin. Ultraviolet (UV) radiation and environmental pollutants, that can be metabolized in skin, cause direct or indirect DNA damage, formation of reactive oxygen species (ROS), and damage to the extracellular matrix. In photoaged skin there is degeneration of collagen and elastin; enhanced MMPs and elastase; and elastin accumulation as solar elastosis. The manifestations are wrinkles, diminished structural integrity, impaired wound healing, and cancer.

The experimental physiology in skin anti-aging is the identification of actives, and their mechanisms of action, by investigating effects of potential agents on various targets including (i) the regulation of gene expression (at protein, mRNA and transcription levels) of elastin, collagen, heat shock proteins, MMPs, and TIMPs in dermal fibroblasts; and growth factors, cytokines, MMPs and TIMPs in keratinocytes, (ii) cellular effects such as viability, metabolism and lipid peroxidation, (iii) keratinocyte-fibroblast modulation via soluble factors (conditioned media) and skin equivalents; and (iv) actives' direct inhibitory effect on MMPs, elastase and reactive oxygen species. These experiments are simultaneously performed in UV irradiated cells to determine photo protective effects.

Several actives have been identified that beneficially regulate the ECM for skin health, the predominant being *Polypodium leucotomos*, lutein, and xanthohumol. The effects of these plant extracts are similar to hormones and TGF-β. In addition, these actives counteract the damaging effects of ultraviolet radiation and environmental pollutants.

Chapter 7 - The potential EU ban on the use of animals in the testing of cosmetic products and their ingredients from 2009 together with the ethical reasons for avoiding tests on humans have recently prompted the development of guidelines on *in vitro* alternative methods and an extensive search for novel validated *in vitro* permeation models. The prediction of the percutaneous absorption by means of *in vitro* methodologies requires good *in vitro-in vivo* correlation. Moreover, due to differences in the type of vehicle (conventional vehicles or particulate carriers) and in the physicochemical properties of a substance such as its solubility, the selection of appropriate *in vitro* conditions is crucial. In particular, the validation of an *in vitro* skin penetration model appears quite difficult for highly lipophilic substances because of their limited rate of transfer between the stratum corneum and the viable epidermis due to their low solubility in most physiological receptor fluids.

This chapter focuses on comparative *in vitro-in vivo* skin permeation of butyl methoxydibenzoylmethane, a highly lipophilic UV-A absorber (log $P_{o/w} = 5.6$); methylbenzylidene camphor (log $P_{o/w} = 4.8$), a less lipophilic sunscreen agent; and glycolic acid, a hydrophilic active substance (log $P_{o/w} < 0$). Special attention is paid to the influence of the *in vitro* receptor medium on the *in vitro-in vivo* correlation. Skin absorption of micro- and nanoparticulate carriers and their suitability for cosmetic formulations are also reviewed.

Chapter 8 - Cutaneous ageing manifests itself as a progressive reduction in maximum function and reserve capacity of its constitutive tissues. The atrophy of collagen is a major factor in skin ageing. The menopause has been shown repeatedly to have a negative effect on the connective tissue of the skin. Such an effect is prevented and in some cases reversed with estrogen therapy. Large-scale clinical trials are necessary to help make informed recommendations regarding postmenopausal estrogen use and its role in prevention of skin ageing.

Chapter 9 - A spatial-temporal framework representing dermal absorption of chemicals is important for toxicological risk assessment. Failure to adequately estimate the amount of chemicals entering the body through the skin may compromise the ability of physiologically-based pharmacokinetic (PBPK) models to predict concentration-time profiles in individual tissue compartments. This contribution considers the conventional PBPK model equations as a boundary condition to a diffusive mass transport problem. The partial differential equation (PDE), representing the uptake of dibromomethane (500 to 10000 ppm) in the skin, is discretized into ordinary differential equations (ODEs) by orthogonal collocation techniques. The resulting system is solved in the Mathematica® environment to evaluate the fate of dibromomethane in the liver, fat, rapidly and slowly perfused compartments and to monitor its evolution in the different layers of the skin. This approach, which uses published physicochemical properties, predicts laboratory data very well. Cumulative amounts of dibromomethane into and out of the skin are also computed and compared to those obtained by applying a perfect sink boundary condition at the skin-capillary interface. Discrepancies between the two model predictions become more pronounced with increased exposure time. The steady-state dibromomethane concentration and the time to reach equilibrium values increased with the exposure level and stratum corneum depth. The proposed methodology may help to explore and elucidate potential links among exposure-time, concentration, skin depth and the onset of skin irritation.

Chapter 10 - Conventional ablative laser resurfacing is still considered the gold standard in the treatment of the sequelae associated with severe facial aging. However, because the post-treatment effects require long recovery periods and patients cannot return to their normal activities during this down time, a technique called fractional laser resurfacing has been proposed as an alternative. Fractional laser resurfacing techniques can offer good results when fighting skin deterioration such as textural changes, tissue laxness and pigmentation occurring with aging while maintaining well-controlled side effects normally associated with laser photothermal action.

With fractional resurfacing, laser radiation does not produce thermal damage to the whole of the cutaneous surface. In this case, therapeutic damage is induced to a small volume of tissue as a result of thousands of microscopic thermal columns. As only partial ablation occurs, the typical, slow wound healing stage of conventional ablative laser resurfacing is shortened and tissue recovery and reepitheliazation occurs quickly due to the active migration of keratinocytes from the neighboring non-treated tissue. In addition, the procedure can be carried out with topical anesthesia, producing only mild discomfort and the side effects, mainly edema and erythema, are milder in intensity and have a much shorter duration than those that occur in conventional ablative laser resurfacing.

Chapter 11 - With the advancement in computer technology, numerical simulation has been a useful tool in assisting the medical field in areas such as skin burns. Successful modeling of the skin can aid doctors in estimating the amount of the damaged skin to be removed to prevent development of poison due to harmful agents that enters the body. This chapter presents a two-dimensional human skin model developed to obtain temperatures within the skin due to heating under thermal steady state conditions. Simulations are carried out using the boundary element method (BEM) and the results are verified against the solutions obtained using the finite element method (FEM). The BEM proved to be a good alternative to using FEM. Advantages of BEM include improved accuracy, less required computer memory and more efficient computation. A parametric study is conducted using six factors: dermis thermal conductivity, subcutaneous fat thermal conductivity, blood perfusion rate, temperature of heating disk, heat transfer coefficient and ambient temperature. Results show that varying the temperature of the heating disk greatly affects the temperature within the affected tissue dominantly as compared to the other five factors.

In: Skin Anatomy and Physiology Research Developments ISBN: 978-1-60741-469-8
Editor: Leon F. Bukowsky

Chapter 1

Nanoemulsions and Lipid Nanoparticles Based Gels for Transdermal Active Pharmaceutical Ingredients Delivery

Eliana B. Souto[1,*] and Prapaporn Boonme[2]
[1]Department of Pharmaceutical Technology, Faculty of Health Sciences, Fernando Pessoa University, Rua Carlos da Maia, 296, Office S.5, P-4200-150 Porto, Portugal
[2]Department of Pharmaceutical Technology, Faculty of Pharmaceutical Sciences, Prince of Songkla University, Thailand

Abstract

Lipid-based colloidal delivery systems are an emerging class of health and beauty formulations that combine the benefits of lipid physiological compounds figuring in their composition with the ability to deliver several active pharmaceutical ingredients (APIs) through the skin. Nanoemulsions and lipid nanoparticles have been exploited to increase skin hydration, to maintain and enhance a healthy skin appearance, associated to their unique properties of carrying APIs, such as sunscreens, antioxidants, anti-agings, antifungals and antimicrobials. In comparison to synthetic polymeric colloidal systems, nanoemulsions and lipid nanoparticles are biotolerable, biodegradable, and have low acute and chronic toxicological profile. To to take advantages these properties, research is being done towards the development of newer approaches, which could improve both the aesthetic appeal and performance of a product for topical, dermal and transdermal API delivery. This chapter describes the latest developments in API delivery using nanoemulsions and lipid nanoparticle when formulated in semi-solid vehicles such as gels. These novel formulations provide several advantages over conventional formulations in terms of skin permeation enhancement. Definitions, preparation procedures, characterization and stability of the formulations have been addressed, as well as their applications for topical, dermal and transdermal API delivery.

* Correspondence author: Phone: +351 22 507 4630, Fax: +351 22 550 4637, E-mail: eliana@ufp.edu.pt

Keywords: Topical, dermal, transdermal API delivery, lipid nanoparticle-based gels, nanoemulsion-based gels, skin permeation enhancement

1. Introduction

The delivery of active pharmaceutical ingredients (APIs) through transdermal route is characterized by their skin passage overcoming several layers, aiming to reach the systemic circulation. In comparison to the oral drug delivery, transdermal route provides several advantages including the avoidance of gastrointestinal tract (GIT) absorption difficulties caused by pH variations, enzymatic activity, API interactions with food, drink or other orally administered API, as well as avoiding the first-pass metabolism [1]. For some specific groups of patients, who have inconveniences of parenteral and oral therapies, transdermal API delivery might be a suitable approach. Furthermore, transdermal delivery provides the possibility to suspend therapy rapidly by removing the application form from the skin and affords easy identification of the medication in emergencies. Controlled release properties are also possible [2].

Although several advantages can be pointed out for transdermal administration, API formulation and delivery through the skin can meet several difficulties due to the skin barrier function [2, 3]. The skin, the largest organ in the human body and functioning as a barrier against external environment, is anatomically divided into stratum corneum (12-20 μm), the living epidermis (60-100 μm) and the underlying dermis (2000-3000 μm) [4]. Beneath the dermis lies the subcutaneous fatty tissue, connecting to the underlying muscular layer. In general, the principal barrier function of the epidermis resides almost entirely in the stratum corneum. For a material absorbed percutaneously, the process is a sequence of deposition onto the stratum corneum, diffusion through the living epidermis and the passage through the upper part of the papillary dermis. The viable tissues may metabolize the API, particularly the epidermis, which contains most of the catabolic enzymes of the skin. The living skin plays an important role as an active metabolizing tissue affecting the API bioavailability when administered cutaneously. The papillary layer of the dermis is characterized by the presence of permeable capillaries which are responsible for driving the API molecules to the microcirculation soon after leaving the epidermis. Thus, the average total residence time of a particular API in the dermal aqueous phase may only be of the order of a minute. The deeper layers of the dermis should not, in general, influence percutaneous absorption. A further problem arises if the API is very lipophilic. After passing the horny layer, the molecule reaches an aqueous interface in which it is poorly soluble. The thermodynamic activity of the API immediately below the barrier may then be relatively high and approach that in the barrier itself. The activity gradient from the stratum corneum to the viable tissues falls and consequently so does the flux. The rate-determining step may become the clearance rate from the barrier rather than the penetration of the barrier. The permeation process to the diffusion of a substance through the horny layer, viable epidermis, and dermis, with the microcirculation can be idealized as an infinite sink. If separate diffusional resistances to the skin layers are apportioned, the total diffusional resistance of the composite skin barrier in steady state permeation can be described using the following equation [5]:

$$\sum R_i = \frac{h_{SC}}{D_{SC} K_{SC}} + \frac{h_E}{D_E K_E} + \frac{h_D}{D_D K_D}$$

where R_i is the diffusional resistance of the ith layer, h is the thickness and D the diffusion coefficient of the stratum corneum (SC), the viable epidermis (E) and the papillary layer of the dermis (D). The dermis and viable epidermis are extensively hydrated and diffusion coefficients are typical of liquid-state diffusion. In the dermis, molecules probably move within water-filled interstices. In contrast, the stratum corneum is a semi-fibrous structure which is characterized by a fibre or semi-solid diffusivity. The diffusional resistance of the stratum corneum to water is approximately 1000 times that of either the viable epidermis of the superficial region of the dermis. Polar and larger molecules usually have smaller diffusion coefficients in comparison to water, and the stratum corneum becomes even more dominant in the total permeation process. Thus, the horny layer will be the rate-limiting barrier for diffusion for the water-soluble API. The viable layers of the skin are relatively more significant barriers to the penetration of non-polar API than of polar ones. Nevertheless, these layers representing only about 4% of the total diffusional resistance will be insignificant for in vivo percutaneous absorption. Thus, for polar and non-polar APIs alike, the stratum corneum provides the rate limiting barrier to percutaneous absorption.

The lipid organization of the stratum corneum is highly responsible for the transport properties of the skin. The stratum corneum is a multicellular, metabolically inactive tissue composed of flattened keratinized cells and lipids surrounding the keratinized cell. On a dry weight basis, it consists of 75%-80% protein, 5%-15% complex lipoid mixture and 5%-10% unidentified material [6]. Its structure has been represented as a brick and mortar model, with the corneocytes (dead keratin filled cells) forming the bricks and the intercellular lipid the mortar. The intracellular space of completely differentiated horny cell is fully packed with semi-crystalline α-keratin and its amorphous keratin counterpart or β-keratin, whereas the intercellular space is composed of lamellar structures with aqueous and lipid layer. A layered structure of epidermal lipids has been proposed [5], being schematically represented in Figure 1.

The polar head groups of the lipids are gathered in layers with the non-polar chains pointed in opposite directions forming layers of methyl groups in the plane where the hydrocarbon ends. Figure 1 shows that not all the lipids are positioned with their polar groups localized in the polar layer. Some of them are in fact actually localized in the region between the methyl groups. These patterns also provide information useful to estimate the penetration by the water molecules into the spaces between the lipid molecules. The diffusion in liquid crystals is highly anisotropic, i.e. the diffusion parallel to these layers is fast similarly as in a liquid, but perpendicularly to the layers the diffusion is one or two magnitudes lower.

This layered structure, characterizing the lipid part of the stratum corneum, is not a perfectly organized array of layers parallel to the skin surface. As a consequence, a series of dislocations always occur. Thus, the diffusion coefficient is the gross one for a partially organized lamellar structure. The stratum corneum or horny layer acts therefore as the main element of the skin barrier function.

The analysis of the possible ways in which a particular API may reach the viable epidermis and the upper dermis after cutaneous application, and in what relative amounts this may occur, is difficult to foreseen. When the API molecule moves onto the intact skin after released from a vehicle, it first contacts with the sebum, cellular debris, bacteria, and other exogenous materials which cover the skin. In general, a molecule may penetrate to the viable tissue below the horny layer (subepidermal tissue) via two potential routes i.e. transepidermal route or transappendageal route.

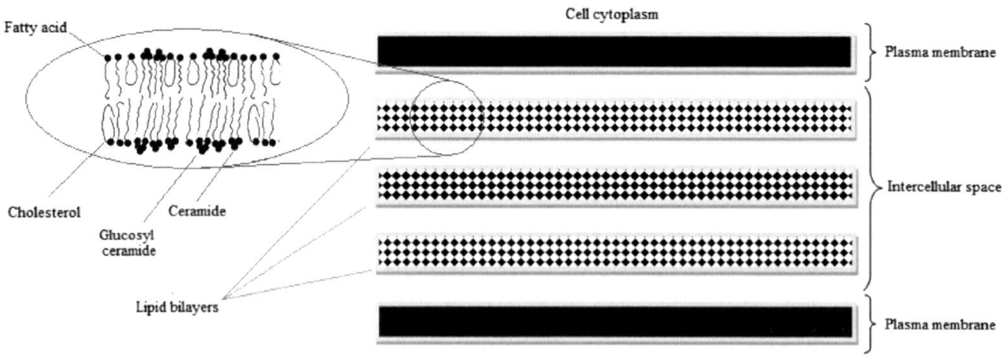

Figure 1. Schematic representation of the layered structure of epidermal lipids (modified after Osborne [5]).

The actual pathway for penetration via pilosebaceous apparatus could be through the hair fibre itself, through the outer root sheath of the hair into the viable cells of the follicle, or through the air-filled canal and into the sebaceous gland [7]. The route for the sweat duct may be through either the lumen or the walls to below the epidermis and through the thin ring of keratinized cells. Dense capillary networks closely envelope the bases of both the sweat ducts and the hair follicles. Most molecules reaching these highly permeable vascular regions would immediately sweep into the systemic circulation. Researchers who favour the appendageal route as the premier mode of entry cite as evidence the rapid diffusion or charged dyes through sweat ducts when they apply a potential gradient, the formation of perifollicular wheals and the preferential staining of hair follicles with dyes. On the other hand, those supporting the diffusion through the unbroken stratum corneum cite the small fraction of surface area of the appendages, the evidence that varying the number of appendages does not affect the steady state permeation and the very large activation energies measured, which would be improbable if the route was the relatively rapid appendageal pathway. Figure 2 shows a schematic representation of the routes by which APIs penetrate the skin, as well as examples of some APIs applied on the skin for particular treatments.

Of all cutaneous formulations, the most characteristic and common are the semi-solids because they are easy to apply. In addition, they are exploited as vehicles for a wide range of APIs in solution or suspension (with little tendency to separation), whether intended solely for topical action or for skin permeation and penetration. Spreading onto the skin may be controlled by adjusting the viscosity either for ease of application over a wide area or to confine the formulation to a circumscribed region. Semi-solids are devoid of mechanical irritant effect manifested by many particulate solids and, as they restrict the evaporation of moisture to a greater or less extent, they are smoothing to dry, fissured or inflamed skin (this property is retained longer with semi-solids than with liquids).

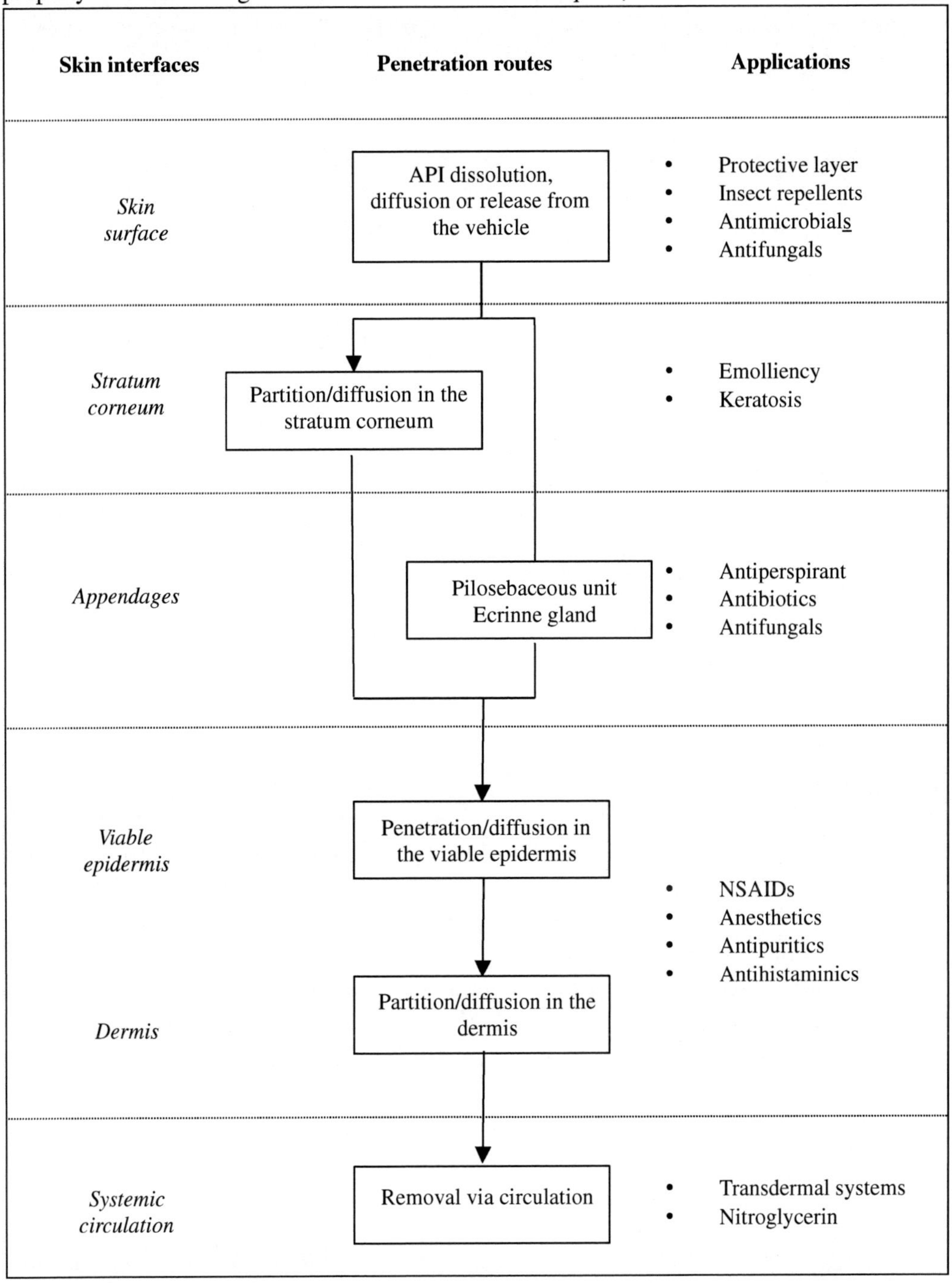

Figure 2. Possible routes by which APIs pass through the different skin layers (modified after Barry [7]).

Several strategies i.e. chemical, physical and synergistic approaches have been proposed in order to increase the skin penetration and permeation of APIs. Formulation development is a kind of chemical approach which can be used as a strategy to overcome the stratum corneum, increasing API penetration and permeation through the skin [8-10]. Nanoemulsion-based gels and lipid nanoparticle-based gels have emerged as useful formulations to modify the skin permeation of several APIs for cosmetic and pharmaceutical applications.

2. Nanoemulsions and Nanoemulsion-Based Gels

Nanoemulsions derive from "microemulsions" which are systems considered optically transparent, of low viscous and thermodynamically stable dispersions of oil and water stabilized by an interfacial film of an amphiphile molecule, such as a surfactant or a phospholipid [11]. Some microemulsion systems are also composed of a co-surfactant such as a polyhydroxy compound, a short-chain and a medium-chain alcohol in order to increase the flexibility of the interfacial film.

The microemulsion concept was introduced in the early 1940s by Hoar and Schulman who generated a clear single-phase solution by titration of a milky emulsion with a medium-chain alcohol. Schulman *et al.* subsequently coined the term "micro emulsion" (now written as "microemulsion") [12, 13]. Nowadays, these are also classified as "nanoemulsions" since they consist of very fine emulsions with a diameter smaller than 100 nm [14]. Thus, the term "nanoemulsion" has been adapted in the present chapter.

Nanoemulsions are metastable systems and can be prepared spontaneously by emulsification, phase inversion techniques or by using high shear homogenization (HSH), allowing a better control of the droplet size and a large choice of compositions. These systems are very fragile being very fluid, thus the slightest sign of destabilization is easily detected, becoming creamy and opaque [15].

Nanoemulsions have been exploited in several fields such as detergency [16], agrochemicals and biodiesels [17], foodstuffs [18, 19], cosmetics and pharmaceutics [15, 20]. In the field of topical, dermal and transdermal delivery, nanoemulsions have been reported as better delivery systems for many APIs through skin in comparison to simple solutions and conventional semi-solid dosage forms [21-27]. Due to their special features, nanoemulsions may modify the degree of skin penetration of APIs having different hydrophilicity [28, 29], they show solubilising properties for hydrophilic and lipophilic APIs, offering as well several advantages for pharmaceutical use, such as ease of preparation, and long-term stability [11]. The advantages associated with nanoemulsions include spontaneous formation, manufacturing facilities, high solubilization capacity, and improved API stability [30]. Nevertheless, skin irritation should be considered for evaluation since nanoemulsions usually require a relatively high concentration of surfactants.

Although it has been reported that nanoemulsions could provide advantages on cutaneous API delivery, application of nanoemulsions directly onto the skin in some cases may not be suitable due to their fluidity. Therefore, nanoemulsions in semi-solid forms i.e. nanoemulsion-based organogels and hydrogels have been proposed. Nanoemulsion-based gels were used as delivery vehicles for sodium salicylate [31], sodium fluorescin [32], triptolide [25, 33], ibuprofen [34] and progesterone [35], to achieve an enhanced skin permeation. In some cases, nanoemulsion-based gels can improve the stability of the loaded-

APIs. Biruss and Valenta reported that 46% of progesterone was degraded in the "pure nanoemulsions" (i.e. without thickeners) after 6 months of storage, whereas progesterone in nanoemulsion-based gels (using polymeric additives) were shown to be more stable [35]. The obtained results have been attributed to the improved stability provided by the polymeric additives which might be caused by an interaction between the nanoemulsion droplets and the polymers.

Kantaria *et al.* reported that gelatine-containing nanoemulsion-based organogels, used in the iontophoretic transdermal delivery of a model hydrophilic API (sodium salicylate), could be formulated using a combination of several polyoxyethylene sorbitans (Tween surfactants), bis-2-(ethylhexyl) sulfosuccinate and the oil isopropyl myristate (IPM) [31]. The preparation of these gels followed a two-step procedure. In the first step, the sodium salicylate-loaded water-in-oil (w/o) nanoemulsions was prepared by injection of an aqueous sodium salicylate solution to a reverse micellar surfactant solution, followed by stirring to obtain clear solutions. These nanoemulsions were composed of 25% w/w surfactant (Tween 21, Tween 81 or Tween 85), 25% w/w water and 50% w/w IPM. In the second step, solid gelatine (acid-hydrolyzed pig-skin gelatine, Bloom 300) was added to the previously prepared w/o nanoemulsions. Subsequently, the mixtures were heated up to 55°C with constant stirring until solubilisation of the gelatine was complete and then cooled to room temperature. The obtained gels were clear, homogeneous and non-birefringent.

Hydrogels are aqueous solutions presented in semi-solid form as a gel, produced by the use of a protective colloid in high concentration. Suitable hydrophilic polymers include xanthan gum, carrageenan, and synthetic molecules such as polyacrylates, and polyoxyethylene glycols.

Chen *et al.* prepared ibuprofen-loaded nanoemulsion-based hydrogels by mixing suitable ratios of ibuprofen, ethyl oleate, Tween 80, propylene glycol and water to obtain oil-in-water (o/w) nanoemulsions [34]. These nanoemulsions were then mixed with xanthan gum. After xanthan gum was entirely dissolved in the nanoemulsion, a clear nanoemulsion-based hydrogel was obtained. In addition to xanthan gum, carrageenan could be used as a jellifying agent in nanoemulsion-based gels. Valenta and Schulz prepared o/w nanoemulsions consisting of polyoxyethylene-10-oleyl ether (Brij 97), water and various oils by mixing the oil with the surfactant, heating up to 70-80°C and then pouring into the hot water (70-80°C) by stirring [32]. Carrageenan was mixed with the obtained nanoemulsions at room temperature. Other thickeners may be used, e.g. polymeric emulsifiers (Brij 97), silicone dioxide [35].

For the production of nanoemulsion-based gels two major steps are usually required. Firstly, nanoemulsions are prepared by mixing oil phase, water phase and surfactant or surfactant mixture at a particular ratio. Suitable ratios between the elements figuring in the nanoemulsion composition can be obtained by means of a ternary or pseudo-ternary phase diagram which is usually constructed by water titration technique [36, 37]. Secondly, a jellifying or thickening agent is added to nanoemulsions (o/w or w/o), being dispersed in the external phase. Due to their external oily phase, w/o nanoemulsions are useful to produce nanoemulsion-based organogels, whereas o/w nanoemulsions provide nanoemulsion-based hydrogels.

Nanoemulsion-based gels have been characterized in terms of rheological behaviour. The viscosity values of nanoemulsion-based gels are much higher than those of their thickener-free nanoemulsions. The optical appearance of nanoemulsion-based gels is transparent semi-solids whereas the original nanoemulsions are transparent liquids. Similarly to original nanoemulsions, nanoemulsion-based gels may be characterized for particle size, appearance under cross-polarized light microscope and conductivity. The droplet sizes of nanoemulsions usually ranges from 10 nm to 140 nm [12]. Birefringence is not typical in nanoemulsions but it is observed in lamellar and hexagonal liquid crystals [38-41]. Generally, o/w nanoemulsions provide higher conductivity than w/o nanoemulsions due to the low conductivity property provided by the oily external pseudophase of the o/w system. In addition, the physical stability can be determined by analysing the changing physical properties during storage time. The chemical stability can be investigated by assessing the amount of API at pre-determined time intervals [31, 32, 34, 35].

The proposed mechanisms to explain the skin permeation enhancement properties of nanoemulsion-based gels should be related to those of nanoemulsions. In nanoemulsion-based gels a large amount of API can be included in the formulation due to their high solubilising properties resulting in high API concentration gradient. The surfactants in the formulations may reduce the diffusional barrier of the stratum corneum. Nanoemulsion-based gels can act as API reservoirs. The inner nanoemulsion droplets of these gels might break down upon administration onto the surface of the stratum corneum and then release their content onto the skin. The enhancement effect can be explained by the nano-sized droplets the nanoemulsion-based gels since they can move easily through the skin carrying the API molecules. If the water content in the formulation is high enough, skin permeation of API can be improved due to the hydration effect of the stratum corneum [42].

3. Lipid Nanoparticles and Lipid Nanoparticle-Based Gels

Solid lipid nanoparticles (SLN) and nanostructured lipid carriers (NLC) are two types of lipid nanoparticles sized between 50 and 1000 nm, composed of physiological lipids, and being solid at body and room temperatures. These submicron carriers can be sorted out according to their inner structure, i.e. SLN consist of pure solid lipids and NLC contain a certain percentage of additional liquid lipid such as medium chain triglycerides (MCT) leading to imperfections in the crystal lattice [43]. The solid and liquid lipid blend also shows a melting point above 40ºC [44, 45]. The production process is identical for both particles, producing SLN and NLC surfaced with a surfactant layer.

SLN and NLC offer unique advantages, being possible their production free from organic solvents and with a wide range of lipid excipients with different properties. Furthermore, these systems can be used to carry APIs requiring high lipid exposure (up to 99% lipid loading), achieving high content uniformity, and high API loading capacity (up to 50% have already been reported) [46].

To overcome the occurrence of large sized particles and high polydispersity in the formulation, researchers often subject the precursor emulsions to large mechanical forces such as HSH, high pressure homogenization (HPH), and ultrasonication [47]. To produce both SLN and NLC, first the solid lipid or lipid blend is melted above 5-10°C its melting point, the active substance is dissolved in the melted lipid phase which is subsequently dispersed by high speed stirring in a hot aqueous surfactant/stabilizer solution of equivalent temperature. The obtained pre-emulsion is homogenized in a high pressure homogenizer yielding a hot o/w nanoemulsion. After cooling the emulsion droplets crystallize forming lipid nanoparticles with solid particle matrix [44, 45]. The high energy input increases operating expenses, increases mechanical contamination risks, and can inhibit the activity of mechanically and thermally sensitive biological molecules. In an effort to avoid the large mechanical energy inputs, some researchers pursue more chemically elegant approaches, namely nanoemulsions [48, 49] and solvent evaporation techniques [50-53]. Nevertheless, these latter require usage of organic solvents.

In both SLN and NLC the solid lipid includes triglycerides (e.g. tristearin), partial glycerides (e.g. Imwitor), fatty acids (e.g. stearic acid), steroids (e.g. cholesterol) and waxes (e.g. cetyl palmitate). All classes of emulsifiers (with respect to charge and molecular weight) have been used to stabilize the lipid dispersion. It has been found that the combination of emulsifiers might prevent particle agglomeration more efficiently [54]. The liquid lipids used in NLC are generally derivatives of caprylic/capric glycerides and triglycerides [55-57]. Alpha-tocopherol was also used in preparation of ketoconazole-loaded NLC [58]. A variety of APIs, including agents for treating cancer, AIDS, fungal infections, high blood pressure, mental illness, skin disease, and imaging have been loaded into lipid particles.

Dermal therapy is still a challenge due to the difficulties in controlling the API fate within the skin. Lipid nanoparticles have shown a great potential as vehicles for topical administration of APIs, mainly owing to the possible targeting effect and controlled release in different skin layers. Intact particles are not considered to permeate the horny layer and, due to the rigid nature of NLC, API penetration mechanism should be similar to that of APIs within gel-state liposomes [8].

The typical bioadhesive properties of lipid nanoparticles may influence the API bioavailability through the skin. In fact, SLN and NLC have proven to show occlusiveness when applied onto the skin, influencing its hydration degree [59]. Wissing *et al.* reported that approximately 4% of lipid nanoparticles with a diameter of 200 nm should theoretically create a monolayered film when ca. 4 mg of formulation is applied per cm^2 [60]. Due to its lipophilic character, this monolayered film has occlusive actions on the skin retarding the loss of moisture due to evaporation. Such moisture barrier properties have shown to influence the occlusion degree of lipid nanoparticles versus microparticles, i.e. depending on the size of the applied particles [61]. In addition, similarities between the composition of the lipid matrix and the skin should also be highlighted. The stratum corneum is mainly composed of three types of lipids, namely ceramides, free fatty acids and cholesterol. In ceramides C_{24}–C_{26} are the most common acyl chain lengths and C_{22}–C_{24} in free fatty acids [8]. These similarities can contribute to the adhesion of lipid nanoparticles onto the skin and even in case of NLC, the presence of liquid lipids, such as MCT, may enhance the NLC ability to mix with the stratum corneum lipids, which are present in the form of liquid crystals and to delay the API permeation on deeper skin strata.

The non-steroidal anti-inflammatory drugs (NSAIDs) ketoprofen and naproxen were loaded into glycerol behenate-based SLN produced either by hot HPH or by and ultrasonication techniques [57]. SLN were able to reduce API penetration increasing, simultaneously, the permeation and the accumulation in the horny layer. A prolonged anti-inflammatory effect was observed in the case of API-loaded SLN in comparison to the API solution.

Due to its liquid state, the presence of oil within a solid lipid matrix (i.e. NLC), may hold higher amounts of API molecules and, behaving as an impurity in the solid lipid, reduces the particle crystallinity conferring better stability and higher suitability for the controlled release [62, 63]. MCT, α-tocopherol and other oils [64] are useful both in NLC formulation optimization [62] and in enhancing the dermal/transdermal API delivery [63]. The presence of oil is also related to an increase of loading capacity (SLN versus NLC) which was shown for both ketoprofen and naproxen [57]. The reason pointed out for such result was the higher solubility of these NSAIDs in MCT, in comparison to their solubility when using solely the solid lipid. In addition, the liquid lipid tends to promote the formation of a small particle population as result of a higher molecular mobility of the matrix. Ketoprofen- and naproxen-loaded NLC showed a decreased permeation through the skin attributed to a possible API accumulation in the horny layer. It is known that nanoparticles can reduce and/or inhibit the permeation through the skin while enhancing the penetration into the upper skin layers [65-71]. This means that depending on the SLN/NLC composition, their size and physicochemical structure, a topical, dermal, or transdermal API delivery can be achieved [72].

The pharmacokinetic and biopharmaceutical differences observed various formulations may also be explained by the different physicochemical characteristics of the entrapped API, namely solubility, pKa and Log P, creating several interactions with the nanoparticle and/or with the stratum corneum lipids [73, 74]. It is estimated that a therapeutic molecule should possess a Log P equal or smaller than 2 to be a potential candidate for transdermal delivery [73]. For instance, in case of corticosteroids, these APIs contribute with their lipophilic character (measured by the partition coefficient between stratum corneum lipids and water) and with their vasoconstriction effect, and thus a higher epidermal accumulation might be observed [75, 76]. On the other hand, NSAIDs may depict a lower epidermal reservoir effect due to the APIs/vehicle physicochemical properties.

Other examples include vitamin A and its derivatives. In comparison to a nanoemulsion of similar composition, vitamin A-loaded SLN revealed a higher API penetration enhancement in the horny layer [65]. Isotretinoin-loaded SLN were also found to increase the amount of API in the skin when compared to the control tincture [68]. Similar findings were reported for prednicarbate- and ubidecarenone-loaded SLN when compared to conventional formulations [63, 77].

When discussing API delivery through the skin for topical, dermal and transdermal application, rheological characterization of the developed formulations is an important issue, which has also been useful to assess the structural characteristics of the lipid matrix [78-80]. Aqueous SLN dispersions composed of glycerol behenate, stearic alcohol or hydrogenated coco-glycerides revealed high storage modulus G' and loss modulus G'', suggesting the presence of a gel-like organization [81]. Moreover, those composed of glycerol behenate and stearic alcohol showed a larger G″ elastic modulus, while hydrogenated coco-glycerides-based SLN revealed a more viscous character (larger G′). Such results were attributed to the supercooled melt of hydrogenated coco-glycerides-based SLN in the opposite higher crystallinity of glycerol behenate and stearic alcohol SLN.

The influence of the particle size on the flow properties of SLN were assessed using cetyl palmitate as solid lipid, showing that both moduli (G′ and G″) increased approximately ten-fold in comparison to microparticles of similar composition [78]. The former shows higher viscoelasticity resembling a gel-like structure, being thereafter suitable for topical application. In comparison to NLC, which are characterized by a spherical-like shape, the gel-like structure of SLN provides higher semi-solid consistency because of their platelet-like arrangement. The platelet structures are created when highly ordered and compact crystalline arrangements occur, while spheroid particles are more likely when the entropy increases followed by a size increase, forcing the system to redistribute into a more thermodynamically stable arrangement. The assumption of a platelet structural assembling of lipid layers has been confirmed by transmission electron microscopy (TEM) [79, 82]. These non-spherical particles offer a much larger surface available for particle–particle interactions thus favouring the formation of a network-like structure. Such structures are naturally occurring especially for pure triglycerides-based SLN [82]. Platelets are defined by a couple of lipid layers forming a 10–18 nm thick structure. Cetyl palmitate SLN tend to crystallize in a platelet-like structure with a step-like surface, which depict an orthorhombic lamellar lattice arrangement [83]. Since the conventional preparation methods imply the SLN formation upon fast cooling from hot melted lipids [84], the lipid crystallization will develop highly ordered matrices.

Aqueous lipid nanoparticle dispersions are usually produced with a lipid content of 20-30%, showing a low consistency, e.g. viscosity is usually 100 mPas [79], similarly to nanoemulsions. And likewise, to develop a suitable formulation for topical, dermal and transdermal API delivery these systems can be added to hydrophilic bases, hydrophobic bases, or alternative producing lipid nanoparticle gels or creams.

For the incorporation of lipid nanoparticles into hydrophilic bases, lipid nanoparticle dispersions can be used as viscosity enhancers in topical hydrophilic formulations [85, 86]. Hydrophilic bases include single phase systems (hydrogels) and biphasic systems (o/w creams and lotions). Examples of suitable hydrogels are polyacrylates [85, 87-91] and polysaccharides, e.g. hydroxyethylcellulose derivatives, chitosan, hyaluronic acid and xantham gum [43, 90, 92]. Whilst similar consistency to the anhydrous o/w emulsifying bases, the hydrogels differ in having substantial water content and thereby exert a distinct cooling effect. For the incorporation of lipid nanoparticles into hydrogels, the gel compounds can be mixed, and a concentrated nanoparticle dispersion added before starting the jellifying process. Usually electrolytes are used to start jellifying process but in case of preparation of polyacrylate gels they may destabilize the lipid nanoparticles thus it is recommended to use neutralising agents such as triethanolamine [92], instead of sodium hydroxide. Electrolytes may change the zeta potential (surface electric charge) of particles reducing it too strongly leading to particle aggregation. To produce o/w creams a highly concentrated lipid nanoparticle dispersion is added, i.e. with 50% solid content. This concentration is enough to create an occlusive effect [60] or to load a cream with chemically unstable compounds which are stabilized by loading them in the lipid nanoparticle matrix [92].

As known, hydrophilic creams or o/w creams are dispersions of two immiscible liquids, the oil of the inner phase and the aqueous external or continuous phase. The presence of emulsifying molecules at the interface of oil and water decreases the interfacial free energy forming a homogeneous and stable semi-solid system. Addition of lipid nanoparticles to creams can be performed during or after the production of the o/w cream. In the first case, a part of the water figuring in the cream formulation is replaced by a highly concentrated dispersion, followed by the usual production process. The lipid nanoparticles are sufficiently stabilized avoiding their coalescence with the oil droplets of the o/w cream. If the production process of the cream is performed at a temperature higher than the melting point of the lipid nanoparticles, these latter will melt but will recrystallize during the cooling at the end of the process. In the second case, the cream is produced as usual, however with reduced water content in order to compensate the water added with the lipid nanoparticle dispersion. After production of the cream, the concentrated dispersion is mixed under stirring at approximately 30ºC or at lower temperatures (e.g. room temperature). This process avoids the melting of the nanoparticles, which could be followed by an undesired change of the internal particle structure.

Rheological behaviour of these semi-solid systems provides qualitative and quantitative information of the internal structure of the developed formulation. In addition, it relates also to the spreading properties during administration onto the skin, e.g. yield value (stress value at which below this, the formulation behaves as elastic solid) should not be too low. Figure 3 depicts the plots of shear rate as a function of shear stress of a conventional hydrophilic cream free of particles, in comparison to a formulation composed of the same hydrophilic cream containing 20% (m/m) of an aqueous SLN dispersion. Both formulations behaved as dilatant systems, revealing extremely low shear rates with the increase of the shear stress. The presence of 20% of SLN in the hydrophilic cream slightly increased the recorded values of shear rate.

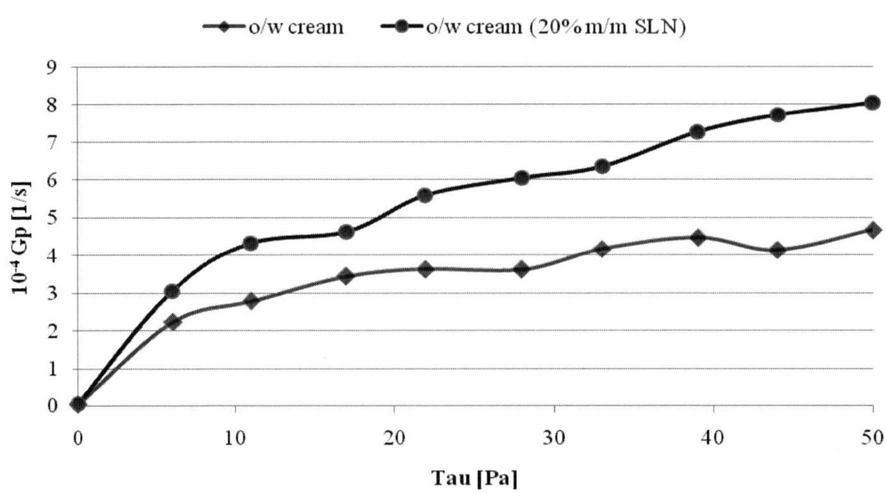

Figure 3. Shear rate as a function of shear stress of a hydrophilic cream (free of particles) and hydrophilic cream containing 20% (m/m) of aqueous SLN dispersion (adapted from Souto and Müller [93]).

When lipid nanoparticles are dispersed in a gel network or in an o/w cream a three dimensional system can be obtained. API can be delivered entrapped into lipid nanoparticles, dissolved in the gel or in both. If the API is present in both phases (i.e. lipid particles and gel network) a supersaturated system can be developed [63, 94]. The principle of supersaturation has been exploited for topical nanoemulsions to increase API penetration into the skin to the tissues underneath the stratum corneum. When applying nanoemulsions saturated with API onto the skin, the water from the skin diffuses into the nanoemulsion increasing its water content. The increase in saturation solubility will lead to an increased diffusion pressure of the API into the skin [63]. Similar systems can be developed when API-loaded lipid nanoparticles are dispersed into semi-solid bases already saturated with API. During storage, the API remains in the lipid matrix because these particles preserve their modification. After application onto the skin, the increase in temperature and water loss observed leads to transformation to a more ordered lipid modification and are responsible for API expulsion from the solid matrix. The API is expelled within the semi-solid vehicle (hydrogel or hydrophilic cream) already saturated with API, leading to supersaturation and API penetration onto the skin.

Incorporation of lipid nanoparticles into hydrophobic bases can be accomplished by using hydrophobic vehicles, such as paraffin, vegetable oils, and fatty alcohols to form w/o systems. These systems are suitable if the aim is to obtain only a topical effect avoiding systemic exposure of the API. Since lipid nanoparticles are oily-soluble constituents, when dispersed in these hydrophobic vehicles skin penetration will be reduced, in comparison to o/w creams. Water evaporation from the skin surface is usually faster from w/o systems than from w/o creams but these are sufficiently occlusive to have good emollient action. Hydrophobic vehicles are usually composed of a w/o emulsifying agent (e.g. cholesterol, white wax) along with a lipophilic diluent. No aqueous phase is usually present except that added by admixture with lipid nanoparticle dispersions. Although a w/o system will take up moderate quantities of water, it is not miscible with a large excess. Residues on the skin will not be easily removed with water alone and these bases are therefore not washable. Advantage of lipid nanoparticles dispersed in hydrophobic vehicles is the reduction of their fatty character nevertheless providing sufficient occlusion without intensive penetration of APIs.

Lipid nanoparticle gels can also be produced, consisting of lipid nanoparticle dispersions jellified by the addition of non-electrolyte jellifying agents, e.g. cellulose derivatives, to avoid particle aggregation. This procedure is relatively fast showing the advantage that the release of API is only controlled by the lipid matrix, and not by the structure of the dispersed vehicle as occurs when using hydrophilic or hydrophobic vehicles. For the production of lipid nanoparticle gels, first the aqueous dispersion is prepared, preferentially as highly concentrated as possible to be diluted to the desired final concentration. Then the jellifying agent is added [92]. For many gel preparations a lipid nanoparticle content of approximately 4-10% is high enough.

Production of lipid nanoparticle creams can be done by enhancing the viscosity of lipid nanoparticle dispersions solely by increasing the concentration of lipid phase usually above 30% (m/m). When using SLN, cream-like systems can be obtained above a maximum concentration of 30% lipid phase, depending on the chemical composition of SLN and NLC.

Nevertheless, when using NLC dispersions, instead of ointment-like systems creamy formulations are still obtained when increasing the concentration up to 50 or 60%. The viscosity of the formulations increases with the lipid concentration, i.e. at about 40-50% the preparations are cream-like, above 50% they become paste-like and when going up to a solid content of 80 or 90% the preparations become definitely solid. When analysing the rheological properties of these systems, a yield value with the increase of solid content is usually measured. The yield value needs to be sufficiently low to be removed from the packaging and sufficiently high to retain the formulation onto the skin area. Formulations containing 80 or 90% of lipid phase cannot be used for topical application but these can be exploited for oral administration [95]. For the production of these creams, firstly a stock lipid nanoparticle dispersion is prepared by high pressure homogenization containing e.g. 40% lipid nanoparticles. Then stepwise additional melted lipid is followed and dispersed again building a concentration of up to 50% of solid content. In the melted state, the preparation is still liquid and thus it has a relatively low viscosity. Under cooling the viscosity will decrease and the system becomes creamy.

4. Nanoemulsions versus Lipid Nanoparticles for Transdermal API Delivery

Depending on the therapeutic purposes, topical and dermatological applications are applied onto the skin to deliver APIs, which can have effect immediately on the local tissues beneath the application site, in deeper regions but near the application site, or far away from the application site if they are intended to reach the systemic circulation. When moving down this way (epidermis $\rightarrow$ dermis $\rightarrow$ blood), the API delivery becomes increasingly more difficult. For example, to reach the circulation through the skin, the API has to be delivered over longer periods of time and in appropriate amounts to exert its pharmacological effect. Therefore, penetration means that the API applied to the skin has made its way into the epithelial layer, possibly only into the outer layer or deeper, whereas absorption means that the API applied has penetrated to the dermis and has been taken into the fluid in the blood or lymphatic capillaries and thus distributed throughout the body.

Cutaneous delivery systems are applied onto the skin in layers which are so thin that compositional changes of the formulation following their application are substantial. By changing the way of formulating conventional topicals and dermatologicals by using nanoemulsions or lipid nanoparticles (SLN and NLC), a modified penetration rate of APIs onto the skin can be observed. This issue has been intensively studied using several different APIs [65, 77, 92, 96-98].

Spin-labelled compounds have been incorporated into lipid nanoparticles to study the possible penetration of particles onto the skin [99]. With this study, it was found that the lipid nanoparticles diffuse into the hair follicle, precisely into the gap surrounding the hair. This study shows the suitability of lipid nanoparticles for the treatment of acne and androgenetic alopecia. Since the layered lipid structure of the stratum corneum is not parallel organized, the particles which are able to penetrate through the pores of the skin will suffer anisotropic diffusion. The pores of the epidermis are of 10-70 μm size, thus lipid nanoparticles with a mean size of 200-400 nm might cross. It was found that liposomes can penetrate intact skin [100], and that the decrease of particle size enhanced skin penetration [101]. This mechanism may be facilitated and enhanced due to the formation of a monolayered film of lipid nanoparticles at the surface of the skin, which exert an occlusive effect and thus increasing the skin hydration. The penetration profiles will depend on the chemical nature of the API, but they are intensively affected by the oil droplets of nanoemulsions or matrix structure of the particles. If assuming the existence of special interactions between the lipids of the formulation with the intercellular lamellar lipids of the epidermis, a pronounced effect on the penetration profile will be observed.

The inner phase of the system (nanoemulsion versus lipid nanoparticle) also affects the release rate of API from the formulation [102]. A burst release followed by a prolonged release rate has been described for NLC [86]. SLN are composed solely of solid lipids thus a sustained released has been observed [102]. Burst release can be useful to improve the penetration of APIs. A controlled release rate becomes important when it is necessary to supply the API over a prolonged period of time, when it is necessary to reduce systemic absorption, and when the API is irritating in high concentrations. The release of incorporated APIs from the lipid nanoparticles can be modulated according to the needs from very fast to very slow [102]. In nanoemulsion formulations oil droplets have a liquid core and API is incorporated in the oil less tightly in comparison to the solid lipid matrix of lipid nanoparticle formulations (Figure 4). In these latter, API molecules are incorporated into the crystalline matrix and their diffusional mobility is decreased [102]. A comparison study has been performed to evaluate the delivery of a NSAID from conventional hydrogels and from lipid nanoparticles. When applying API-loaded lipid nanoparticles-based gels the anti-inflammatory effect was over two fold higher than of conventional hydrogels [85]. An improved API uptake has also been observed for the topical corticosteroid prednicarbate when delivered by means of SLN [77]. Due to their occlusive properties, lipid nanoparticles can increase skin penetration of corticosteroids. This is of major importance since these substances are associated to severe side effects when applied topically. Skin atrophy is frequently reported and may be minimized if a lower dose of API can be used maintaining the therapeutic efficiency.

Triptolide has been formulated in nanoemulsions and in lipid nanoparticles, and their ability for transdermal delivery of this anti-inflammatory, immunosuppressive, anti-fertility and anti-neoplastic API has been evaluated [33]. Both systems were suitable for enhancing triptolide penetration into the skin. Nevertheless, lipid nanoparticles depicted stronger anti-inflammatory activity than nanoemulsion in carrageenan induced rat paw edema, whereas nanoemulsions induced enhanced anti-inflammatory effects in complete Frenud's adjuvant induced paw edema. The release studies revealed higher ability of tristearin glyceride-based lipid nanoparticles to prolong the release of triptolide in comparison to IPM-based nanoemulsions.

5. Conclusions and Future Trends

The enhanced activity attributed to nanoemulsions and lipid nanoparticles seems to be associated to a variety of factors depending on the composition and the resulting microstructure of the topical, dermal and transdermal formulations. The exploitability of these systems in the practice depends on the choice of well-tolerated ingredients, mainly surfactants, and the restriction of their amounts in order to guarantee skin compatibility. Lipid-based colloidal carriers intended for topical, dermal and transdermal applications should be biocompatible and physically stable. Local irritancy is one of the primary concerns associated with the API and/or the delivery system. Nanoemulsions and lipid nanoparticles are composed of biodegradable, well tolerated and physiological lipids, usually the same used in the pharmaceutical and cosmetic industry. Therefore, it can be foreseen that cutaneous application of these systems reduces the risk of acute and chronic toxicity.

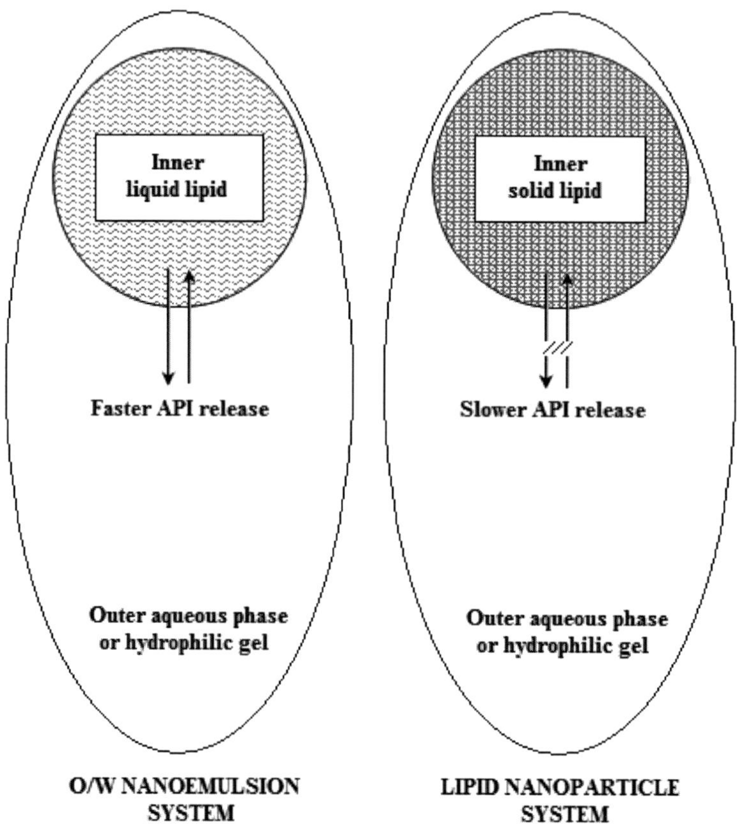

Figure 4. Schematic representation of morphological differences between nanoemulsions and lipid nanoparticles systems.

From the data of skin permeation enhancement and API stability improvement, nanoemulsion and lipid nanoparticle based gels can be suitable alternative API carrier systems for transdermal API delivery. When formulated as e.g. semi-solid gels, they provide better application on skin areas compared to their initial liquid formulations.

References

[1] Kaestli, LZ; Wasilewski-Rasca AF; Bonnabry P; Vogt-Ferrier N. Use of transdermal drug formulations in the elderly. *Drugs Aging,* 2008, 25, 269-280.

[2] Cevc, G. Lipid vesicles and other colloids as drug carriers on the skin. *Adv Drug Deliv Rev.,* 2004, 56, 675-711.

[3] Brown, MB; Traynor, MJ; Martin, GP; Akomeah, FK. Transdermal drug delivery systems: skin perturbation devices. *Methods Mol Biol,* 2008, 437, 119-139.

[4] Gambichler, T; Boms, S; Stucker, M; Moussa, G; Kreuter, A; Sand, M; Sand, D; Altmeyer, P; Hoffmann, K. Acute skin alterations following ultraviolet radiation investigated by optical coherence tomography and histology. *Arch Dermatol Res.,* 2005, 297, 218-225.

[5] Osborne, DW; Amann, AH. *Topical drug delivery formulations.* New York and Basel: Marcel Dekker; 1990.

[6] Marjukka Suhonen, T; Bouwstra, JA; Urtti, A. Chemical enhancement of percutaneous absorption in relation to stratum corneum structural alterations. *J Control Release,* 1999, 59, 149-161.

[7] Barry, BW. Dermatological formulations. In *Percutaneous absorption.* Edited by Barry BW. Marcel Dekker, New York and Basel: Marcel Dekker; 1983

[8] Bouwstra, JA; Honeywell-Nguyen, PL; Gooris, GS; Ponec, M. Structure of the skin barrier and its modulation by vesicular formulations. *Prog Lipid Res,* 2003, 42, 1-36.

[9] Hadgraft, J. Skin, the final frontier. *Int J Pharm,* 2001, 224, 1-18.

[10] Hadgraft, J. Modulation of the barrier function of the skin. *Skin Pharmacol Appl Skin Physiol,* 2001, 14 Suppl 1, 72-81.

[11] Heuschkel, S; Goebel, A; Neubert, RH. Microemulsions--modern colloidal carrier for dermal and transdermal drug delivery. *J Pharm Sci.,* 2008, 97, 603-631.

[12] Eccleston, GM. Microemulsions. In *Encyclopedia of Pharmaceutical Technology.* Volume 9. Edited by Boylan JC: Marcel Dekker: New York, pp. 375-421; 1988

[13] Lawrence, MJ; Rees, GD. Microemulsion-based media as novel drug delivery systems. *Adv Drug Deliv Rev.,* 2000, 45, 89-121.

[14] Sarker, DK. Engineering of nanoemulsions for drug delivery. *Curr Drug Deliv,* 2005, 2, 297-310.

[15] Sonneville-Aubrun, O; Simonnet, JT; L'Alloret, F. Nanoemulsions: a new vehicle for skincare products. *Adv Colloid Interface Sci.,* 2004, 108-109, 145-149.

[16] Bonini, M; Lenz, S; Giorgi, R; Baglioni, P. Nanomagnetic sponges for the cleaning of works of art. *Langmuir,* 2007, 23, 8681-8685.

[17] Wellert, S; Karg, M; Imhof, H; Steppin, A; Altmann, HJ; Dolle, M; Richardt, A; Tiersch B; Koetz, J; Lapp, A; Hellweg, T. Structure of biodiesel based bicontinuous microemulsions for environmentally compatible decontamination: A small angle neutron scattering and freeze fracture electron microscopy study. *J Colloid Interface Sci.,* 2008, 325, 250-258.

[18] Patel, N; Schmid, U; Lawrence, MJ. Phospholipid-based microemulsions suitable for use in foods. *J Agric Food Chem.,* 2006, 54, 7817-7824.

[19] Flanagan, J; Singh, H. Microemulsions: a potential delivery system for bioactives in food. *Crit Rev Food Sci Nutr.,* 2006, 46, 221-237.

[20] Tenjarla, S. Microemulsions: an overview and pharmaceutical applications. *Crit Rev Ther Drug Carrier Syst.,* 1999, 16, 461-521.

[21] Junyaprasert, VB; Boonsaner, P; Leatwimonlak, S; Boonme, P. Enhancement of the skin permeation of clindamycin phosphate by Aerosol OT/1-butanol microemulsions. *Drug Dev Ind Pharm,* 2007, 33, 874-880.

[22] Kreilgaard, M; Pedersen, EJ; Jaroszewski, JW. NMR characterisation and transdermal drug delivery potential of microemulsion systems. *J Control Release,* 2000, 69, 421-433.

[23] Paolino, D; Ventura, CA; Nistico, S; Puglisi, G; Fresta, M. Lecithin microemulsions for the topical administration of ketoprofen: percutaneous adsorption through human skin and in vivo human skin tolerability. *Int J Pharm.,* 2002, 244, 21-31.

[24] Peltola, S; Saarinen-Savolainen, P; Kiesvaara, J; Suhonen, TM; Urtti, A. Microemulsions for topical delivery of estradiol. *Int J Pharm.,* 2003, 254, 99-107.

[25] Chen, H; Chang, X; Weng, T; Zhao, X; Gao, Z; Yang, Y; Xu, H; Yang, X. A study of microemulsion systems for transdermal delivery of triptolide. *J Control Release,* 2004, 98, 427-436.

[26] Hua, L; Weisan, P; Jiayu, L; Hongfei, L. Preparation and evaluation of microemulsion of vinpocetine for transdermal delivery. *Pharmazie,* 2004, 59, 274-278.

[27] Hua, L; Weisan, P; Jiayu, L; Ying, Z. Preparation, evaluation, and NMR characterization of vinpocetine microemulsion for transdermal delivery. *Drug Dev Ind Pharm.,* 2004, 30, 657-666.

[28] Junyaprasert, VB; Boonme, P; Wurster, DE; Rades, T. Aerosol OT microemulsions as carriers for transdermal delivery of hydrophobic and hydrophilic local anesthetics. *Drug Deliv,* 2008, 15, 323-330.

[29] Junyaprasert, VB; Boonme, P; Songkro, S; Krauel, K; Rades, T. Transdermal delivery of hydrophobic and hydrophilic local anesthetics from o/w and w/o Brij 97-based microemulsions. *J Pharm Pharm Sci.,* 2007, 10, 288-298.

[30] Date, AA; Patravale, VB. Microemulsions: applications in transdermal and dermal delivery. *Crit Rev Ther Drug Carrier Syst.,* 2007, 24, 547-596.

[31] Kantaria, S; Rees, GD; Lawrence, MJ. Gelatin-stabilised microemulsion-based organogels: rheology and application in iontophoretic transdermal drug delivery. *J Control Release,* 1999, 60, 355-365.

[32] Valenta, C; Schultz, K. Influence of carrageenan on the rheology and skin permeation of microemulsion formulations. *J Control Release,* 2004, 95, 257-265.

[33] Mei, Z; Chen, H; Weng, T; Yang, Y; Yang, X. Solid lipid nanoparticle and microemulsion for topical delivery of triptolide. *Eur J Pharm Biopharm,* 2003, 56, 189-196.

[34] Chen, H; Chang, X; Du, D; Li, J; Xu, H; Yang, X. Microemulsion-based hydrogel formulation of ibuprofen for topical delivery. *Int J Pharm.,* 2006, 315, 52-58.

[35] Biruss, B; Valenta, C. The advantage of polymer addition to a non-ionic oil in water microemulsion for the dermal delivery of progesterone. *Int J Pharm.,* 2008, 349, 269-273.

[36] Boonme, P; Krauel, K; Graf, A; Rades, T; Junyaprasert, VB. Characterisation of microstructures formed in isopropyl palmitate/water/Aerosol OT:1-butanol (2:1) system. *Pharmazie,* 2006, 61, 927-932.
[37] Boonme, P; Krauel, K; Graf, A; Rades, T; Junyaprasert, VB. Characterization of microemulsion structures in the pseudoternary phase diagram of isopropyl palmitate/water/Brij 97:1-butanol. *AAPS PharmSciTech.,* 2006, 7, E45.
[38] Kayali, I; Suhery, T; Friberg, SE; Simion, FA; Rhein, LD. Lyotropic liquid crystals and the structural lipids of the stratum corneum. *J Pharm Sci.,* 1991, 80, 428-431.
[39] Friberg, SE; Kayali, I; Beckerman, W; Rhein, LD; Simion, A. Water permeation of reaggregated stratum corneum with model lipids. *J Invest Dermatol,* 1990, 94, 377-380.
[40] Friberg, SE; Kayali, I. Water evaporation rates from a model of stratum corneum lipids. *J Pharm Sci.,* 1989, 78, 639-643.
[41] Shah DO; Hamlin, RM. Jr. Structure of Water in Microemulsions: Electrical, Birefringence, and Nuclear Magnetic Resonance Studies. *Science,* 1971, 171, 483-485.
[42] Boonme, P. Applications of microemulsions in cosmetics. *J Cosmet Dermatol,* 2007, 6, 223-228.
[43] Souto, EB; Wissing, SA; Barbosa, CM; Muller, RH. Evaluation of the physical stability of SLN and NLC before and after incorporation into hydrogel formulations. *Eur J Pharm Biopharm.* 2004, 58, 83-90.
[44] Souto, EB; Müller, RH. Lipid nanoparticles (SLN and NLC) for drug delivery. In *Nanoparticles for Pharmaceutical Applications.* Edited by Domb AJ, Tabata, Y., Ravi Kumar, M.N.V., Farber, S. (Eds.): American Scientific Publishers, Chapter 5; 2007, 103-122
[45] Souto, EB; Müller, RH. Challenging cosmetics: Solid lipid nanoparticles (SLN) and nanostructured lipid carriers (NLC). In *Science and Applications of Skin Delivery Systems.* Edited by Wiechers J, Kozlowski, A., (Eds.): Allured Publishing, Carol Stream, Chicago, USA, Chapter 13; 2008, 227-250
[46] Jannin, V; Musakhanian, J, Marchaud, D. Approaches for the development of solid and semi-solid lipid-based formulations. *Adv Drug Deliv Rev.,* 2008, 60, 734-746.
[47] Hou, D; Xie, C; Huang, K; Zhu, C. The production and characteristics of solid lipid nanoparticles (SLNs). *Biomaterials,* 2003, 24, 1781-1785.
[48] Gasco, MR. Method for producing solid lipid microspheres having a narrow size distribution. *US Patent 5 250 236: Italy*; 1993.
[49] Sjostrom, B; Kaplun, A; Talmon, Y; Cabane, B. Structures of nanoparticles prepared from oil-in-water emulsions. *Pharm Res.,* 1995, 12, 39-48.
[50] Sjostrom, B; Bergenstahl, B; Kronberg, B. A method for the preparation of submicron particles of sparingly water-soluble drugs by precipitation in oil-in-water emulsions. II: Influence of the emulsifier, the solvent, and the drug substance. *J Pharm Sci.,* 1993, 82, 584-589.
[51] Battaglia, L; Trotta, M; Gallarate, M; Carlotti, ME; Zara, GP; Bargoni, A. Solid lipid nanoparticles formed by solvent-in-water emulsion-diffusion technique: development and influence on insulin stability. *J Microencapsul,* 2007, 24, 660-672.
[52] Shah, KA; Date, AA; Joshi, MD; Patravale, VB. Solid lipid nanoparticles (SLN) of tretinoin: potential in topical delivery. *Int J Pharm.,* 2007, 345, 163-171.

[53] Yuan, H; Huang, LF; Du, YZ; Ying, XY, You, J; Hu, FQ; Zeng, S. Solid lipid nanoparticles prepared by solvent diffusion method in a nanoreactor system. *Colloids Surf B Biointerfaces,* 2008, 61, 132-137.

[54] Mehnert, W; Mader, K. Solid lipid nanoparticles: production, characterization and applications. *Adv Drug Deliv Rev.,* 2001, 47, 165-196.

[55] Hu, FQ; Jiang, SP; Du, YZ; Yuan, H; Ye, YQ; Zeng, S. Preparation and characteristics of monostearin nanostructured lipid carriers. *Int J Pharm.,* 2006, 314, 83-89.

[56] Teeranachaideekul, V; Souto, EB; Junyaprasert, VB; Muller, RH. Cetyl palmitate-based NLC for topical delivery of Coenzyme Q(10) - development, physicochemical characterization and in vitro release studies. *Eur J Pharm Biopharm,* 2007, 67, 141-148.

[57] Puglia, C; Blasi, P; Rizza, L; Schoubben, A; Bonina, F; Rossi, C; Ricci, M. Lipid nanoparticles for prolonged topical delivery: an in vitro and in vivo investigation. *Int J Pharm.,* 2008, 357, 295-304.

[58] Souto, EB; Muller, RH. SLN and NLC for topical delivery of ketoconazole. *J Microencapsul,* 2005, 22, 501-510.

[59] Souto, EB; Muller, RH. Cosmetic features and applications of lipid nanoparticles (SLN, NLC). *Int J Cosmet Sci.,* 2008, 30, 157-165.

[60] Wissing, S; Lippacher, A; Muller, R. Investigations on the occlusive properties of solid lipid nanoparticles (SLN). *J Cosmet Sci.,* 2001, 52, 313-324.

[61] Wissing, SA; Muller, RH. Cosmetic applications for solid lipid nanoparticles (SLN). *Int J Pharm.,* 2003, 254, 65-68.

[62] Muller, RH; Radtke, M; Wissing, SA. Nanostructured lipid matrices for improved microencapsulation of drugs. *Int J Pharm.,* 2002, 242, 121-128.

[63] Muller, RH; Radtke, M; Wissing, SA. Solid lipid nanoparticles (SLN) and nanostructured lipid carriers (NLC) in cosmetic and dermatological preparations. *Adv Drug Deliv Rev.,* 2002, 54 Suppl 1:S131-155.

[64] Souto, EB; Muller, RH. Investigation of the factors influencing the incorporation of clotrimazole in SLN and NLC prepared by hot high-pressure homogenization. *J Microencapsul* 2006, 23, 377-388.

[65] Jenning, V; Gysler, A; Schafer-Korting, M; Gohla, SH. Vitamin A loaded solid lipid nanoparticles for topical use: occlusive properties and drug targeting to the upper skin. *Eur J Pharm Biopharm,* 2000, 49, 211-218.

[66] De Jalon, EG; Blanco-Prieto, MJ; Ygartua, P; Santoyo, S. Topical application of acyclovir-loaded microparticles: quantification of the drug in porcine skin layers. *J Control Release,* 2001, 75, 191-197.

[67] Chen, HB; Chang, XL; Du, DR; Liu, W; Liu, J; Weng, T; Yang, YJ; Xu, HB; Yang, XL. Podophyllotoxin-loaded solid lipid nanoparticles for epidermal targeting. *Journal of Controlled Release,* 2006, 110, 296-306.

[68] Liu, J; Hu, W; Chen, H; Ni, Q; Xu, H; Yang, X. Isotretinoin-loaded solid lipid nanoparticles with skin targeting for topical delivery. *Int J Pharm.,* 2007, 328, 191-195.

[69] Lombardi Borgia, S; Regehly, M; Sivaramakrishnan, R; Mehnert, W; Korting, HC; Danker, K; Roder, B; Kramer, KD; Schafer-Korting, M. Lipid nanoparticles for skin penetration enhancement-correlation to drug localization within the particle matrix as

determined by fluorescence and parelectric spectroscopy. *J Control Release,* 2005, 110, 151-163.

[70] Alvarez-Roman, R; Naik, A; Kalia, YN; Guy, RH; Fessi, H. Enhancement of topical delivery from biodegradable nanoparticles. *Pharm Res.,* 2004, 21, 1818-1825.

[71] Alvarez-Roman, R; Naik, A; Kalia, YN; Guy, RH; Fessi, H. Skin penetration and distribution of polymeric nanoparticles. *J Control Release,* 2004, 99, 53-62.

[72] Jacobi, U; Tassopoulos, T; Surber, C; Lademann, J. Cutaneous distribution and localization of dyes affected by vehicles all with different lipophilicity. *Arch Dermatol Res.,* 2006, 297, 303-310.

[73] Beetge, E; Du Plessis, J; Muller, DG; Goosen, C; Van Rensburg, FJ. The influence of the physicochemical characteristics and pharmacokinetic properties of selected NSAID's on their transdermal absorption. *Int J Pharm.,* 2000, 193, 261-264.

[74] Schafer-Korting, M; Mehnert, W; Korting, HC. Lipid nanoparticles for improved topical application of drugs for skin diseases. *Adv Drug Deliv Rev.,* 2007, 59, 427-443.

[75] Hadgraft, J. The epidermal reservoir: a theoretical approach. *Int J Pharm* 1979, 2, 265-274.

[76] Malkinson, FD; Ferguson EH. Percutaneous absorption of hydrocortisone-4-C14 in two human subjects. *J Invest Dermatol* 1955, 25, 281-283.

[77] Santos Maia, C; Mehnert, W; Schaller, M; Korting, HC; Gysler, A; Haberland, A; Schafer-Korting, M. Drug targeting by solid lipid nanoparticles for dermal use. *J Drug Target,* 2002, 10, 489-495.

[78] Lippacher, A; Muller, RH; Mader, K. Preparation of semisolid drug carriers for topical application based on solid lipid nanoparticles. *Int J Pharm.,* 2001, 214, 9-12.

[79] Lippacher, A; Muller, RH; Mader, K. Investigation on the viscoelastic properties of lipid based colloidal drug carriers. *Int J Pharm.,* 2000, 196, 227-230.

[80] Illing, A; Unruh, T. Investigation on the flow behavior of dispersions of solid triglyceride nanoparticles. *Int J Pharm.,* 2004, 284, 123-131.

[81] Souto, EB; Wissing, SA; Barbosa, CM; Muller, RH. Comparative study between the viscoelastic behaviors of different lipid nanoparticle formulations. *J Cosmet Sci.,* 2004, 55, 463-471.

[82] Jores, K; Mehnert, W; Drechsler, M; Bunjes, H; Johann, C; Mader, K. Investigations on the structure of solid lipid nanoparticles (SLN) and oil-loaded solid lipid nanoparticles by photon correlation spectroscopy, field-flow fractionation and transmission electron microscopy. *J Control Release,* 2004, 95, 217-227.

[83] Lukowski, G; Kasbohm, J; Pflegel, P; Illing, A; Wulff, H. Crystallographic investigation of cetylpalmitate solid lipid nanoparticles. *Int J Pharm.,* 2000, 196, 201-205.

[84] Wissing, SA; Kayser, O; Muller, RH. Solid lipid nanoparticles for parenteral drug delivery. *Adv Drug Deliv Rev.,* 2004, 56, 1257-1272.

[85] Mei, Z; Wu, Q; Hu, S; Li, X; Yang, X. Triptolide loaded solid lipid nanoparticle hydrogel for topical application. *Drug Dev Ind Pharm.,* 2005, 31, 161-168.

[86] Joshi, M; Patravale, V. Formulation and evaluation of Nanostructured Lipid Carrier (NLC)-based gel of Valdecoxib. *Drug Dev Ind Pharm.,* 2006, 32, 911-918.

[87] Joshi, M; Patravale, V. Nanostructured lipid carrier (NLC) based gel of celecoxib. *Int J Pharm.,* 2008, 346, 124-132.

[88] Bhaskar, K; Krishna Mohan, C; Lingam, M; Jagan Mohan, S; Venkateswarlu, V; Madhusudan Rao, Y; Anbu, J; Ravichandran, V. Development of SLN and NLC Enriched Hydrogels for Transdermal Delivery of Nitrendipine: In Vitro and In Vivo Characteristics. *Drug Dev Ind Pharm.,* 2008, 1-16.

[89] Liu, W; Hu, M; Xue, C; Xu, H; Yang, X. Investigation of the carbopol gel of solid lipid nanoparticles for the transdermal iontophoretic delivery of triamcinolone acetonide acetate. *Int J Pharm.,* 2008.

[90] Shahgaldian, P; Quattrocchi, L; Gualbert, J; Coleman, AW; Goreloff, P. AFM imaging of calixarene based solid lipid nanoparticles in gel matrices. *Eur J Pharm Biopharm.,* 2003, 55, 107-113.

[91] Souto, EB; Muller, RH. The use of SLN and NLC as topical particulate carriers for imidazole antifungal agents. *Pharmazie,* 2006, 61, 431-437.

[92] Jenning, V; Schafer-Korting, M; Gohla, S. Vitamin A-loaded solid lipid nanoparticles for topical use: drug release properties. *J Control Release,* 2000, 66, 115-126.

[93] Souto, EB; Muller, RH. Rheological and in vitro release behaviour of clotrimazole-containing aqueous SLN dispersions and commercial creams. *Pharmazie* 2007, 62, 505-509.

[94] Souto, EB; Almeida, AJ; Muller, RH. Lipid nanoparticles (SLN (R), NLC (R)) for cutaneous drug delivery: Structure, protection and skin effects. *Journal of Biomedical Nanotechnology,* 2007, 3, 317-331.

[95] Muller, RH; Keck, CM. Challenges and solutions for the delivery of biotech drugs--a review of drug nanocrystal technology and lipid nanoparticles. *J Biotechnol,* 2004, 113, 151-170.

[96] Gysler, A; Kleuser, B; Sippl, W; Lange, K; Korting, HC; Holtje, HD. Skin penetration and metabolism of topical glucocorticoids in reconstructed epidermis and in excised human skin. *Pharm Res.,* 1999, 16, 1386-1391.

[97] Gysler, A; Lange, K; Korting, HC; Schafer-Korting, M. Prednicarbate biotransformation in human foreskin keratinocytes and fibroblasts. *Pharm Res.,* 1997, 14, 793-797.

[98] Lange, K; Gysler, A; Bader, M; Kleuser, B; Korting, HC; Schafer-Korting, M. Prednicarbate versus conventional topical glucocorticoids: pharmacodynamic characterization in vitro. *Pharm Res.,* 1997, 14, 1744-1749.

[99] Munster, U; Nakamura, C; Haberland, A; Jores, K; Mehnert, W; Rummel, S; Schaller, M; Korting, HC; Zouboulis Ch, C; Blume-Peytavi, U; Schafer-Korting M. RU 58841-myristate--prodrug development for topical treatment of acne and androgenetic alopecia. *Pharmazie,* 2005, 60, 8-12.

[100] Cevc, G; Schatzlein, A; Richardsen, H. Ultradeformable lipid vesicles can penetrate the skin and other semi-permeable barriers unfragmented. Evidence from double label CLSM experiments and direct size measurements. *Biochim Biophys Acta,* 2002, 1564, 21-30.

[101] Verma, DD; Verma, S; Blume, G; Fahr, A. Particle size of liposomes influences dermal delivery of substances into skin. *Int J Pharm.,* 2003, 258, 141-151.

[102] Souto, EB; Wissing, SA; Barbosa, CM; Muller, RH. Development of a controlled release formulation based on SLN and NLC for topical clotrimazole delivery. *Int J Pharm.*, 2004, 278, 71-77.

In: Skin Anatomy and Physiology Research Developments ISBN: 978-1-60741-469-8
Editor: Leon F. Bukowsky

Chapter 2

Non-Fourier Thermal Behaviour of Skin Tissue and Its Role in Skin Thermal Pain Sensation

F. Xu[1], T. J. Lu[2,*] and E.Y.K. Ng[3]

[1]Engineering Department, Cambridge University, Cambridge CB2 1PZ, UK

[2]MOE Key Laboratory of Strength and Vibration, School of Aerospace, Xi'an Jiaotong University, Xi'an 710049, P.R. China

[3]School of Mechanical and Aerospace Engineering, Nanyang Technological University, 50 Nanyang Avenue, Singapore 639798

Abstract

Skin thermal pain is one of the most common problems for humans in everyday life and in thermal therapies, a process in which the thermal behaviour of skin tissue is critical. In spite of its importance, the underlying physical and neural mechanisms of skin thermal pain are not clearly understood, and there are few attempts to model it. Besides, due to the lengthy thermal relaxation time in biological tissue, non-Fourier thermal behaviour has been experimentally observed, attracting increasingly more attention to this phenomenon. In this study, a new thermal-neural model is developed in order to investigate the possible role of non-Fourier thermal behaviour of skin tissue and its role in the transduction process of skin thermal pain sensation. In the model, the non-Fourier thermal behaviour of skin tissue is coupled to the neural response of the nociceptor (special receptor for pain sensation). The results demonstrate that the predicted thermal-neural responses of nociceptors from different bioheat transfer models can deviate substantially under constant surface temperature heating, implying that the non-Fourier thermal feature may play an important role in the nociceptor transduction process of skin thermal pain.

* Corresponding author: Fax: +86-29-83234781; E-mail address: tjlu@mail.xjtu.edu.cn

Keywords: skin tissue, non-Fourier thermal behaviour, neural response, thermal pain, modeling, nociceptor

1. Introduction

Skin is generally composed of several layers with different microstructures, as shown in Figure 1(a), and plays a variety of roles including sensory, thermoregulation and host defense, etc. The most important role of skin is thermoregulation, enabling the skin to act as an important barrier for the human body to various outside conditions. However, when exposed to extreme heat or cold, people feel uncomfortable or even pain: obviously, the skin fails to protect the body when the temperature moves out of the normal physiological range. On the other hand, in medicine, various thermal-based therapies are widely used to cure disease/injury involving skin tissue, with thermal injury induced precisely within the diseased tissue but without affecting the surrounding healthy tissue. The effectiveness of these treatments is governed by the coupled thermal, mechanical, biological and neural responses of the affected tissue: a favorable interaction results in a procedure with relatively little pain and no lasting side effects. The associated problem of pain relief has nonetheless limited the further application and development of these thermal treatments.

1.1. Non-Fourier Thermal Behaviour of Skin Tissue

In many situations, heat conduction in materials has been treated according to the classic Fourier's law, which assumes that any thermal disturbance on a body is instantaneously felt throughout the body or, equivalently, the propagation speed of the thermal disturbance is infinite. Although this assumption is reasonable for the majority of practical applications, it fails in particular thermal conditions or heat conduction media, such as materials with non-homogeneous inner structure [1]. The non-homogeneous inner structure of biological tissue suggests the existence of non-Fourier heat conduction behavior, as temperature oscillation (an unusual oscillation of tissue temperature with heating) and wave-like behaviour are commonly observed. Temperature oscillation in living tissue was first observed by Richardson et al. [2] and later by Roemer et al. [3]. Subsequently, Mitra et al. [4] carried out four different experiments with processed meat for different boundary conditions and also observed the wave-like behavior (i.e., temperature jumps that can be regarded as the wave front). On the other hand, Davydov et al. [5] experimentally observed that heat transfer in a muscle tissue under local strong heating exhibits substantial anisotropy, which cannot be explained by the standard Fourier-theory based heat diffusion model. Banerjee et al. [6] measured the thermal response of meat under laser irradiation, and found that the non-Fourier hyperbolic heat conduction equation is a better approximation than the classical parabolic Fourier heat conduction formulation.

From a therapeutic viewpoint, the high-intensity short duration heating scheme can efficiently produce an appropriate and precise dose of heat during thermal therapies. In addition, reducing the overall treatment time is important, especially when the treatment target volume is large. A rapid heating scheme with a good strategy is therefore essential for an effective thermal therapy. However, the possible non-Fourier nature of heat transfer in living tissue, as described above, may play an important role during rapid heating, such as thermal ablation/thermal surgery, when a high-intensity thermal source such as focused laser, ultrasound or radiofrequency ablation is used. For example, it has been shown that the thermal relaxation of tissue will delay the appearance of peak temperature during thermal treatments, leading to a lower thermal dose level [7].

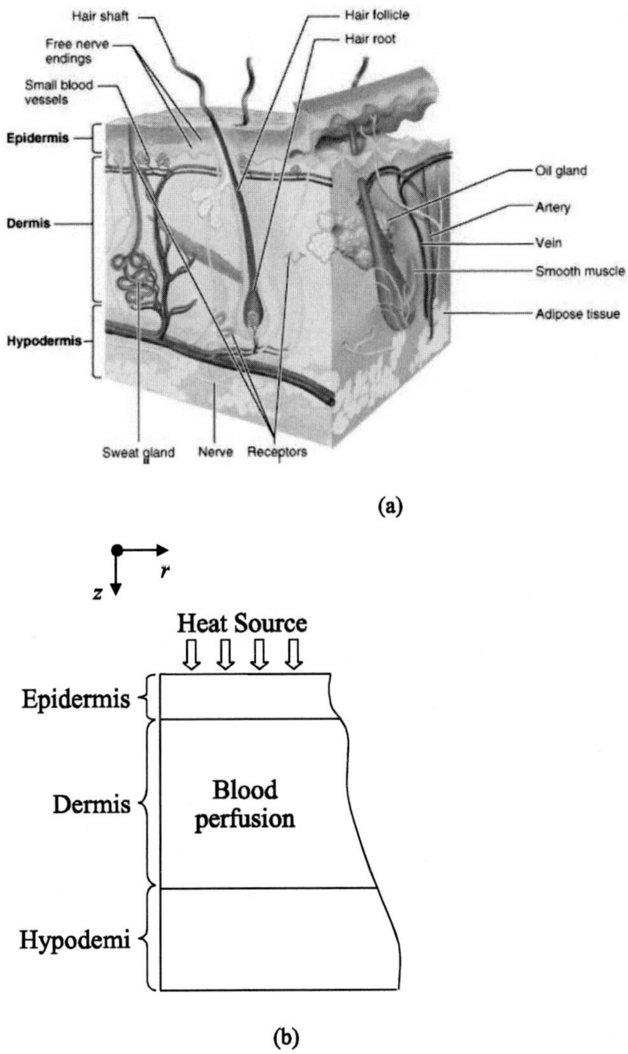

Figure 1. (a) Skin structure [104] and (b) corresponding idealized skin model

In our previous study [8], the dual-phase-lag model is introduced for the first time to bioheat transfer of skin tissue due to its ability to characterize the microstructural interactions effect in heat transport. Together with the thermal wave model of bioheat transfer proposed by other researchers, the non-Fourier thermo-mechanical behaviour of skin tissue is analyzed under surface heating boundary conditions. Exact solutions for thermal stresses with single-layer skin model and full numerical simulations with multi-layer skin model are then used to examine the non-Fourier process and its influence on the mechanical response of skin tissue. The results demonstrate that non-Fourier feature may play an important role in the thermal behavior of skin tissue, particularly under rapid heating/cooling conditions.

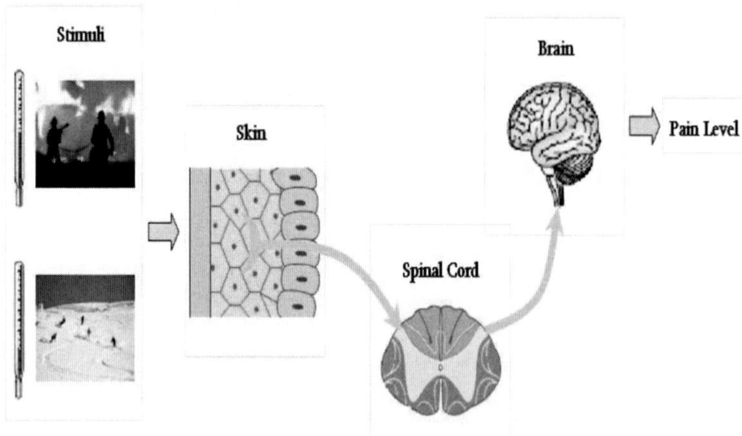

Figure 2. Skin thermal pain pathway: stimulus **(hot/cold)** → **skin** (the energy of thermal stimulus is converted into electrical energy via nerve impulses) → spinal cord & brain (the signals are transmitted to the dorsal horn of the spinal cord and brain, where they are modulated and perceived as pain sensation)

1.2. Skin Thermal Pain

When the skin temperature rises above (or drops below) a critical value, an uncomfortable or pain sensation is induced. Pain can in general be classified as nociceptive pain, inflammatory pain and neuropathic pain.

1.2.1. Pain pathway

The physiology of nociceptive pain has been studied extensively [9-12]. The pain pathway is schematically shown as Figure 2, which is mainly composed of four processes. 1) Transduction. When a stimulus is applied to the skin tissue, the nociceptors located there will trigger action potentials by converting the physical energy from a noxious thermal, mechanical, or chemical stimulus into electrochemical energy via nerve impulses. 2) Transmission. The signals are subsequently transmitted in the form of chains of action potentials similar to pulse trains via nerve fibers from the site of transduction (peripheral site, e.g., skin) to the dorsal horn[1] of the spinal cord and brain, which then activates the associated

[1] The dorsal horn of the spinal cord is the dorsal (more towards the back) grey matter of the spinal cord. It receives several types of sensory information from the body, including light touch, proprioception, and vibration. This information is sent from receptors of the skin, bones, and joints through sensory neurons whose cell bodies lie in the dorsal root ganglion. [13] M. Patestas, L.P. Gartner, *A Textbook of Neuroanatomy*, p. Blackwell Publishing Ltd., Oxford (2006).

transmission neuron. 3) Modulation. This is when descending inhibitory and facilitory input from the brain influences, or modulates, nociceptive transmission at the level of the spinal cord. 4) Perception. This is the appreciation of signals arriving in higher level structures of the neural system such as the brain, as pain.

1.2.2. Nociceptors for pain

Nociceptors, as special receptors for pain sensation, are the first cells in the series of neurons leading to the sensation of nociceptive pain [14]. Nociceptors transduct mechanical, chemical and/or thermal energy to ionic current leading to action potentials: these potentials are conducted from the peripheral sensory site to the synapse in the central nervous system, and converted into neurotransmitter release at the presynaptic terminal (frequency modulation) [15].

Peripheral nerves include myelinated afferent $A\delta$, $A\alpha$ and $A\beta$ fibers, as well as unmyelinated afferent C fibers. However, $A\beta$ fibers only respond to non-noxious, low density mechanical stimuli. Most nociceptors are either $A\delta$ or C fibers, while thermal pain sensations are mediated by both thin myelinated $A\delta$ and unmyelinated C fibers [16]. In addition, there are so-called "silent" nociceptors, which cannot be activated at normal conditions [17-20]. For example, in the survey of cutaneous C fibers, Bessou & Perl [21] found that 10% of the neural fibers in the skin sample was inexcitable while Lynn & Carpenter [22] and Pini & Baranowski [23] found that up to 28% of the nerve units in rat skin tissue were inexcitable. Under conditions of inflammation or tissue injury, however, these silent nociceptors are sensitized and activated by a variety of chemical mediators [19, 24, 25]. This recruitment of previously silent nociceptors under pathological states may contribute to temporal and spatial summation of pain and considerably enhances the C fiber afferent barrage to the dorsal horn. It may also contribute both to primary hyperalgesia due to heat and pressure after chemical irritation, and secondary hyperalgesia as a consequence of central sensitization [11, 19, 20].

According to their response character to different stimulations, nociceptors can be further classified as: C and $A\delta$ mechanoheat nociceptors (CMH, AMH); C and $A\delta$ high threshold mechanoreceptors (CM, AM); C and $A\delta$ chemoreceptors; C and $A\delta$ polymodal nociceptors; C and $A\delta$ cold nociceptors; C and $A\delta$ mechanoinsensitive (silent) nociceptors. Furthermore, C fibers, which respond only to heating and known as CH, have also been found [19]. In the study of cutaneous sensory receptors in the skin tissue of rat hindpaw, Leem et al. [26] found that $\sim$70% of the $A\delta$ nociceptors were mechanical nociceptors, 20% were mechanoheat nociceptors, and 10% were mechanocold nociceptors. The cutaneous nociceptors responding to thermal stimulations are largely polymodal, as they can be activated by thermal, mechanical and/or chemical stimuli [27, 28].

1.2.3. Distribution of nociceptors in skin tissue

The skin is a large organ which senses the external environment. Numerous encapsulated and free sensory nerve endings within the skin tissue respond to stimulations by temperature, pressure and touch. Their perceptions are cultivated by variable combinations of three types of sensory receptor: mechanoreceptors for touch, vibration, and pressure; thermal receptors for temperature; and nociceptors for pain.

Nociceptors with sensory terminals in skin tissue have been widely studied since Burgess & Perl [29] and Bessou & Perl [21]. As for nociceptors in skin tissue, C, $A\delta$ and $A\beta$ fibers are typically present in respective proportions of, approximately, 70%, 10% and 20%, but these ratios may vary [11]. Each of these fibers is attached to a receptor in the skin tissue which may be a Meissner's corpuscle, a Pacinian corpuscle, a Ruffini or Krause end-organ or, for the great majority (60–70%), a free nerve ending. Many unmyelinated C fibers can be traced far into the epidermal layer. Vertical sections reveal that free nerve endings emerge from superficial dermal nerve plexuses running into epidermis [30], as shown by the green points in Figure 3. The study of myelinated mechanical nociceptor endings in hairy cat skin tissue showed that the free nerve endings for pain receptors exist around a depth of $50\ \mu m$ from the skin surface [31], while the receptors responsible for mediating the pain sensation are found to be at a depth of approximately $200\ \mu m$ [32]. In comparison, the receptor depth in the hairy skin tissue of monkeys, which has been estimated from responses to ramped stimuli, ranged from 20 to $570\ \mu m$, with a mean of $201\ \mu m$ [33, 34].

It has been also found that there are more C fibers in the skin tissue than $A\delta$ fibers [35, 36]. Depending on the species and the methods for quantification, the density of C terminals is approximately 2–8 per mm^2, while that of $A\delta$ fibers is less than 1 per mm^2 [37].

1.2.4. Ion channels of nociceptors

The essential function of nociceptors depends on ion channels [9, 15], which are integral membrane proteins found in all cells. They mediate the selective passage of specific ions or molecules across a cell membrane [38]. Although there are many different ion channels belonging to nociceptors, these channels are generally converted from closed to open states, or "gated", by three types of stimulus: thermal (hot or cold), mechanical, and chemical stimuli, with thresholds of 43 °C and ~ 0.2 MPa for the first two, as shown in Figure 3. Although not directly gated by stimuli, channels that are gated by changes in transmembrane voltage form a very important class of channels. These voltage-gated channels respond to membrane depolarization or hyperpolarization, and are central to the generation and transmission of electrical signals (action potential) along nerve axons [39].

The working mechanism of a nociceptor can be simply described as follows. When a large noxious stimulus is applied to the nociceptor, the corresponding ion channels will be opened, as shown in Figure 3, inducing a heat current through the nociceptor membrane and increasing the membrane voltage. When the voltage increases more than its threshold, the current will then open more channels in a positive feedback mode that results in the depolarization of the membrane, eventually generating the action potential. In our previous study [40], an analytical model of nociceptor transduction in skin thermal pain has been developed by introducing the skin thermomechanical model and incorporating the biophysical and neurological mechanisms of pain sensation. The concepts of bioengineering are coupled with established methods in neuroscience, and the biological behavior of skin is re-casted in engineering systems parlance. The model development has been made consistent with the known morphology and physiology of skin tissue. It has been demonstrated that the model is capable of capturing the essential properties of experimentally measured frequency responses.

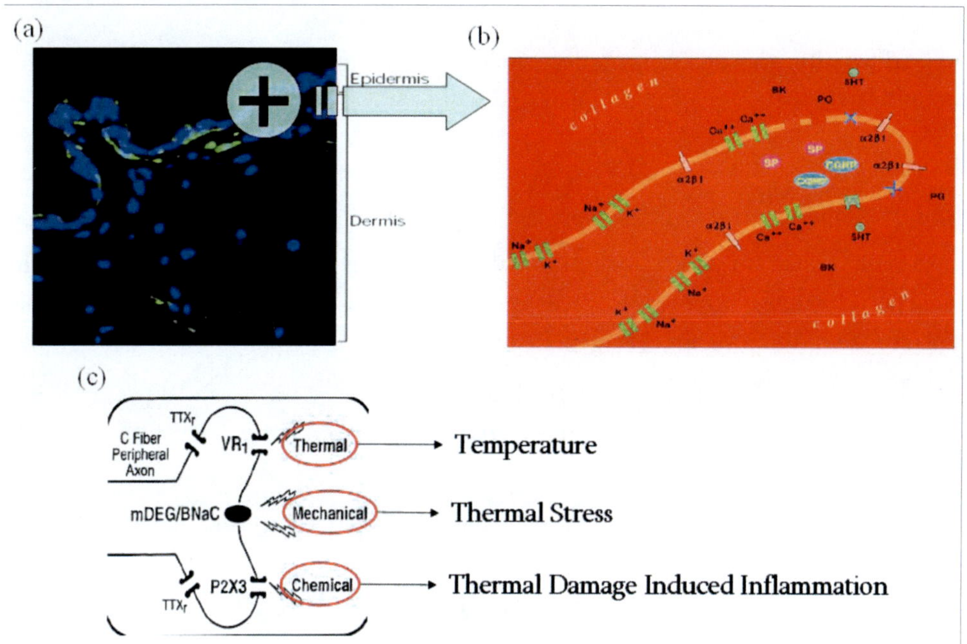

Figure 3. Schematic of nociceptor transduction: if the thermal stimulus overpasses the thermal threshold of nociceptors (green points in (a)), the heat current will be induced due to the opening of the corresponding ion channels in (b) and action potential is triggered; the thermal stress and thermal damage induced release of some chemical mediators may also open corresponding mechanical- and chemical-gated channels in (c) if it is larger than the mechanical threshold 37

1.3. Aims and Structure of This Chapter

The aim of this paper is to investigate the possible role of non-Fourier thermal behaviour of skin tissue in skin thermal pain sensation, by combining the non-Fourier skin bioheat transfer model with the nociceptor transduction model of skin thermal pain. The paper is structures as follows: the development of skin bioheat transfer model and nociceptor transduction model are first presented, which are then used to calculate the temperature, membrane voltage variation and frequency response of nociceptors under surface heating; discussion and conclusions are given at the end to highlight the role of non-Fourier thermal response of skin tissue.

2. Model Development

2.1. Skin Bioheat Transfer Model

2.1.1. Pennes bioheat transfer equation

Traditionally, the analysis of heat conduction in materials is based on the classical Fourier's law:

$$q(\vec{r},t) = -k\nabla T(\vec{r},t) \tag{1}$$

where q is the heat flux vector representing heat flow per unit time, per unit area of the isothermal surface in the direction of the deceasing temperature; k is the thermal conductivity which is a positive, scalar quantity; ∇T is the temperature gradient; and $\vec{r}$ stands for the position vector. The general bioheat transfer equation is given as:

$$\rho c\frac{\partial T}{\partial t} = -\nabla q + \varpi_b \rho_b c_b (T_a - T) + q_{met} + q_{ext} \tag{2}$$

Combination of Eqs. (1) and (2) leads to the Pennes bioheat transfer equation [41]:

$$\rho c\frac{\partial T}{\partial t} = k\nabla^2 T + \varpi_b \rho_b c_b (T_a - T) + q_{met} + q_{ext} \tag{3}$$

where ρ, c and k are the density, specific heat and thermal conductivity of tissue, respectively; ρ_b and c_b are the density and specific heat of blood, ϖ_b is the blood perfusion rate; T_a and T are the temperatures of blood and tissue, respectively; q_{met} is metabolic heat generation and q_{ext} is heat generation due to external heating sources.

Although the Fourier assumption has been employed extensively and successfully, some doubts have been cast on its completeness [42]. In the Fourier law, it is assumed that any temperature disturbance or thermal wave will propagate at an infinite speed through the medium. However, this assumption has been shown to be physically unrealizable since, in reality, any equilibrium state in thermodynamic transition needs time to establish [43, 44]. Fourier's law has been shown to fail during the short duration of an initial transient, or when the thermal propagation speed of thermal wave is not high [45], as observed in micro laser heating of thin metal films and in laser surgery techniques [46-48]. Liu & Lu [49] and Lu et al. [50, 51] reported that some thermal wave effects of changing power on bioheat transfer in tissue cannot be described by the Pennes equation.

2.1.2. Thermal wave model

Since the experimental observation of a finite thermal wave speed in liquid helium [52], the fundamental wave behavior in heat conduction has been argued from various physical view points [53-55]. Using the concept of a finite heat propagation velocity, Cattaneo [54] and Vernott [55] independently formulated a modified unsteady heat conduction equation, which is a linear extension of the unsteady Fourier equation, where an additional parameter, τ_q, is added to Eq.(1) in order to account for the thermal wave behavior not captured by Fourier's theory:

$$q(\vec{r}, t+\tau_q) = -k\nabla T(\vec{r}, t) \tag{4}$$

where $\tau_q = \alpha / C_t^2$ is defined as the thermal relaxation time, α is the thermal diffusivity, and C_t is the speed of thermal wave in the medium. The first order Taylor expansion of Eq.(4) gives:

$$q(\vec{r}, t) + \tau_q \, \partial q(\vec{r}, t) / \partial t = -k\nabla T(\vec{r}, t) \tag{5}$$

Due to its similarity in formulation compared to an acoustic wave, the proposed propagation mode of thermal signals is also termed the "second sound wave" [52, 56].

A direct integration of (5) leads to [57]:

$$\begin{aligned} &\int_0^t \left[q(\vec{r}, t) + \tau_q \, \partial q(\vec{r}, t) / \partial t \right] dt = \int_0^t \left[-k\nabla T(\vec{r}, t) \right] dt \\ &\Rightarrow q(\vec{r}, t) = -\frac{k}{\tau_q} \exp\left(-\frac{t}{\tau_q} \right) \int_0^t \exp\left(\frac{t}{\tau_q} \right) \nabla T(\vec{r}, t) \, dt \end{aligned} \tag{6}$$

According to this equation, the heat flux $q(\vec{r}, t)$ at a certain time t depends on the entire history of the temperature gradient established from time 0 to t. In other words, the heat flux now has a memory that keeps track of the time-history of temperature gradient due to the appearance of τ_q [1, 58]. The thermal wave theory ensures a strong path dependency for the temperature gradient rather than the point value depicted by Fourier's law [57, 59].

Substituting the bioheat conduction equation (2) into the thermal wave theory, Eq.(5), one can get thermal wave model of bioheat transfer, as:

$$\begin{aligned} \tau_q \rho c \frac{\partial^2 T}{\partial t^2} &= k\nabla^2 T - \varpi_b \rho_b c_b T - (\tau_q \varpi_b \rho_b c_b + \rho c) \frac{\partial T}{\partial t} + \\ &\left(\varpi_b \rho_b c_b T_b + q_m + q_{ext} + \tau_q \frac{\partial q_m}{\partial t} + \tau \frac{\partial q_{ext}}{\partial t} \right) \end{aligned} \tag{7}$$

The above equation is known as a hyperbolic bioheat equation because there appears a two double-derivative term (called the wave term) that modifies the parabolic Fourier heat equation into a hyperbolic partial differential equation [60].

Physical meaning and experimental determination of the relaxation time

Various physical points of view have been proposed for the thermal relaxation time τ_q [58]: τ_q results from the rate equation within the mainframe of the second law in non-equilibrium, irreversible thermodynamics; mechanically, τ_q arises due to the phase-lag between the heat-flux vector and temperature gradient in a high-rate response; when considering diffusion behavior and wave propagation, τ_q is the physical constant at which the intrinsic length scales merge together.

The value of the relaxation time for homogeneous materials can be calculated theoretically [61, 62], which is, however, not suitable for materials having non-homogeneous inner structures such as skin tissue. At present, no direct experimental method exists for the determination of τ_q. It has been suggested that τ_q can be determined by fitting experimental temperature data with theoretical predictions from the hyperbolic equation, by using τ_q as a variable parameter [63-67]. In view of the relation $\tau_q = \alpha / C_t^2$, τ_q for non-homogenous materials can also be determined based on the measurement of thermal wave speed C_t (which can be derived from the penetration time[2] and the distance of this point to the heat source) and the measurement of the thermal diffusivity α.

Kaminski [1] proposed that τ_q represents the interaction of different inner structural elements of a material during heat transfer. For homogeneous materials, this interaction occurs at the molecular or crystal lattice level, and τ_q has a value in the range of 10^{-8}-10^{-14} s. For heterogeneous materials, the structural heat transfer interaction takes place at a different scale and τ_q characterizes the thermal inductance, defined as the time needed for accumulating the thermal energy required for propagative transfer between different elements internally. Accordingly, it may take a much larger value (in the range of 10^{-3}-10^{3} s) in heterogeneous materials [68].

Most biological materials that contain cells, superstructures, liquids, and solid/soft tissue are non-homogeneous, resulting in higher thermal relaxation times compared to engineering materials. Vedavarz et al. [47] found that τ_q for biological tissues lies in the range of 10~1000 s at cryogenic temperature and 1~100 s at room temperature. Brazhnikov et al. [65] and Kaminski [1] found τ_q = 20-30 s for meat products; Mitra et al. [4] found that τ_q for processed meat was about 15.5 s while Roetzel et al. [69] found it to be 1.77 s.

Problems associated with the thermal wave model

Although the thermal wave model has been used to explain many interesting phenomena [59] and the predicted relaxation behavior has been shown to be admissible within the

---

[2] The penetration time is the period between the appearance of temperature jump (thermal wave front) and start of heating at a measurement point.

framework of the second law of extended irreversible thermodynamics [58], its validity can be questionable. For example, it is not built upon the details of energy transport in the material; material properties may not be regarded as constant (e.g., the relaxation time τ_q is generally temperature-dependent) [58]; although the thermal wave model can capture the microscale response in time [57, 70], the wave concept does not capture the microscale response in space [71, 72] and the thermal wave model can lead to unusual solutions [62, 73, 74]; due to the assumption of a macroscopic behavior averaged over many grains, the validity of the thermal wave model becomes debatable in view of the fast-transient response with microstructural interaction effects [75].

2.1.3. Dual-phase-lag (DPL) model

In order to account for deviations from the classical approach involving Fourier conduction and to consider the effect of microstructural interactions in the fast transient process of heat transport, an effect absent in the thermal wave model, namely, phase lag for temperature gradient, τ_T, is introduced [57, 70, 75]. Together with τ_q, the corresponding equation is called the dual-phase-lag (DPL) equation, and is stated as:

$$q\ \vec{r},t+\tau_q\ = -k\nabla T\ \vec{r},t+\tau_T \tag{8}$$

where τ_q and τ_T can be interpreted as periods arising from "thermal inertia" and "microstructural interaction", respectively [76]. More specifically, τ_q is the phase-lag in establishing the heat flux and associated conduction through a medium, while τ_T accounts for the diffusion of heat ahead of sharp wave fronts that would be induced by τ_q, representing the phase-lag in establishing the temperature gradient across the medium during which conduction occurs through its small-scale structures. Equation (8) reduces to the thermal wave model by setting $\tau_T = 0$ and reduces to Fourier's heat equation by also setting $\tau_q = 0$.

With the first and second order Taylor expansions, the DPL model can be developed into several pertinent models. Since these DPL models give similar results [8], only the simplest is discussed here. The simplest example of the DPL model is its first order expansions for both q and T, given as:

$$q\ \vec{r},t\ +\tau_q\frac{\partial q\ \vec{r},t}{\partial t} = -k\left[\nabla T\ \vec{r},t\ +\tau_T\frac{\partial \nabla T\ \vec{r},t}{\partial t}\right] \tag{9}$$

Substitution of the bioheat conduction equation (2) into this equation leads to the so-called type 1 DPL model of bioheat transfer:

$$\tau_q \rho c \frac{\partial T^2}{\partial t^2} = k\nabla^2 T + \tau_T k \nabla^2 \frac{\partial T}{\partial t} - \varpi_b \rho_b c_b T - \tau_q \varpi_b \rho_b c_b + \rho c \frac{\partial T}{\partial t} + \left(\varpi_b \rho_b c_b T_a + q_{met} + q_{ext} + \tau_q \frac{\partial q_{met}}{\partial t} + \tau_q \frac{\partial q_{ext}}{\partial t} \right) \tag{10}$$

Applying first-order and second-order Taylor series expansion for q and T, respectively, we have:

$$q + \tau_q \frac{\partial q}{\partial t} = -k\left(\nabla T + \tau_T \frac{\partial \nabla T}{\partial t} + \frac{\tau_T^2}{2} \frac{\partial^2 \nabla T}{\partial t^2} \right) \tag{11}$$

Substitution of (2) into this equation leads to the type 2 DPL model of bioheat transfer:

$$\tau_q \rho c \frac{\partial T^2}{\partial t^2} = k\nabla^2 T + \tau_T k \nabla^2 \frac{\partial T}{\partial t} + k \frac{\tau_T^2}{2} \frac{\partial^2}{\partial t^2} \nabla^2 T - \varpi_b \rho_b c_b T - \tau_q \varpi_b \rho_b c_b + \rho c \frac{\partial T}{\partial t} + \left(\varpi_b \rho_b c_b T_a + q_{met} + q_{ext} + \tau_q \frac{\partial q_{met}}{\partial t} + \tau_q \frac{\partial q_{ext}}{\partial t} \right) \tag{12}$$

Taking second-order Taylor series expansion for both q and T, respectively, we have:

$$q + \tau_q \frac{\partial q}{\partial t} + \frac{\tau_q^2}{2} \frac{\partial^2 q}{\partial t^2} = -k\left(\nabla T + \tau_T \frac{\partial \nabla T}{\partial t} + \frac{\tau_T^2}{2} \frac{\partial^2 \nabla T}{\partial t^2} \right) \tag{13}$$

Substituting (2) into this equation we obtain the type 3 DPL model of bioheat transfer:

$$\begin{aligned} \frac{\tau_q^2}{2} \rho c \frac{\partial^3 T}{\partial t^3} &= k\nabla^2 T + k\tau_T \frac{\partial}{\partial t} \nabla^2 T + k \frac{\tau_T^2}{2} \frac{\partial^2}{\partial t^2} \nabla^2 T + -\varpi_b \rho_b c_b \ T + \\ & -\tau_q \varpi_b \rho_b c_b - \rho c \ \frac{\partial T}{\partial t} + \left(-\frac{\tau_q^2}{2} \varpi_b \rho_b c_b - \tau_q \rho c \right) \frac{\partial^2 T}{\partial t^2} + \\ & \left(\varpi_b \rho_b c_b T_b + q_m + q_{ext} + \tau_q \frac{\partial q_m}{\partial t} + \tau_q \frac{\partial q_{ext}}{\partial t} + \frac{\tau_q^2}{2} \frac{\partial^2 q_m}{\partial t^2} + \frac{\tau_q^2}{2} \frac{\partial^2 q_{ext}}{\partial t^2} \right) \end{aligned} \tag{14}$$

2.2. Skin Thermal Pain Model

2.2.1. Model of current generation

A pain signal is created by the current induced by the opening of ion channels in nociceptor as described in Section 1.2. Since ion channels are generally gated by three different stimuli (thermal, mechanical and chemical), there are correspondingly three different currents. The total stimulation induced current, I_{st}, may be calculated as the sum of the three currents in view of the parallel distributions of ion channels in the membrane of nociceptors which can be treated as a parallel circuit, given as:

$$I_{st} = I_{heat} + I_{chem} + I_{mech} \tag{15}$$

where I_{heat}, I_{chem} and I_{mech} are the currents due to the opening of thermally-, chemically-, and mechanically-gated ion channels, respectively. In the present study, only heat-gated ion channels are considered for the generation of stimulation current for the main stimulation is induced by thermal stimuli. Since the gating of the ion channels is a threshold process, the heat current, I_{heat}, is assumed to be a function, f_h, of temperature at the location of nociceptor, T_{noci}. The thermal pain threshold, T_{thr}, can therefore be denoted by:

$$I_{heat} = f_h \; T_{noci}, T_{thr} \tag{16}$$

where T_{thr} is assumed to be the usual value of 43°C.

Unfortunately, there is no empirical relationship between stimuli and current available and no consensus of any standard model. However, it has been shown that the current is exponentially proportional to the stimulus [77], so that the following qualitative relation may be assumed [40]:

$$I_{st} = I_{heat} = \left(\left[C_{h1} \exp\left(\frac{T_{noci} - T_{thr} \; / T_{thr}}{C_{h2}} \right) + C_{h3} \right] + I_{shift} \right) \times \mathrm{H} \; T_{noci} - T_{thr} \tag{17}$$

where the inherent threshold current for action potential generation for the original the Hodgkin-Huxley (H-H) model [78] itself is considered; C_{h1}, C_{h2} and C_{h3} are constants; **exp** is the exponential function accounting for the experimentally-observed current variation with stimulus intensity; I_{shift} is a shift current; $\mathrm{H} \;\; x$ is the Heaviside function accounting for the threshold process. With the current range as reported in literature [77, 79, 80], the constants are chosen as $C_{h1} = 0.382\ \mu\text{A/cm}^2$, $C_{h2} = 0.064$, $C_{h3} = -0.355\ \mu\text{A/cm}^2$.

2.2.2. Model of frequency modulation

When the evocated current, I_{st}, surpasses the threshold of nociception, I_{thr_noci}, an action potential is generated. It is now accepted that the intensity of external stimulation is carried through the frequency of these impulses, $freq_s$, not the exact magnitude or shape of the signal, which can be calculated as a function of I_{st}, given as:

$$freq_s = f_{\text{mod}} \ I_{st} \tag{18}$$

The subscript 'mod' denotes modulation.

Unfortunately, no study has attempted to quantify the current-frequency relation. We need, therefore, to choose a model for the generation of action potential. Although there has been no analysis of the response kinetics of nociceptor, all neurons have been found to behave qualitatively similar to that described by the H-H model [78]. In our previous study [40], a revised H-H model has been developed by changing the rates of existing channels in the H-H equations themselves, considering the temperature influence, and adding transient K^+ channels. The revised model has been shown to be capable capturing the frequency response characteristics as experimentally observed [40]. The modified H-H model is schematically shown in Figure 4 and can be mathematically described as:

$$C_m \frac{dV_m}{dt} = I_{st} + I_{Na} + I_K + I_L + I_{K2} \tag{19}$$

where V_{mem} is the membrane potential (mV), which is positive when the membrane is depolarized and negative when the membrane is hyperpolarized; t is time (ms); C_{mem} is membrane capacity per unit area ($\mu\mathrm{F/cm^2}$); I_{st} is the stimuli-induced current density, as defined by Eq.(17), which is positive when the current is outward ($\mu\mathrm{A/cm^2}$); I_{Na}, I_K and I_L are the sodium, potassium and leakage current components ($\mu\mathrm{A/cm^2}$), respectively, while I_{K2} is an additional current for the second potassium channel. The various current components, I_{Na}, I_K, I_L, and I_A, are given as:

$$I_{Na} = g_{Na} m^3 h \ E_{Na} - V_{mem} \ , I_K = g_K n^4 \ E_K - V_{mem} \ ,$$
$$I_L = g_L \ E_L - V_{mem} \ , I_A = g_A A^3 B \ V_A - V_{mem} \ . \tag{20}$$

where m, n and h are gating variables, while A and B are factors having the same functional significance as factors m and h; E_{Na}, E_K and E_L are the corresponding reversal potentials (at which there is no net flow of ions from one side of the membrane to the other) for sodium, potassium and leakage current components given by the Nernst equation (all in mV), respectively; g_{Na}, g_K and g_L are the maximal ionic conductance through sodium, potassium and leakage current components (all in $\mathrm{mS/cm^2}$), respectively.

Each of the above four ionic currents is driven by an electrical potential difference and a permeability coefficient, or conductance [78]. The conductances of the ionic currents are regulated by voltage dependent activation and inactivation variables, known as gating variables, which are given by:

$$\frac{dx}{dt} = C_{Tx\_rc} \frac{x_\infty \; V_{mem} \; - x}{\tau_x \; V_{mem}} \tag{21}$$

This equation is sometimes also presented in another format, given as:

$$\frac{dx}{dt} = C_{Tx\_rc}\left[\alpha_x \; 1 - x \; - \beta_x x\right] \tag{22}$$

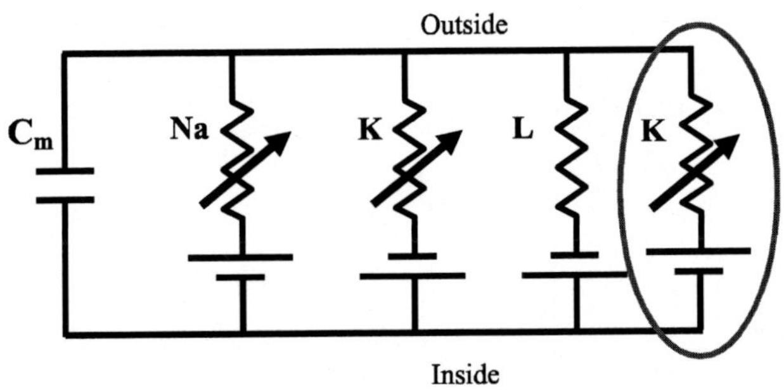

Figure 4. Revised Hodgkin-Huxley model [40] 38

Here, x is the gating variable and can be any one of the three gating variables, m, n and h; $\tau_x = x_{fac}\left[1/ \; \alpha_x + \beta_x \;\right]$ and $x_\infty = \alpha_x / \; \alpha_x + \beta_x$, where α_x and β_x are rate constants (in sec^{-1}); $x_\infty \; V_m$ is a steady-state voltage dependent (in)activation function of x, and $\tau_x \; V_m$ is a voltage-dependent time constant; x_{fac} is a scaling factor introduced to allow greater flexibility in adjusting the firing frequency; and C_{Tx_rc} is the coefficient of temperature dependence. Note that $x_\infty \; V_{mem}$ and $\tau_x \; V_{mem}$ can be calculated as [81]:

$$x_\infty \; V_{mem} \; = 1/ \; 1 + \exp\left[\; V_{mem} - \vartheta_x \; / \sigma_x\right] \tag{23}$$

$$\tau_x \; V_{mem} \; = x_{fac} \; \tau_x / \cosh\left[\; V_{mem} - \vartheta_x \; / \; 2\sigma_x \;\right] \tag{24}$$

C_{Tx_rc} depends on the difference between actual temperature T and reference temperature T_0, defined as:

$$C_{Tx\_rc} = \; Q_{rc}^{\; T - T_0 \; /10} \tag{25}$$

where Q_{rc} is a constant accounting for the increase of membrane behaviour when the temperature is increased by 10ºC; T_0 = 32°C is chosen as the reference temperature since it coincides with the lower temperature limits in most neurophysiological experiments and lies within the reasonable physiological range of human body [81].

The dependence of the maximum conductances (g_{Na}, g_K and g_L) on temperature can be accounted for by the coefficient of temperature dependence, C_{Tx_mc}, given as [82]:

$$C_{Tx\_mc} = Q_{mc}^{\ (T-32)/10} \tag{26}$$

The temperature-dependent reversal membrane potential E_{Na} and E_K can be calculated as [83]:

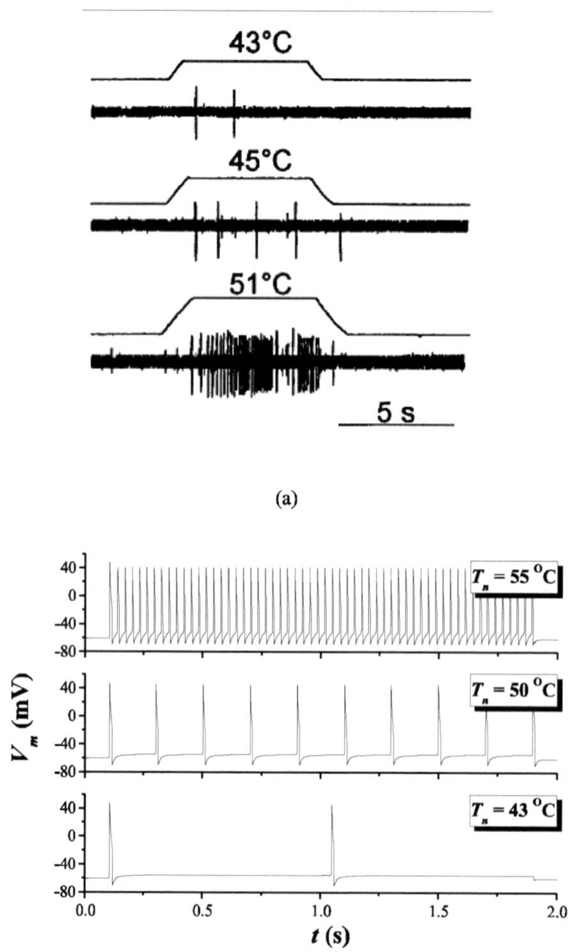

Figure 5. (a) Experimental observations of the responses of nociceptors in mouse glabrous skin evoked by heat stimuli of 43, 45, and 51°C (Response threshold to heat was 43°C) [85]; (b) Predicted membrane potential from our model 39

$$E_{Na} = 10^3 \times \frac{R\ (T + 273.15)}{F} \ln\left([Na]_e / [Na]_i\right) \tag{27}$$

$$E_K = 10^3 \times \frac{R\ T + 273.15}{F} \ln\ K_e / K_i \tag{28}$$

where K_e and K_i are the external and internal concentration of potassium ions, given as $K_e = 20$ mM and $K_i = 400$ mM [84]; Na_e and Na_i are the external and internal concentration of sodium ions, given as $Na_e = 440$ mM and $Na_i = 50$ mM [84]; $F = 9.6485 \times 10^4$ C/mol is the Faraday constant; and $R = 8.314$ J/mol K is the universal gas constant. Thus, for the normal temperature condition of T = 32°C, one obtains that $E_{Na} = 57.19$ mV and $E_K = -78.78$ mV. The reversal potential of leakage current $E_L = -63.79$ mV is obtained by adjusting E_L so that the equilibrium membrane potential is achieved.

The predicted membrane potential and frequency responses under stimulus of different nociceptor temperatures (T_{noci}), as shown in Figure 5(b), have been compared with experimental observations of nociceptors [85], reproduced in Figure 5(a). A good agreement between model predictions and test data is observed for the intensity-response relationship although, because of the various assumptions introduced to simplify the analytical model, higher temperatures are required to mirror the corresponding intensities. In particular, with the revised model, the predicted neural impulse rate is comparable to that of the actual nociceptors.

3. Case Studies

In this section, a case study of skin heating with constant surface temperature is carried out to illustrate the possible role of non-Fourier thermal behaviour of skin tissue in skin thermal pain sensation.

3.1. Thermal Behaviour of Skin Tissue

3.1.1. Description of the problem

The skin is initially cooled by natural convection using environmental air. At $t = 0$, the skin surface is suddenly taken into contact with a hot source of constant temperature 100°C (e.g., that of boiling water); after contacting for 15 s, the hot source is removed and the skin is cooled with water ice mixture of 0 °C for 30 s.

According to the real biological structure of skin, as shown in Figure 1(a), it is divided into three layers with different properties: epidermis, dermis and subcutaneous fat, as shown in Figure (b). Blood perfusion is only considered in the dermis layer while metabolic heat generation is considered in all three layers. The relevant parameters used for the heat transfer analysis are summarized in Tables 1 and 2. As for the thermal relaxation time, τ_q and τ_T, unfortunately, there exists yet no relevant experimental data of skin tissue. However, existing experimental measurements on other biological tissues and important cutaneous structures show that their magnitudes are in the order of seconds [4, 69, 86]. Therefore, in this study, τ_q and τ_T are chosen as constants varying in the range of 0–10 s.

3.1.2. Results and discussion

The problem is solved by using different models: Pennes model, thermal wave model and three types of dual-phase lag models (DPL1MBT, DPL2MBT and DPL3MBT). The results and discussion are given below.

Table 1. Thermophysical properties of blood

Parameters		References
Blood density $\left[kg/m^3\right]$	1060.0	[97]
Blood specific heat J/kgK	3770.0	[98]
Arterial blood temperature °C	37	
Core temperature °C	37	

Table 2. Thermophysical properties of skin tissue used in three-layer model

Parameters		Value	References
Skin density $\left[kg/m^3\right]$	Epidermis	1190.0	[97]
	Dermis	1116.0	[97]
	Subcutaneous fat	971.0	[97]
Skin thermal conductivity W/mK	Epidermis	0.235	[99]
	Dermis	0.445	[99]
	Subcutaneous fat	0.185	[99]
Skin specific heat J/kgK	Epidermis	3600.0	[100]
	Dermis	3300.0	[100]
	Subcutaneous fat	2700.0	[100]
Metabolic heat generation $\left[W/m^3\right]$	Epidermis	368.1	[101]
	Dermis	368.1	[101]
	Subcutaneous fat	368.3	[101]
Thickness mm	Epidermis	0.1	[102]
	Dermis	1.5	[103]
	Subcutaneous fat	4.4	Assumption

For the multi-layer skin model, the temperature fields predicted by different bioheat transfer models are compared in Figure 6(a)-(d). The temperature distributions in the skin at the end of heating ($t = 15$ s) and cooling ($t = 45$ s) are shown separately in Figure 6(c)-(d), whilst Figure 6(a)-(b) plot the corresponding temperature at the ED interface and DF interface as functions of time, respectively.

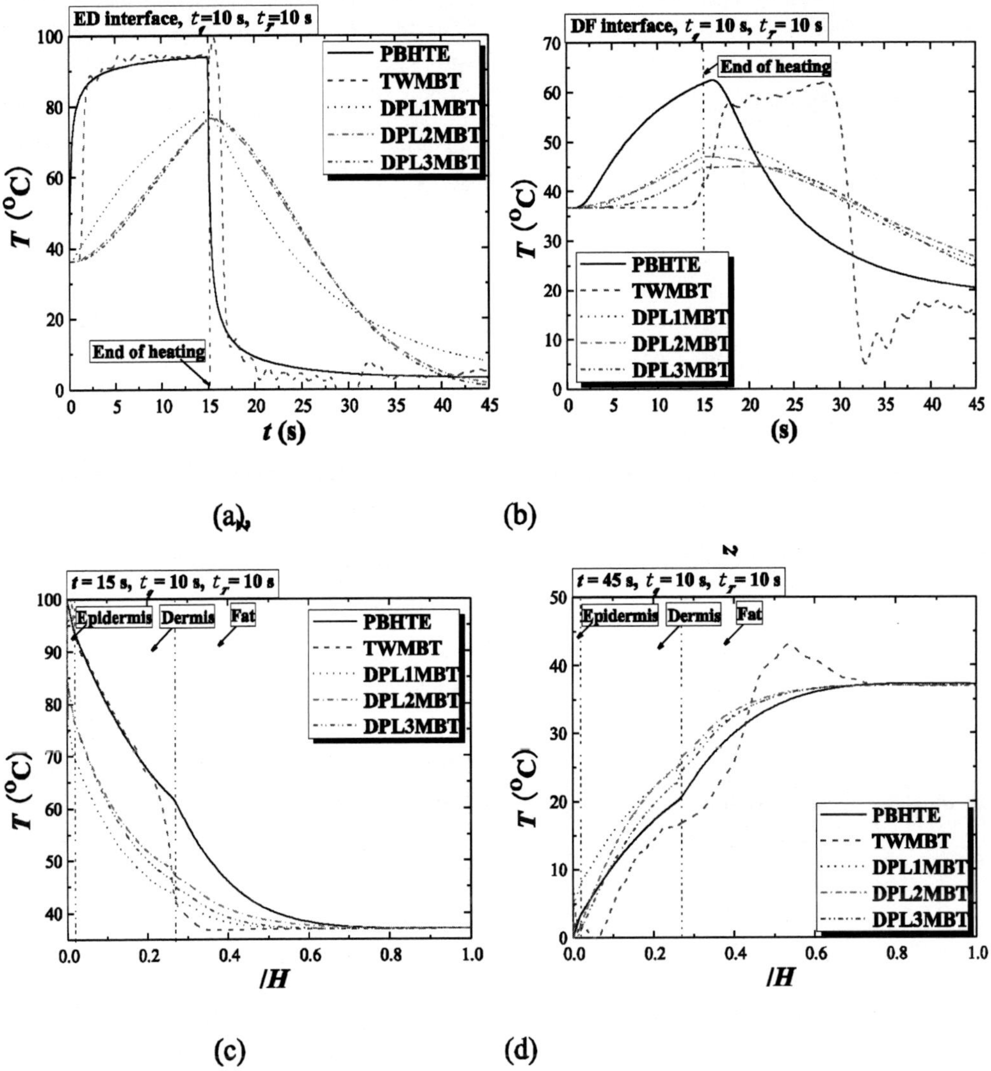

Figure 6. Comparison of predictions of temperature from different models for the case of surface contact heating in non-Fourier analysis (Section 5.4.2): (a) variation with time at epidermis-dermis (ED) interface, (b) variation with time at DF interface, (c) distribution along skin depth at , and (d) distribution along skin depth at (PBHTE: Pennes model; TWMBT: thermal wave model; DPL: dual-phase-lag model). Note that indicate the epidermis-dermis (ED) and dermis-fat (DF) interfaces, respectively 40

The results of Figure6 demonstrate that tissue temperature calculated from different bioheat transfer models can deviate substantially under constant surface temperature heating. With the thermal wave model, the tissue temperature inside the body was undisturbed during the initial stage of heating before jumping instantaneously, Figure 6(b); this may be viewed as the wave front emerging from the finite propagation of the thermal wave or the existence of the relaxation time τ_q. The unchanged tissue temperature initially may be attributed to the nonthermally consumption related biological activities [87]. The results from the three DPL models exhibit similar behaviors, and all differ from the results of both Pennes model and thermal wave model. Unlike the thermal wave model, no wave behavior is observed in the DPL models as expected, but a non-Fourier diffusion-like behavior exists due to the second thermal relaxation time τ_T, the effect of which is to weaken the thermal wave, thereby destroying the sharp wave front. It is noticed that a sudden temperature drop for heating or a step for cooling at the skin surface occurs with the DPL models, as shown in Figure 6(c)-(d).

3.2. Thermo-Neural Behaviour of Skin Tissue

3.2.1. Description of the problem

The skin is initially kept at constant temperature. At $t = 0$, its surface initially at normal temperature is suddenly taken into contact with a hot source of constant temperature T_s = 60°C (i.e., the surface temperature is instantaneously raised to T_s); after contacting for 5s, the hot source is removed and the skin is cooled by cold water (T_s = 15°C) for 10s. The depth of nociceptor is assumed to be $z_{noci} = 50\,\mu\text{m}$, which is in the reasonable range of experimental measurement [33, 34]. Using the skin bioheat transfer model, the temperature history of the nociceptor is obtained first, which is then used as input for the neural model.

For the analysis of neural response, the various voltage- and time-dependent parameters (*m, n, h*) are defined as shown in Eqs. (21) and (22), where α_x and β_x can be approximated from voltage clamp experiments [78], as:

$$\alpha_n = -0.01\ V_{mem} + 50 \Big/ \exp\left[-\ V_{mem} + 50\ /10\right] - 1$$

$$\beta_n = 0.125 \exp\left[-\ V_{mem} + 60\ /80\right], \tag{29}$$

$$\alpha_m = -0.1\ V_{mem} + 35 \Big/ \exp\left[-\ V_{mem} + 35\ /10\right] - 1\ ,$$

$$\beta_m = 4 \exp\left[-\ V_{mem} + 60\ /18\right], \tag{30}$$

$$\alpha_h = 0.07 \exp\left[-\ V_{mem} + 60\ /20\right],\ \beta_h = 1\big/\ \exp\left[-\ V_{mem} + 30\ /10\right] + 1 \tag{31}$$

The factors A and B appearing in Eq. (20) are determined according to [88]:

$$\tau_A \frac{dA}{dt} + A = A_\infty, \; A_\infty = \left(0.0761 \frac{\exp\left[V_{mem} + 94.22 / 31.84 \right]}{1 + \exp\left[V_{mem} + 1.17 / 28.93 \right]} \right)^{1/3}$$

$$\tau_A = A_{fac} \left(0.3632 + \frac{1.158}{1 + \exp\left[V_{mem} + 55.96 / 20.12 \right]} \right) \tag{32}$$

$$\tau_B \frac{dB}{dt} + B = B_\infty, \; B_\infty = \left(\frac{1}{1 + \exp\left[V_{mem} + 53.3 / 14.54 \right]} \right)^4$$

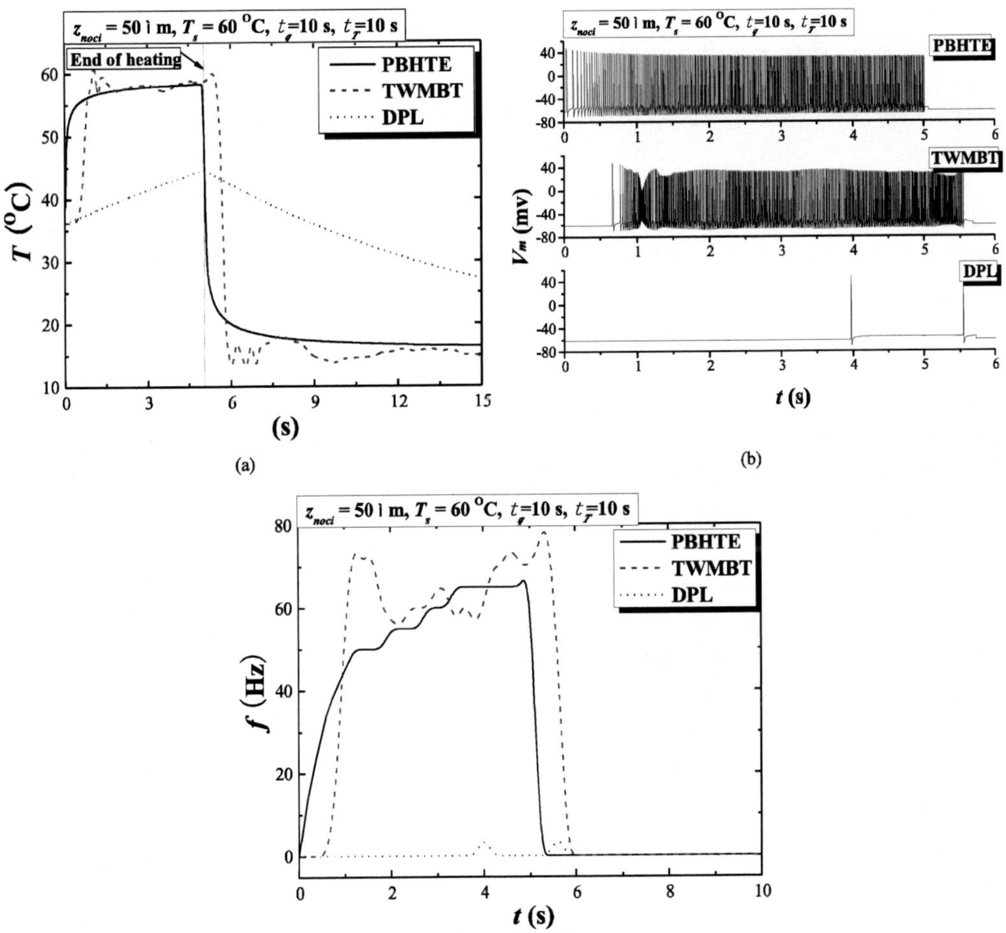

(c)

Figure 7. Comparison of predictions of the thermal-neural response of nociceptors from different models: (a) temperature, (b) membrane voltage variation, and (c) frequency response. (PBHTE: Pennes model; TWMBT: Thermal wave model; DPL: dual-phase lag model) 42

$$\tau_B = B_{fac}\left(1.24 + \frac{2.678}{1+\exp\left[\;V_{mem}+50\;/16.027\right]}\right) \tag{33}$$

Since there are at present no reported data on skin nociceptors, the parameters used for the current model are based on those for a squid axon [88-90]: $g_A = 47.7\ \text{mS/cm}^2$, $C_m = 2.8\ \mu\text{F/cm}^2$, $g_{Na} = 120\ \text{mS/cm}^2$, $g_K = 36\ \text{mS/cm}^2$, $G_L = 0.3\ \text{mS/cm}^2$, $A_{fac} = B_{fac} = 7.0$, $m_{fac} = h_{fac} = 0.263$ and $n_{fac} = 2.63$.

The whole group of governing equations, Eqs. (1)–(28), are solved using an explicit Runge-Kutta formula and the Dormand-Prince pair [91] with MATLAB (Version 6.5.1, The Mathworks, Natick, MA, USA).

3.2.2. Results and discussions

Comparison of the thermal-neural responses

Comparison between the thermal-neural responses of nociceptors predicted with different models is presented in Figure 7(a) for temperature, in Figure 7(b) for membrane voltage variation, and in Figure 7(c) for frequency response. From Figure 7(a), it can be seen that the nociceptor temperature increases nearly exponentially during heating, tending eventually to a constant value with time. With the thermal wave model, the tissue temperature inside the body is undisturbed during the initial stage of heating before jumping instantaneously. The large differences amongst the predicted temperatures from different models can cause significant deviations in membrane voltage variation and frequency response of nociceptors, as can be seen from Figure 7(b)–(c). For the results predicted from both the Pennes model and the thermal wave model, the generation frequency of action potential spikes increases with time and, similar to temperature, it tends to a constant value. Note that there is a clear latency (about 0.6 s) for neural response predicted by the thermal wave model, as shown in Figure 7 (b)–(c). Similar results have also been experimentally observed [92]. This means that non-Fourier thermal behaviour may play a role in the latency phenomenon, which has previously been attributed to signal transmission along nerve fibers [93]. However, with the DPL model, only two action potentials can be observed. This can be explained by the corresponding temperature as shown in Figure 7 (a), where the nociceptor temperature is less than the threshold (43°C) during most of the heating period. It has been established that pain level is decided by signal frequency [94]. Therefore, it can be seen from our results that, for the same heating condition, both the Pennes model and the thermal wave model predict relatively high levels of pain (frequency), and there is little pain predicted from the DPL model.

Effect of thermal relaxation time

To investigate the effect of τ_q and τ_T on the thermal-neural response of nociceptors, calculations with different values of thermal relaxation time have been performed with the

DPL model. The results are presented in Figure 8(a) for temperature, in Figure 8(b) for membrane voltage variation, and in Figure 8(c) for frequency response. As can be seen from Figure 8(a), no obvious wave-fronts are found in all the cases studied: the sharp wave-fronts due to τ_q are smoothed by the promoting conduction of τ_T, and the effect is more noticeable with increasing values of τ_T. This is attributable to the stronger dissipation from the mixed derivative term ($\tau_T k \nabla^2 \partial T / \partial t$) due to the existence of τ_T, as shown in Eq.(9), which leads to the non-Fourier diffusion-like conduction.

From the membrane voltage variation and frequency response shown in Figure 8 (b)-(c), it can be seen that, with τ_T fixed at 1 s, the latency of neural response increases with increasing τ_q: when $\tau_q = 1\ \text{s}$, the time for the generation of the first action potential is $t \approx 0.5\ \text{s}$, which delays to $t \approx 0.8\ \text{s}$ when $\tau_q = 10\ \text{s}$. This suggests that it is τ_q, rather than τ_T, that dominates the wave-like behaviour of the thermal-neural response of nociceptors in skin tissue.

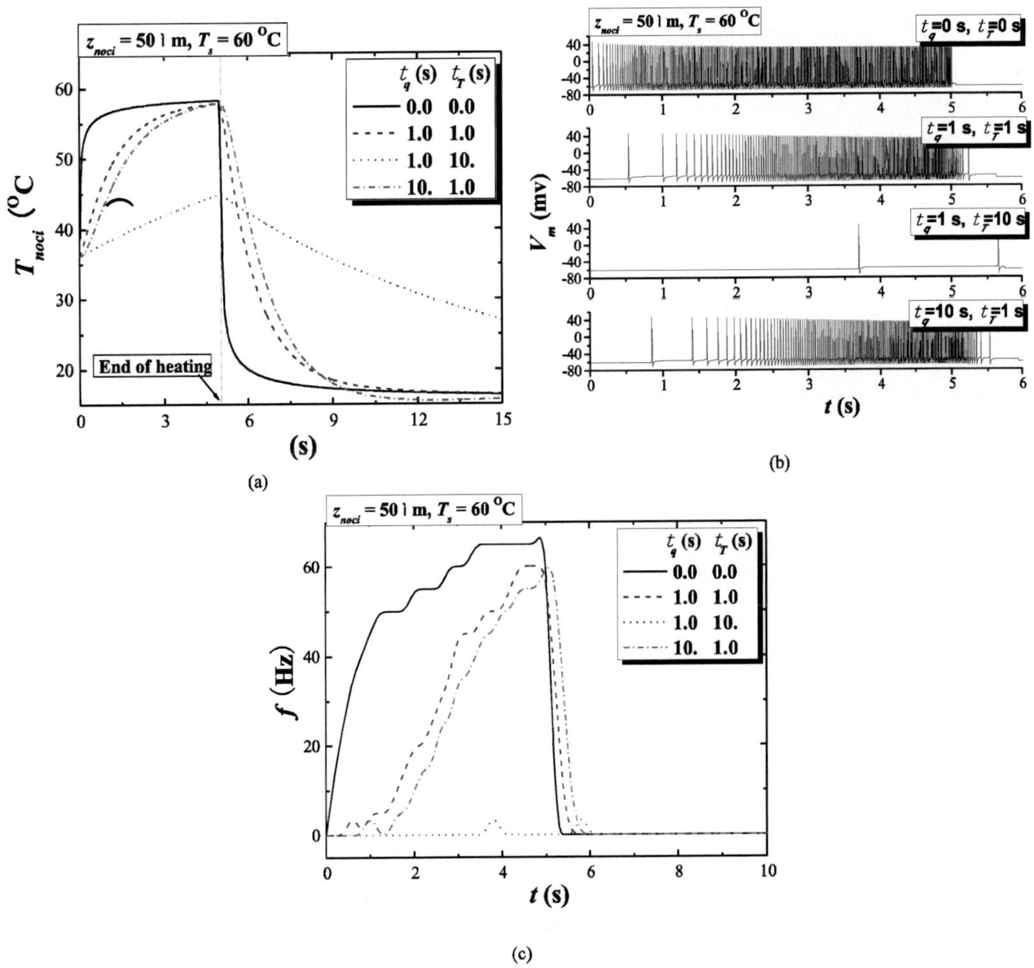

Figure 8. Effect of and on the predictions of thermal-neural response of nociceptors from DPL model: (a) temperature, (b) membrane voltage variation, and (c) frequency response 44

4. Conclusions

A mathematical model has been developed to characterize the effect of non-Fourier thermal behaviour in skin tissue upon the thermal-neural response of thermally sensitive nociceptors. For illustration, the model is used to calculate the temperature, membrane voltage variation and frequency response of nociceptors under surface heating. The following main conclusions are drawn: a non-Fourier feature may play an important role in the thermal-neural behaviour of skin tissue; the wave behaviour of thermal-neural response may play a role in the phenomenon of latency; it is τ_q, rather than τ_T, that dominates the wave-like behaviour.

There are nonetheless several limits of the proposed model. The first is the thermal relaxation time: there exists no reported data for skin tissue. Further experimental verification is therefore necessary to measure the transport of energy in living systems at the micro-scale level, from which detailed data on the relaxation time of tissue may be obtained. Another deficiency is that constant thermal properties of skin tissue have been assumed. As temperature is increased, the denaturation of collagen (the major component of skin) occurs, which has been shown to have great influence on skin properties. However, more experiments are needed to quantify the variation of skin properties with temperature (for existing test data are scarce) so that these properties can be reliably used in future models. Besides, in the current study only thermally-gated ion channels have been considered in the generation of through- membrane current. However, when skin is heated to a temperature beyond the thermal threshold (~ 43°C), thermal damage of skin tissue starts to accumulate. The thermal damage will cause the cells to break down and release a number of tissue byproducts and mediators, activating and sensitizing accordingly the nociceptors [95]. Further, thermally-induced stresses due to non-uniform temperature distributions may also lead to the sensation of thermal pain, in addition to the pain generated by heating alone [96]. There is also no consideration of spatial summation effects either peripherally or centrally, and it is assumed that the response at the periphery determines sensation—clearly at variance with the vast literature on pain perception, which demonstrates the primacy of central neural processes in pain sensation. All of these issues will be addressed in our future work.

Acknowledgments

This work is supported by the Overseas Research Studentship (ORS) and Overseas Trust Scholarship of Cambridge University, the National Natural Science Foundation of China (10572111, 10632060), the National 111 Project of China (B06024), and the National Basic Research Program of China (2006CB601202).

References

[1] Kaminski, W. Hyperbolic heat conduction equation for materials with a nonhomogeneous inner structure, *Journal of Heat Transfer, Transactions ASME*, 1990, 112 (3), 555-560.

[2] Richardson, AW; Imig, CG; Feucht, BL; Hines, HM. Relationship between deep tissue temperature and blood flow during electromagnetic irradiation, *Arch. Phys. Med. Rehabil.*, 1950, 31, 19-25.

[3] Roemer, RB; Oleson, JR; Cetas, TC. Oscillatory Temperature Response to Constant Power Applied to Canine Muscle, *American Journal of Physiology*, 1985, 249 (2), R153-R158.

[4] Mitra, K; Kumar, S; Vedavarz, A; Moallemi, MK. Experimental evidence of hyperbolic heat conduction in processed meat, *Journal of Heat Transfer, Transactions ASME*, 1995, 117 (3), 568-573.

[5] Davydov, EV; Lubashevsky, IA; Milyaev, VA; Musin, RF. *Nondiffusive heat transfer in muscle tissue*, 2001, 1 (1), Preliminary results, arXiv: cond-mat/0102006.

[6] Banerjee, A; Ogale, AA; Das, C; Mitra, K; Subramanian, C. Temperature distribution in different materials due to short pulse laser irradiation, *Heat Transfer Engineering*, 2005, 26 (8), 41-49.

[7] Shih, TC; Kou, HS; Liauh, CT; Lin, WL. The impact of thermal wave characteristics on thermal dose distribution during thermal therapy: A numerical study, *Medical Physics*, 2005, 32 (9), 3029-3036.

[8] Xu, F; Seffen, KA; Lu, TJ. Non-Fourier analysis of skin biothermomechanics, *International Journal of Heat and Mass Transfer*, 2008, in press.

[9] Caterina, MJ; Julius, D; Sense and specificity: a molecular identity for nociceptors, *Current opinion in Neurobiology*, 1999, 9, 525-530.

[10] Julius, D; Basbaum, AI. Molecular mechanisms of nociception, *Nature*, 2001, 413 (6852), 203-10.

[11] Millan, MJ. The induction of pain: an integrative review, *Prog. Neurobiol.*, 1999, 57, 1-164.

[12] Brooks, J; Tracey, I. From nociception to pain perception: imaging the spinal and supraspinal pathways, *J. Anat.*, 2005, 207 (1), 19-33.

[13] Patestas, M; Gartner, LP. *A Textbook of Neuroanatomy*, 2006, p. Blackwell Publishing Ltd., Oxford.

[14] Sherrington, CS. *The Integrative Action of the Nervous System*, 1906, p. Scribner, New York.

[15] McCleskey, EW; Gold, MS. Ion Channels of Nociception, *Annu. Rev. Physiol.*, 1999, 61, 835-856.

[16] Meyer, RA; Campbell, JN; Raja, SN. Peripheral neural mechanisms of nociception, in *Textbook of Pain*, 1994, P.D. Wall and R. Melzack, Eds. London: Churchill Livingstone, pp. 13-44.

[17] Treede, RD; Meyer, RA; Campbell, JN. Myelinated mechanically insensitive afferents from monkey hairy skin: heat-response properties, *J Neurophysiol*, 1998, 80 (3), 1082-93.

[18] Torebjork, E. Subpopulations of human C-nociceptors and their sensory correlates, in 9th World Congress on Pain, p.^pp. 2000, 199-206, Seattle.

[19] Schmidt, R; Schmelz, M; Forster, C; Ringkamp, M; Torebjork, E; Handwerker, H. Novel classes of responsive and unresponsive C nociceptors in human skin, *J Neurosci*, 1995, 15 (1 Pt 1), 333-41.

[20] Schmidt, R; Schmelz, M; Torebjork, HE; Handwerker, HO. Mechano-insensitive nociceptors encode pain evoked by tonic pressure to human skin, *Neuroscience*, 2000, 98 (4), 793-800.

[21] Bessou, P; Perl, ER. Response of cutaneous sensory units vith unmnvelinated fibers to noxious stimuli, *J. Neurophysiol.*, 1969, 32 1025-1043.

[22] Lynn, B; Carpenter, SE. Primary afferent units from the hairy skin of the rat hind limb, *Brain Research*, 1982, 238 (1), 29-43.

[23] Pini, A; Baranowski, R; Lynn, B. Long-term reduction in the number of C-fibre nociceptors following capsaicin treatment of a cutaneous nerve in adult rats, *Eur. J. Neurosci.*, 1990, 2, 89-97.

[24] Sengupta, JN; Gebhart, GF. Characterization of mechanosensitive pelvic nerve afferent fibers innervating the colon of the rat, *J Neurophysiol*, 1994, 71 (6), 2046-60.

[25] Dmitrieva, N; McMahon, SB. Sensitisation of visceral afferents by nerve growth factor in the adult rat, *Pain*, 1996, 66 (1), 87-97.

[26] Leem, JW; Willis, WD; Chung, JM. Cutaneous sensory receptors in the rat foot, *J Neurophysiol* 1993, 69 (5), 1684-99.

[27] Simone, DA; Kajander, KC. Responses of cutaneous A-fiber nociceptors to noxious cold, *J. Neurophysiol*, 1997, 77 (4), 2049-2060.

[28] Arendt-Nielsen, L; Chen, ACN. Lasers and other thermal stimulators for activation of skin nociceptors in humans, *Neurophysiologie Clinique/Clinical Neurophysiology*, 2003, 33 (6), 259-268.

[29] Burgess, PR; Perl, ER. Myelinated afferent fibres responding specifically to noxious stimulation of the skin, *J. Physiol.*, 1967, (Lond), 90 541-562.

[30] Patapoutian, A; Peier, AM; Story, GM; Viswanath, V. Thermo TRP channels and beyond: mechanisms of temperature sensation, *Nat. Rev. Neurosci.*, 2003, 4(8), 529-539.

[31] Kruger, L; Perl, ER; Sedivec, MJ. Fine structure of myelinated mechanical nociceptor endings in cat hairy skin, *J Comp Neurol*, 1981, 198 (1), 137-54.

[32] Stoll, AM; Greene, LC. Relationship between pain and tissue damage due to thermal radiation, *J Appl Physiol*, 1959, 14 (3), 373-82.

[33] Tillman, DB; Treede, RD; Meyer, RA; Campbell, JN. Response of C fibre nociceptors in the anaesthetized monkey to heat stimuli: correlation with pain threshold in humans, *J.Physiol*, 1995, 485 (Pt 3), 767-774.

[34] Tillman, DB; Treede, RD; Meyer, RA; Campbell, JN. Response of C fibre nociceptors in the anaesthetized monkey to heat stimuli: estimates of receptor depth and threshold, *J Physiol*, 1995, 485 (Pt 3), 753-65.

[35] Ochoa, J; Mair, WG. The normal sural nerve in man. I. Ultrastructure and numbers of fibres and cells, *Acta Neuropathol*, 1969, (Berl), 13(3), 197-216.

[36] Tran, TD; Inui, K; Hoshiyama, M; Lam, K; Kakigi, R. Conduction velocity of the spinothalamic tract following CO2 laser stimulation of C-fibers in humans, *Pain*, 2002, 95 (1-2), 125-31.

[37] Lynn, B; Baranowski, RA. Relative numbers and properties of cutaneous nociceptors in different species, in *Fine afferent nerve fibers and pain*, 1987, R.F. Schmidt, H.G. Schaible, and C. Vahle-Hinz, Eds.: Weinheim: VCH, pp. 86-94.

[38] Alberts, B; Bray, D; Lewis, J; Raff , M; Roberts, K; Watson, JD. *Molecular biology of the cell*, 1994, p. Garland, New York.

[39] Elmore, DE. *Investigations of Ion Channel Structure-Function Relationships Using Molecular Modeling and Experimental Biochemistry*, 2004, vol, PhD California Institute of Technology.

[40] Xu, F; Wen, T; Lu, TJ; Seffen, KA. Modelling of nociceptor transduction in skin thermal pain sensation, *Journal of Biomechanical Engineering* in press, 2008.

[41] Pennes, HH. Analysis of tissue and arterial blood temperatures in the resting human forearm, *J. Appl. Physiology*, 1948, 1 93-122.

[42] Herivel, J. Joseph Fourier: *face aux objections contre sa theorie de la chaleur*, 1980, p. Bibliotheque Nationale, Paris.

[43] Herwig, H; Beckert, K. Fourier versus non-Fourier heat conduction in materials with a nonhomogeneous inner structure, *Journal of Heat Transfer-Transactions of the Asme*, 2000, 122 (2), 363-365.

[44] Ozisik, MN; Tzou, DY. On the wave theory in heat conduction, p.^pp. 13-27, Anaheim, CA, USA, 1992.

[45] Glass, DE; Ozisik, MN; Vick, B. Hyperbolic heat conduction with surface radiation, *International Journal of Heat and Mass Transfer*, 1985, 28 (10), 1823-1830.

[46] Qiu, TQ; Tien, CL. Short-pulse laser heating on metals, *International Journal of Heat and Mass Transfer*, 1992, 35 (3), 719-726.

[47] Vedavarz, A; Kumar, S; Moallemi, MK. Significance of non-Fourier heat waves in conduction, *Journal of Heat Transfer*, 1994, 116 (1), 221-224. Transactions ASME.

[48] Antaki, PJ. Importance of nonFourier heat conduction in solid-phase reactions, *Combustion and Flame*, 1998, 112 (3), 329-341.

[49] Liu, J; Lu, WQ. Dual Reciprocity Boundary Element Method for Solving Thermal Wave Model of Bioheat Transfer, *Space Medicine & Medical Engineering*, 1997, 10 (6), 391-395.

[50] Lu, WQ; Liu, J; Zeng, Y. Simulation of the thermal wave propagation in biological tissues by the dual reciprocity boundary element method, *Engineering Analysis with Boundary Elements*, 1998, 22 (3), 167-174.

[51] Lu, WQ; Liu, J; Zeng, Y. Extension of the dual reciprocity boundary element method to simulate thermal wave propagation in biological tissu, *Journal of Engineering Thermophysics*, 1998, 19 (6), 728-731.

[52] V. Peshkov, Second sound in helium II, *J. Phys.*, 1944, VIII, 381.

[53] Morse, PM; Feshbach, H. *Methods of Theoretical Physics*, 1953, vol. 1, p. McGraw-Hill, New York.

[54] Cattaneo, C. A form of heat conduction equation which eliminates the paradox of instantaneous propagation, *Comp. Rend.*, 1958, 247, 431-433.

[55] Vernotte, P. Les paradoxes de la theorie continue de l'equation de la chaleur, *Comp. Rend.*, 1958, 246, 3154-3155.

[56] Chester, M. Second sound in solid, *Phys. Rev.*, 1963, 131, 2013-2015.

[57] Ozisik, MN; Tzou, DY. On the wave theory in heat conduction, ASME *J. Heat Transfer*, 1994, 116, 526-535.

[58] Tzou, DY. An engineering assessment to the relaxation time in thermal wave propagation, *International Journal of Heat and Mass Transfer*, 1993, 36(7), 1845-1851.

[59] Tzou, DY. Thermal Shock Phenomena Under High-Rate Response in Solids, in Annual Review of Heat Transfer, C.L. Tien, Ed. Washington, D.C.: *Hemisphere*, 1992, pp. 111-185.

[60] Tang, DW; Araki, N. *The wave characteristics of thermal conduction in metallic films irradiated by ultra-short laser pulses.*, 1996, vol. 29, p. 2527.

[61] Sieniutycz, S. The variational principles of classical type for non-coupled non-stationary irreversible transport processes with convective motion and relaxation, *International Journal of Heat and Mass Transfer*, 1977, 20 (11), 1221-1231.

[62] Taitel, Y. On the parabolic, hyperbolic and discrete formulation of the heat conduction equation, *International Journal of Heat and Mass Transfer*, 1972, 15 (2), 369-371.

[63] Antonishyn, NV; Geller, MA; Parnas, AL. Hyperbolic heat conduction equation for disperse system, *Inzhenerno Fizicheskij Zhurnal*, 1974, 26 (3), 503-508.

[64] Raspopov, BM. Control of Some Transfer Processes, *Inzhenerno Fizicheskij Zhurnal*, 1967, 12 444.

[65] Brazhnikov, AM; Karpychev, VA; Luikova, AV. One engineering method of calculating heat conduction processes, *Inzhenerno Fizicheskij Zhurnal*, 1975, 28 (4), 677-680.

[66] Michalowski, S; Mitura, E; Kaminski, W. The Application of Mathematical Method to Describe the Kinetics of Drying, *Hungarian Journal of Industrial Chemistry*, 1982, 10 387.

[67] Mitura, E; Michalowski, S; Karnlnski, W. A mathematical model of convection drying in Falling drying rate period, *Drying Technology*, 1988, 6, 113-137.

[68] Luikov, AV. Application of irreversible thermodynamics methods to investigation of heat and mass transfer, *International Journal of Heat and Mass Transfer*, 1966, 9 (2), 139-152.

[69] Roetzel, W; Putra, N; Das, SK. Experiment and analysis for non-Fourier conduction in materials with non-homogeneous inner structure, *International Journal of Thermal Sciences*, 2003, 42 (6), 541-552.

[70] Tzou, DY. *Macro- to Micro-scale Heat Transfer: The Lagging Behavior*, 1997, p. Taylor and Francis, Washington, DC.

[71] Bayazitoglu, Y; Peterson, GP. Fundamental issues in hyperbolic heat conduction, ASME HTD, 1992, 227.

[72] Tzou, DY; Ozisik, MN; Chiffelle, RJ. The lattice temperature in the microscopic two-step model, *J. Heat Transfer*, 1994, 116, 1034-1038.

[73] Koerner, C; Bergmann, HW. Physical defects of the hyperbolic heat conduction equation, *Applied Physics A: Materials Science & Processing*, 1998, 67 (4), 397-401.

[74] Godoy, S; García-Colín, LS. Nonvalidity of the telegrapher's diffusion equation in two and three dimensionsfor crystalline solids, *Phys. Rev. E*, 1997, 55, 2127-2131.

[75] Tzou, DY. A unified field approach for heat conduction from macro- to micro-scales, *Journal of Heat Transfer, Transactions ASME*, 1995, 117 (1), 8-16.

[76] Tzou, DY. Experimental support for the lagging behavior in heat propagation, *Journal of Thermophysics and Heat Transfer*, 1995, 9, 686-693.

[77] Cesare, P; Moriondo, A; Vellani, V; McNaughton, PA. Ion channels gated by heat, *Proc Natl Acad Sci U S A*, 1999, 96 (14), 7658-63.

[78] Hodgkin, AL; Huxley, AF. A quantitative description of membrane current and its application to conduction and excitation in nerve, *The Journal of Physiology*, 1952, 117 500-544.

[79] Caterina, MJ; Rosen, TA; Tominaga, M; Brake, AJ; Julius, D. Capsaicin-receptor homologue with a high threshold for noxious heat, *Nature*, 1999, 398 (6726), 436-441.

[80] Caterina, MJ; Schumacher, MA; Tominaga, M; Rosen, TA; Levine, JD; Julius, D. The capsaicin receptor: a heat-activated ion channel in the pain pathway, *Nature*, 1997, 389 (6653), 816-24.

[81] Wechselberger, M; Wright, CL; Bishop, GA; Boulant, JA. Ionic channels and conductance-based models for hypothalamic neuronal thermosensitivity, *Am J Physiol Regul Integr Comp Physiol*, 2006, 291 (3), R518-29.

[82] Hodgkin, AL; Huxley, AF; Katz, B. Measurement of current-voltage relations in the membrane of the giant axon of Loligo, *J Physiol*, 1952, 116 (4), 424-48.

[83] Lv, YG; Liu, J. Interpretation on thermal comfort mechanisms of human bodies by combining Hodgkin-Huxley neuron model and Pennes bioheat equation, *Forschung im Ingenieurwesen*, 2005, 69 101-114.

[84] Hodgkin, AL. *The conduction of the nervous impulses*, 1964, p. Liverpool University Press, Livepool.

[85] Cain, DM; Khasabov, SG; Simone, DA. Response properties of mechanoreceptors and nociceptors in mouse glabrous skin: an in vivo study, *J Neurophysiol*, 2001, 85 (4), 1561-74.

[86] Stratigos, AJ; Dover, JS. *Overview of lasers and their properties.*, 2000, vol. 13, pp. 2-16.

[87] Liu, J; Chen, X; Xu, LX. New thermal wave aspects on burn evaluation of skin subjected to instantaneous heating, *IEEE Transactions on Biomedical Engineering*, 1999, 46 (4), 420-428.

[88] Connor, JA; Walkter, D; McKown, R. Neural repetitive firing modifications of the hodgkin-huxley axon suggested by experimental results from crustacean axons, *Biophysical Journal*, 1977, 18 81-102.

[89] Hille, B. *Ionic Channels of Excitable Membranes*, 1992, p. Sinauer Associates Inc.

[90] Connor, JA; Stevens, CF. Prediction of repetitive firing behaviour from voltage clamp data on an isolated neurone soma, *J Physiol*, 1971, 213 (1), 31-53.

[91] JR; Dormand, PJ. Prince, A family of embedded Runge-Kutta formulae, *J. Comp. Appl. Math*, 1980, 6, 19-26.

[92] Campbell, JN; LaMotte, RH. Latency to Detection of First Pain, *Brain Research*, 1983, 266, 203-208.

[93] Plaghki, L; Mouraux, A. How do we selectively activate skin nociceptors with a high power infrared laser? Physiology and biophysics of laser stimulation, *Neurophysiol Clin*, 2003, 33 (6), 269-77.

[94] Torebjork, HE; LaMotte, RH; Robinson, CJ. Peripheral neural correlates of magnitude of cutaneous pain and hyperalgesia: simultaneous recordings in humans of sensory judgments of pain and evoked responses in nociceptors with C-fibers, *J. Neurophysiol*, 1984, 51 (2), 325-339.

[95] Junger, H; Moore, AC; Sorkin, LS. Effects of full-thickness burns on nociceptor sensitization in anesthetized rats, *Burns*, 2002, 28 (8), 772-777.

[96] Xu, F; Wen, T; Lu, TJ; Seffen, KA. Skin biothermomechanics under medical treatments, *Journal of the Mechanical Behavior of Biomedical Materials*, 2008, in press.

[97] Duck, FA. *Physical properties of tissue: A comprehensive reference book*, 1990, p. Academic Press.

[98] Torvi, DA; Dale, JD. A finite element model of skin subjected to a flash fire, *J Biomech Eng.*, 1994, 116 (3), 250-5.

[99] Elkins, W; Thomson, JG. Instrumented Thermal Manikin, Acurex Corporation, Aerotherm Division Report, 1973, AD-781, 176.

[100] Henriques, FC; Moritz, AR. Studies of thermal injury, 1. The conduction of heat to and through skin and the temperatures attained therein. A theoretical and an experimental investigation, *A. J. Pathol.*, 1947, 23 531-549

[101] Roetzel, W; Xuan, Y. Transient response of the human limb to an external stimulus, *International Journal of Heat and Mass Transfer*, 1998, 41 (1), 229-239.

[102] Sejrsen, P. Measurement of cutaneous blood flow by freely diffusible radioactive isotopes, *Dan. Med. Bull.*, 1972, 18 1-38.

[103] Dahan, S; Lagarde, JM; Turlier, V; Courrech, L; Mordon, S. Treatment of neck lines and forehead rhytids with a nonablative 1540-nm Er:glass laser: a controlled clinical study combined with the measurement of the thickness and the mechanical properties of the skin, *Dermatol. Surg.*, 2004, 30 (6), 872-879.

In: Skin Anatomy and Physiology Research Developments ISBN: 978-1-60741-469-8
Editor: Leon F. Bukowsky

Chapter 3

Discovering Novel Photoprotective Compounds For Dermal Administration By Use Of Skin Lipid Model Systems And Modern Analytical Methods

Hagen Trommer* and Reinhard H. H. Neubert
Martin-Luther-University Halle-Wittenberg,
Institute of Pharmacy, Pharmaceutical Technology and Biopharmaceutics Group,
Leipzig, Germany

Abstract

Ultraviolet radiation and oxygen together can cause severe damage to biological tissues. The outermost layer of the human skin, the stratum corneum, is of particular interest because of its constant exposure to these irritants. The effects of both noxious factors were examined to learn more about the molecular processes of damage, which may lead to the development of potential protective agents. Furthermore, the mechanisms of action of the molecules already applied to human skin as photoprotectives should be revealed completely. Skin lipid models are introduced as in vitro screening systems for the antioxidative properties of several test substances. Three lipid systems of variable complexity with increasing similarity to human skin were established. Ferrous sulfate, an electron donator and catalyst of the Haber-Weiss reaction, was added to the samples to trigger the formation of reactive oxygen species via a Fenton-like reaction. The amount of lipid peroxidation was quantified by the thiobarbituric acid assay detecting malondialdehyde. Investigations on a molecular level were carried out by use of the instrumental analytical methods mass spectrometry and electron paramagnetic resonance spectroscopy. The findings show that lipid model systems represent a useful approach in drug screening for powerful UV protectors. Hyaluronic acid was found to act

* Correspondence address: Dr. H. Trommer, Bernhard-Kellermann-Str. 16, D - 04279 Leipzig, Germany, Phone: +49 341 / 3303202, Fax: +49 341 / 3303202, E-mail: hagen.trommer@pharmazie.uni-halle.de

antioxidatively in the skin lipid models, ascorbic acid acted as a prooxidant in all lipid model systems. Further investigations of both substances revealed the molecular mechanisms of the observed effects. The topical administration of ascorbic acid, therefore, needs critical re-consideration. Human skin has constant exposure to UV light and oxygen. Therefore, the administration of protectors in pharmaceutical formulations or sunscreens, as found in this study, may be helpful for the protection of the human skin against UV induced damage. In vivo experiments with hyaluronan and its fragments should follow to allow in vitro-in vivo correlation and clinical interpretation of the data.

Keywords: Skin lipid models, Oxidative stress, UV irradiation, Antioxidants, Dermal application, Thiobarbituric acid assay, Mass spectrometry, Electron paramagnetic resonance spectroscopy, Hyaluronic acid, Ascorbic acid

Introduction

Ultraviolet radiation is able to damage all important biomolecules, such as lipids, DNA, carbohydrates and proteins severely [1, 2]. The reason is the initiation of free radical reactions [3]. This process can be catalysed by transition metal ions as electron donors for molecular oxygen [4]. The reaction products of these reductions are highly reactive radical species, such as superoxide ion radicals and the most reactive hydroxyl radicals [5]. If the amount of these oxidative influences is higher than the amount of the components of the human antioxidative defense system a condition called oxidative stress is reached [6, 7]. This imbalance and oxidative dysfunction can lead to oxidative damages of physiological structures in the entire organism [8].

The human skin is of particular interest, because it is constantly exposed to ultraviolet radiation, oxygen and other noxious environmental influences [9]. These factors can lead to premature skin ageing and mutation [10, 11]. The outermost layer of the human skin, the stratum corneum, determines its barrier function [12]. Peroxidation of the intercellular lipid matrix of this layer caused by UV radiation is harmful and causes loss of function [13].

Transition metal catalysts play a key role in UV induced lipid peroxidation and skin damage. UV radiation is able to increase the skin pool of non-heme iron (Fe^{II}) in dermis and epidermis significantly. Authors have measured 18 ppm/dry weight of unexposed body parts (buttocks, thigh) versus 53 ppm/dry weight in epidermis biopsies of exposed parts such as cheek, forehead and neck [14]. This is an indirect pathway leading to dangerous oxygen radicals in addition to the direct damage of biomolecules by UV. Furthermore, Green et al. demonstrated that human skin plays a significant role in iron ion excretion [15]. In a collaborative study a total iron ion content in the epidermal skin of 22.5 (±17.8) mg was calculated from material obtained from eccrine areas. The involvement of iron ions in UV irradiation induced free radical formation in the skin was confirmed by Buettner and Jurkiewicz [16]. The treatment of skin samples with the iron chelator Desferal® resulted in a significant reduction of a spin adduct after irradiation giving evidence to support the key role of iron in UV mediated free radical formation.

Lipid model systems of different complexity were developed as *in vitro* counterparts of the intercellular lipid matrix of the stratum corneum [17, 18]. For the ultraviolet irradiation experiments an irradiation chamber, allowing selective well-defined UV exposure, was used.

For the evaluation of the amount of the oxidative damage the thiobarbituric acid (TBA) assay detecting malondialdehyde (MDA) as a classic lipid peroxidation secondary product was employed [19, 20]. It is the most widely used method for the quantification of peroxidative lipid damage [21].

Sixteen different substances were tested in this study for their properties to prevent stratum corneum lipids from UV induced oxidative damage in the *in vitro* lipid model screening systems.

The qualitative changes of selected substances were studied on a molecular level by electrospray ionisation mass spectrometry (ESI-MS). ESI as a soft ionisation method enables the analysis of screening substances and their degradation products without artificial fragmentation. However, structural elucidation is possible using the capabilities of an ion trap mass analyser [22], namely tandem mass spectrometry (MS/MS) and multiple stage mass spectrometry (MS^n).

To elucidate the nature of free radical involvement electron paramagnetic resonance (EPR) studies were carried out. EPR spectroscopy is being used more frequently in pharmaceutical research [23, 24] because of the unique information which can be obtained by EPR spectra of both *in vivo* and *in vitro* experiments [25]. The spin trapping method with 5,5-dimethyl-1-pyrroline-1-oxide (DMPO) was used to detect the highly reactive hydroxyl radicals [26]. The influence of screening substances on the concentration of these free radicals generated by the Fenton system, as well as the properties of the molecules regarding the stable 2,2-diphenyl-1-picrylhydrazyl hydrate (DPPH) radical were studied in this work.

Development Of Model Systems For Antioxidative Screening And Inclusion Criteria For The Screening Substances

For the investigations to find new, unknown antioxidants for topical application suitable model systems were required. There were two standards these model systems should meet. These systems should be simple to avoid an overlapping of effects which would make data interpretation difficult or impossible. Despite this simplicity the main properties of the stratum corneum intercellular lipid matrix should be present to assure the similarity to the horny layer of human skin. Beginning with simple systems containing only one stratum corneum lipid the systems were made more complex by stratum corneum lipid addition becoming more similar to the real horny layer.

Substances belonging to the horny layer lipid matrix physiologically were chosen as model lipids for the experiments. Cholesterol (CHOL), α-Linolenic acid (LLA) and L-α-Dipalmitoylphosphatidylcholine (DPPC) as a liposome generator were used for system modeling. The simple system was an oil in water dispersion of LLA. The samples were obtained by shaking the system for 120 minutes using a laboratory flask shaker.

The complex systems were prepared as liposomes. For liposome preparation the thin layer method was applied. The lipids were dissolved in chloroform. The solvent was removed by use of a rotation vaporizer. To make sure to obtain a thin and homogeneous lipid film a fast rotation was chosen (150 rpm). The remaining lipid film was dispersed in double distilled water by shaking intensively for 360 minutes. To achieve the final concentration the remaining double distilled water was added.

The stock solution was passed through a 400 nm polycarbonate filter under nitrogen pressure using an extruder device to obtain vesicles of a uniform size. This step was repeated five times. The exact composition of the model systems as well as an overview of the manufacturing processes are shown in Table 1.

Table 1. The systems used for screening (additionally 10 µM $FeSO_4$ were added to each sample)

System	Lipids	Concentration	Manufacturing Process
1. Simple system (LLA)	α-Linolenic acid	100 µM	Shaking for 120 min
2. Complex system (LLA/CHOL/DPPC)	α-Linolenic acid DPPC Cholesterol	100 µM 200 µM 100 µM	Liposomes prepared by the thin film method
3. Complex system with ceramides			
a) Ceramide III (C III)	α-Linolenic acid DPPC Cholesterol Ceramide III	100 µM 200 µM 100 µM 100 µM	Liposomes prepared by the thin film method
b) Ceramide IV (C IV)	α-Linolenic acid DPPC Cholesterol Ceramide IV	100 µM 200 µM 100 µM 100 µM	Liposomes prepared by the thin film method

UV-B irradiation experiments were carried out using a UV irradiation chamber enabling a selective exposure to UV-B because of special lamps with a main emission range of 290 – 320 nm. Prior to irradiation, 5.0 ml sample were transferred to 55 mm open glass dishes. The optical pathlength was 2.1 mm and a homogeneous exposure was assumed in spite of light scattering.

The samples were treated with an UV-B dose of 0.25 J/cm^2 which corresponds approximately with the 10fold of the minimal erythema dose (MED) for averaged pigmented (type II in the skin pigmentation classification) caucasians [27]. This high dosage was required to provoke stress conditions.

10 μM Ferrous sulfate were added to the samples as an electron donator and catalyst of the Haber-Weiss reaction to initiate reactive oxygen species (ROS) generation via a Fenton type reaction. Previous investigations have shown that there is no effect when irradiating lipid model systems without transition metal catalysts [17].

All the liposome suspensions, fatty acid dispersions and test substance solutions were freshly prepared just before use.

There were conditions the test substances had to meet to be used for the screening experiments as well. They had to be classed to at least one of the following groups:

(a) the exact mechanism of action of the substance is not known in detail yet,
(b) the substance is present in the skin organ physiologically,
(c) the substance may act antioxidatively because of structural properties,
(d) the incorporation into modern semisolid formulations for topical application is possible from a pharmaceutical and technological point of view,
(e) although the substance has got another main effect antioxidative behavior can be assumed and therefore testing in the screening is worthwhile.

Analytical Methods Used For The Screening Studies And For The Investigations On A Molecular Level

Thiobarbituric Acid Assay

The TBA test is a quantitative assay for the detection of MDA, and is the most widely used technique to determine lipid peroxidation products.

Here, the Buege-Aust method of the TBA assay was applied [28]. Briefly, 2.0 ml of a stock TBA reagent containing 15 % (w/v) trichloroacetic acid in 0.25 M HCl and 0.37 % (w/v) thiobarbituric acid in 0.25 M HCl was added to 1.0 ml of the UV-B treated sample. After heating at 90° C for 15 minutes and cooling down, the red TBA:MDA-complex (2:1) appears allowing fluorescence measurement. A HPLC system (Merck-Hitachi, Darmstadt, Germany) was used to quantify the pigment. A reversed phase column was used with a mobile phase methanol/water for HPLC procedure. The excitation wavelength was 515 nm and the emission measurement was performed at 555 nm.

Mass Spectrometry

ESI-MS was used as a modern analytical tool for the experiments. The electrospray interface allowed a soft ionisation without instant fragmentation. The ion trap analyser enabled tandem MS and multiple MS experiments, facilitating structure identification.

The mass spectrometric analysis was carried out using a Finnigan LCQ ion trap mass spectrometer with ESI interface and integrated syringe pump (Thermo Finnigan, San Jose, CA, USA). Electrospray ionisation mass spectrometry was performed in the negative and positive ion mode with an ESI voltage of 4.0 kV and a heated capillary temperature of 220 °C. The aqueous samples were mixed with methanol to guarantee a stable electrospray during flow injection via a syringe pump (10 μl/min). The ion optics of the LCQ mass spectrometer were tuned to the lipid peaks to allow recordings in the best resolution mode at maximum intensity.

Electron Paramagnetic Resonance Spectroscopy

EPR studies were carried out in the X-Band using a Bruker ESP 380 E FT-EPR spectrometer (Bruker, Rheinstetten, Germany). Quantitative investigations were performed using the double resonator technique in a rectangular cavity with corresponding aqueous sample cells (Rototec Spintec, Spektroskopie Vertriebs-GmbH, Remshalden). For evaluating the hydroxyl radical scavenging activity, the spin trapping method was used. Therefore, the reactive hydroxyl radicals were produced via the Fenton system consisting of hydrogen peroxide and iron (II) ions and trapped by DMPO. Before transferring the specimen into the cavity 1 ml of each stock solution was added in the following order:

I) Adenosine 5'-diphosphate sodium salt (ADP) as a chelating agent (2 mM),
II) Ferrous sulfate (0.5 mM),
III) Test substance or double distilled water as a blank control,
IV) The spin trap DMPO (40 mM), V) H_2O_2 (0.3 %).

Exactly 120 s after the addition of hydrogen peroxide the recording of the spectrums was started measuring the specimen in the resonator 1 of the cavity and 2,2,6,6-Tetramethyl-1-piperidyl-N-oxyl (TEMPO) as the reference (50 μM in methanol) in the resonator 2 of the double resonator.

The double resonator technique is a method to study aqueous samples in a reproducibly quantitative manner. Every measured signal was set in proportion to a reference signal of TEMPO to avoid analytical artifacts due to changes in the Q factor of the resonator.

All signals are the results of 5 time accumulations. The quantitative analysis of the EPR spectrums were carried out by double integration of the EPR signals using the WinEPR software (Bruker, Rheinstetten, Germany).

Screening Results

Figure 1 shows the results of the TBA assay of the simple stratum corneum lipid model system when adding different drugs as test substances [29]. The effects of 100 μM screening substance on a LLA dispersion are shown.

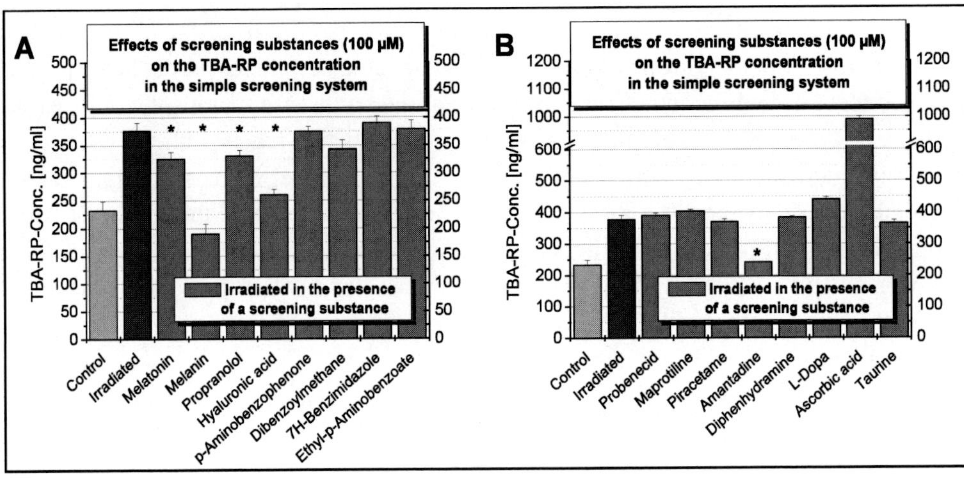

Figure 1. Concentration of the thiobarbituric acid reaction products (TBA-RP Conc.) and influences of ultraviolet irradiation and different test drugs (100 µM each) in the simple screening system [29].

Figure 1A shows significant lipid protection after UV irradiation when adding melatonin, melanin, propranolol and hyaluronic acid to the LLA dispersion. The results for melanin should be due to its filter properties for UV radiation because the complex tyrosine derivative is responsible for the protection of the DNA after its *in vivo* synthesis in the melanocytes of the skin. It is also considered to be a radical scavenger [30, 31]. A very interesting result is the failing of the substances usually utilised in sunscreens to protect the lipids from UV induced peroxidation. The substances which were used as a representation of these UV filter molecules were the following: dibenzoylmethane, 7H-benzimidazole and ethyl-p-aminobenzoate. All three chemicals were ineffective in significant lipid protection after UV irradiation in this study. Antioxidative properties of propranolol [32] and melatonin [33, 34] can be found in the literature. Melatonin has been found to protect human skin from UV induced erythema in an *in vivo* study when topically used on its own or applied in combination with the vitamins E and C [35].

The antioxidative properties of hyaluronic acid can be explained by transition metal scavenging [19]. Lipid peroxidation reducing effects for other glycosaminoglycans are also described [36]. The mechanism of the lipid protecting effects of these polysaccharides seems to be the chelation of transition metal ions as well. Sipos and co-workers suggested complexes of the kind $L[Fe(OH)_3]_n$ where L is the polysaccharide monomer [37]. This chelation can lead to anti- and prooxidative effects and therefore, has to be tested in every isolated case [38]. Recently the effects of different metal ions including Zn, Co, Mn etc. on the oxidative damage and the antioxidant capacity of hyaluronan have been investigated and compared with iron [39].

Figure 1B shows surprising effects for ascorbic acid and amantadine. When adding ascorbic acid secondary lipid peroxidation products (measured as MDA units) are significantly increased.

Conflicting data concerning the interactions of vitamin C with ROS has lead to controversy in the literature as both antioxidant and prooxidant properties have been reported

[40, 41]. Genotoxic effects were found and suggested to be a result of the ability of ascorbic acid to decompose lipid hydroperoxides to DNA damaging secondary products [42].

The effect of the drug amantadine used for Parkinson disease treatment can be explained by a Schiff base reaction where the aminogroup of amantadine reacts with the carboxylgroup of malondialdehyde giving the azomethine. So the analyte is masked and cannot be quantified properly by the TBA assay. This is in correspondency with the results of Albrecht-Goepfert et al. [43]. Several aminoadamantane derivatives have been tested for their influences on ROS. Neither radical scavenging nor singlet oxygen quenching was observed. On the other hand the topical application of amantadine could be of advantage because skin damaging carboxyls would be neutralised this way.

Further investigations should be carried out to check the compounds found as protectives in the screening for its *in vivo* influences, for example, on the MED after topical application with test persons. This is of importance for *in vivo* evaluation of the generated data and its clinical interpretation. Preformulation studies testing the stability of the potential antioxidants in several formulations and examinations of the penetration behavior of the test substances should follow as well.

Elucidation Of The Molecular Mechanisms

The interesting screening results obtained by the experiments with hyaluronic acid and with ascorbic acid were the motive to expand the investigations with these two molecules. Aim of the further studies was to reveal the mechanisms which were responsible for the results in the screening system on a molecular level. Furthermore, the effects of hyluronic acid derivatives with lower molecular weights on the TBA levels in the lipid systems were of interest.

Hyaluronic Acid

Hyaluronic acid is a polysaccharide existing in many parts of the human organism. Besides many well-known and well investigated functions of the glycoaminoglycan (e.g. as a joint lubricant, a viscoelastic filling substance and a wound healing stimulator) there are other tasks of the macromolecule which are not clarified in detail yet [44].

Hyaluronic acid and the fragments from enzymatic degradation were a gift from the Institute of Experimental Microbiology Jena (Germany). The source of the polysaccharides was the highly productive microorganism *Streptococcus zooepidemicus.* The biotechnological production of the hyaluronan was carried out via fermentation after a cyclic batch high performance procedure. A detailed description of this method as well as the parameters influencing the fermentation process are published [45]. For the enzymatic degradation 10.0 g of Hyaluronan were preincubated in 5.0 l pH 6 acetate buffer (0.05 mM) at 37°C. Afterwards 0.5 l acetate buffer (37°C) containing 10 000 units hyaluronate lyase from *Streptococcus agalactiae* were added. The termination of the enzymatic reaction was attained by fast heating (90°C) for 10 minutes after the desired incubation times. The non enzymatically exposed macromolecul was heated as well. After cooling the fragments were lyophilised. Molecular weight determinations were carried out by laser light scattering (Table 2).

Table 2. Characterisation of Hyaluronic acid and its fragments used for the experiments (additionally a fragment with the molecular weight of 22 kDa was used for the mass spectrometric investigations)

Abbreviation	Incubation with Hyaluronate lyase [min]	Molecular weight [g/mol]
HYA 0	0	1×10^6
HYA 15	15	6×10^5
HYA 30	30	$3{,}3 \times 10^5$
HYA 60	60	$3{,}2 \times 10^5$
HYA 120	120	$2{,}2 \times 10^5$

For mass spectrometric investigations a fragment of a molecular weight of 22 kDa from the same source as described above has been used. The smaller fragments resulting from the enzymatic degradation process were not separated to allow detection in the mass range of the spectrometer used between m/z = 50 – m/z = 2000.

The high viscosity of the native hyaluronic acid and the fragments with high molecular weights was narrowing the choice of the concentrations for the experiments. MDA determinations via the TBA assay were carried out using 0.1 μM hyaluronan or hyaluronan fragment solutions.

Figure 2 shows the results of the thiobarbituric acid assay of the stratum corneum lipid systems [19]. The effects of 0.1 μM hyaluronan or hyaluronan fragments on a LLA dispersion are shown in figure 2A. Secondary lipid peroxidation products (measured as MDA units) are significantly decreased. The TBA reaction product concentration level is decreased by hyaluronan from 675 ng/ml for the irradiated sample to 260 ng/ml for the sample containing 0.1 μM of HYA 0.

Figure 2B shows the effects of the polysaccharide measured using the complex system including the phospholipid DPPC, CHOL and LLA. Hyaluronan and its fragments are acting antioxidatively as well, but the level of peroxidative damage after irradiation is increased. Only LLA is sensitive to UV light, transition metals and ROS because it is the only compound of the lipid system containing allylic double bonds. The enhanced sensitivity of unsaturated compounds when encapsulated into liposomes has been reported [17].

The addition of C III and C IV to the lipid systems made the models more complex, making them more similar to the lipid matrix of the human stratum corneum (Figures 2C and 2D). The addition of the sphingolipids caused nearly no additional effect on the TBA level of the complex system. This can be explained by the lack of conjugated or allylic double bonds, and the relative stability against oxidative attack arising from the sphingolipid structure.

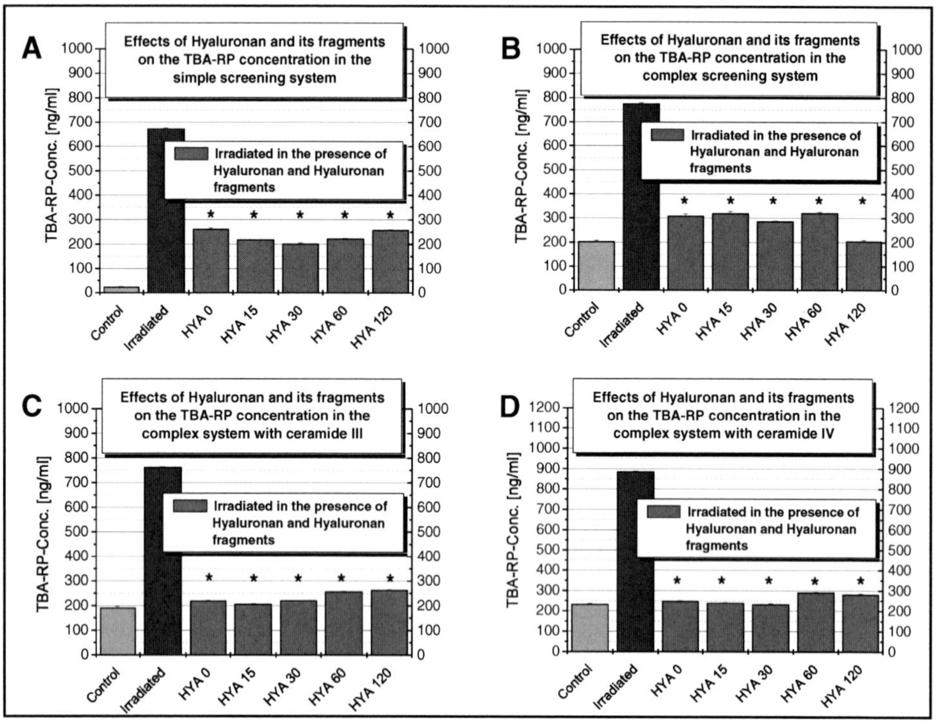

Figure 2. Concentration of the thiobarbituric acid reaction products (TBA-RP Conc.) and influences of ultraviolet irradiation and hyaluronan and its fragments from enzymatic degradation in the systems used [19]. A) Simple system. B) Complex system. C) Complex system with ceramide III. D) Complex system with ceramide IV.* $P < 0.05$, UV exposed samples in the presence of hyaluronan or fragments (light grey columns) vs. samples irradiated without hyaluronan (dark grey columns), two-tailed test. All data represent the mean values ± SD of sextuple measurements (n = 6).

Hyaluronan and its fragments from enzymatic degradation decrease the amount of lipid peroxidation products measured as MDA content in all skin lipid model systems studied. Interestingly, the different fragments of hyaluronan show nearly similar effects on the level of the generated lipid peroxidation products. A dependence between polysaccharide molecular weight and the degree of the antioxidative action was not detectable. This is of importance when interpreting the mechanism of the protection behavior.

For the qualitative characterisation of the UV irradiation effects on hyaluronan mass spectrometric investigations were performed using an ESI-MS device. Figure 3A shows the negative ion mode spectrum of the 22 kDa hyluronan fragment with non separated smaller fragments from enzymatic degradation in the m/z range 50 – 1500.

The single charged tetramer at m/z = 757, the sodium adduct of the double charged tetramer at m/z = 779, the sodium adduct of the triple charged sixmer with m/z = 579, the single charged dimer with m/z = 378 (the hyalobiuronic acid), the single charged trimer with m/z = 554 as well as the single charged glucuronic acid anion at m/z = 175 were detected as the six main signals in the range of m/z = 0-1000 [46, 47]. One has to consider that the peaks in the mass spectrum can be assigned to more than one carbohydrate structure [48, 49]. So the peak at m/z = 378 can not only be interpreted as the single charged dimer. It can also be assigned to the double charged tetramer which can be proved by the distance between the main peak and its C13 satellite of 0.5 mass units instead of 1 mass unit. Another structural explanation for the 378 peak is the triple charged hexamer.

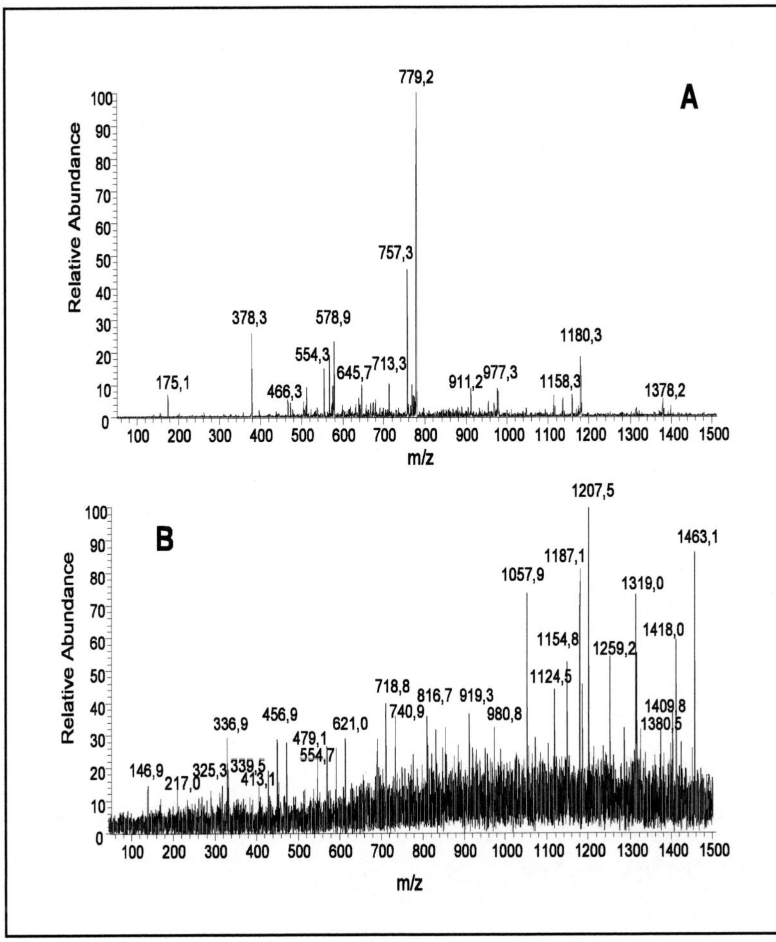

Figure 3. A) Negative ion mode ESI mass spectrum of the 22 kDa hyaluronan fragment with non separated smaller degradation products [19]. B) Negative ion mode ESI mass spectrum of the 22 kDa hyaluronan fragment irradiated with 0.25 J/cm^2 UV-B [19].

Figure 3B shows the negative ion mode mass spectrum of the 22 kDa fragment after UV irradiation. The treatment was very effective leading to many additional ion signals which are due to a photo degradation of the macromolecule. As a result smaller fragments are generated which are visible in the m/z range of the mass spectrometer used (m/z = 50 – 2000).

In 1996 Hawkins and Davies carried out EPR experiments and could detect hyaluronan radicals as intermediates of hydroxyl radical induced degradation of hyaluronic acid [50]. Photo degradation products of hyaluronan has been visualised by EPR spin trapping [51].

Using EPR spectroscopy it was possible to elucidate the radical processes involved in the systems studied. For the EPR investigations a concentration range consisting of 0.02 μM, 0.04 μM, 0.06 μM, 0.08 μM and 0.1 μM solutions was used. Experiments with hydroxyl radicals using the spin trapping technique with DMPO as a trap for the ROS were carried out. Hydroxyl radicals are the most reactive oxygen species, hence it is impossible to detect them directly even by EPR because of their high reaction constants. An indirect determination can be achieved by the reaction with spin traps such as DMPO. The decrease in the signal intensity is regarded as a measure of the antioxidative potential of compounds.

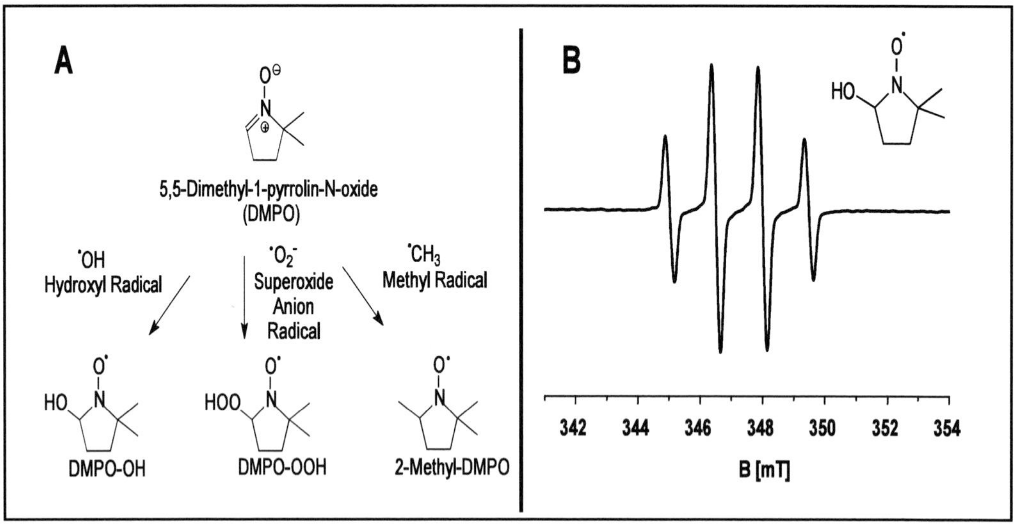

Figure 4. A) Reactions of the spin trap DMPO with several free radicals. B) X-Band EPR spectrum of hydroxyl radicals trapped by DMPO.

Figure 4A shows examples for reactions of the spin trap with different free radicals. Figure 4B shows the EPR spectrum of the DMPO-OH adduct with its characteristic spin hamiltonian hfs parameter $a^H = a^N = 1.49$ mT [52]

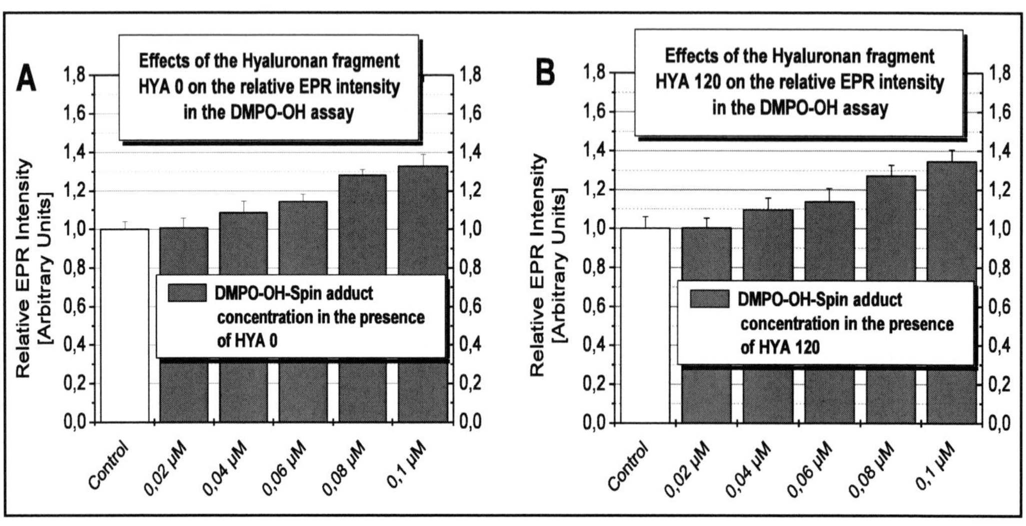

Figure 5. Effect of hyaluronan and fragments on the concentration of the DMPO-OH spin adduct measured using the EPR double resonator technique in relation to the TEMPO reference [19]. A) Fragment HYA 0. B) Fragment HYA 120. The error bars represent the standard deviation (± SD) obtained by quadruple measurements (n = 4) which was always below 5 % (SD < 5%).

Figure 5 shows the results of the DMPO-OH spin adduct quantification using the double resonator technique. As examples for all fragments investigated the data for native hyaluronan HYA 0 (Figure 5A) and the fragment HYA 120 (Figure 5B) are shown. Hyaluronan and all its fragments from enzymatic degradation showed prooxidative effects in the DMPO-OH assay quantifying Fenton generated hydroxyl radicals via spin trapping. The effect was dependent on the polysaccharide concentration. These results are helpful to interprete the mechanism of the antioxidative effects observed in the TBA assay. The prooxidative behavior in the Fenton assay can be explained by the chelation of iron ions, a theoretical approach which has been proposed also for other glycosaminoglycanes and proteoglycanes [35]. There are prooxidative and antioxidative effects of iron chelators described in the literature [37]. Davies et al. could show that uric acid as another polyhydroxy compound was able to form stable co-ordination complexes with iron ions and inhibit lipid peroxidation in liposomes by this [53]. Transition metal chelation has been classified along with direct radical scavenging, reduction by electron donation and enzymatic antioxidativity as an important part of antioxidative behavior of compounds [54]. In the lipid model systems the iron complexation leads to a lipid protection and a decrease of the amount of lipid peroxidation products. In the Fenton system used for EPR investigations an iron ion chelation showed opposite results. The addition of a second transition metal chelator besides ADP had an additional prooxidative effect. Apparently, an iron chelation in the Fenton system increased the availability or rather the transfer of the transition metal electron to oxygen resulting in increased hydroxyl radical concentrations. This interpretation is supported by the results of Agren et al. The affinity between hyaluronan and iron ions has been proved by adding superoxide dismutase, catalase and Detapac (Diethylenetriaminepentaacetic acid) to skin explants [55]. The iron chelator Detapac was the most effective compound in preventing ^{3}H labelled hyaluronan from degradation which shows the interaction between the polysaccharide and iron before hyaluronan degradation. This transition metal chelation theory also explains the similarity of the protective effects of hyaluronan and its fragments observed in the TBA assay. Assuming iron chelation as the main reason for the antioxidative behavior of hyaluronan and transition metal catalysis as the key step in lipid peroxidation the similarity is easily explained. All samples contain the same concentrations of iron ions and the chelation of them leads to a similar protection from UV induced lipid peroxidation.

It was shown that hyaluronan and hyaluronan fragments from enzymatic degradation exhibit antioxidative effects on lipid model systems of differing complexity. The polysaccharide`s degradation after UV irradiation was demonstrated by mass spectrometry.

The results of EPR investigations were useful for detailed studies regarding the mechanism of hyaluronan protecting stratum corneum lipids from UV irradiation. Iron chelation is suggested to be an important part of the mechanism of the antioxidative properties of hyaluronan and its fragments. Recently data were presented that suggest that the initiation of repair and regeneration mechanisms in human skin may be physiological key tasks of hyalronan in response to UV-B irradiation [56].

Ascorbic Acid

Ascorbic acid or vitamin C is an important water soluble vitamin and part of the so-called non enzymatic antioxidative defence system of humans. Vitamin C is involved in many physiological functions of living organisms, for example the regulation of the collagen synthesis, the synthesis of muscle carnitine and enzyme stimulation in the tyrosin metabolism.

However, there are a lot of controversies regarding the health benefits of ascorbic acid.

Figure 6 shows the results of the TBA acid assay in the skin lipid model systems and the influences of ascorbic acid addition [18]. The effects of 1 – 100 μM ascorbic acid on a LLA dispersion are shown in figure 6A. Secondary lipid peroxidation products (measured as MDA units) are significantly increased in a concentration dependent manner. The TBA reaction product concentration level is increased by ascorbic acid from 250 ng/ml for 1μM ascorbic acid to 1100 ng/ml for 100 μM vitamin C.

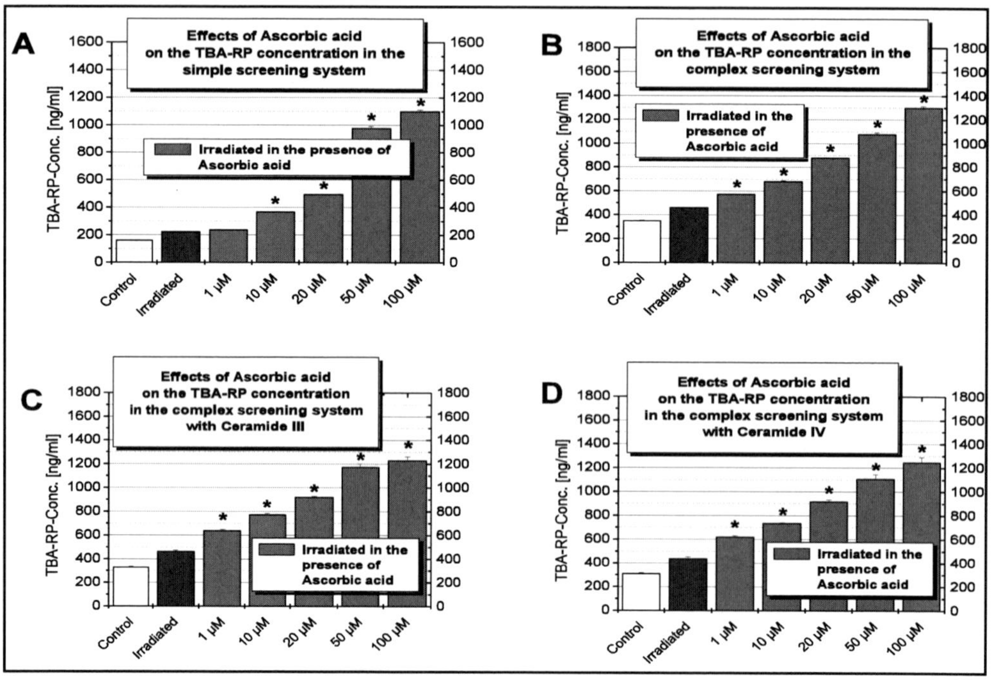

Figure 6. Concentration of the thiobarbituric acid reaction products (TBA-RP Conc.) and influences of ultraviolet irradiation and ascorbic acid in the systems used [18]. A) Simple system. B) Complex system. C) Complex system with ceramide III. D) Complex system with ceramide IV. * $P < 0.05$, UV exposed in the presence of ascorbic acid vs. irradiated without ascorbic acid (light grey column), two-tailed test. All data represent the mean values ± SD of sextuple measurements ($n = 6$).

Figure 6B shows the effects of the vitamin measured using the complex system including the phospholipid DPPC, CHOL and LLA. Ascorbic acid is acting prooxidatively as well and the level of peroxidative damage is increased.

The addition of the sphingolipids ceramide III and ceramide IV (Figures 6C and 6D) caused no additional effect on the TBA level of the complex system as already observed at the experiments with hyaluronic acid. Ascorbic acid increases the amount of lipid peroxidation products measured as malondialdehyde content in all skin lipid systems in a concentration dependent manner. The level of the thiobarbituric acid assay reaction products is higher in lipid systems that are more complex. This provides evidence supporting the EPR results of Buettner et al.: Catalytic metals, ascorbate and free radicals are combinations to avoid [16].

Figure 7 shows that α-Tocopherol protects lipids from UV induced oxidative damage catalysed by iron ions, while ascorbic acid was found to increase oxidative damage. A mixture of both vitamins is able to decrease the amount of lipid peroxidation caused by ascorbic acid, UV and transition metal catalysts. This may reflect the redox cycling abilities of ascorbic acid; as a molecule with strong reducing properties it is able to regenerate used α-Tocopherol from its oxidized radical form.

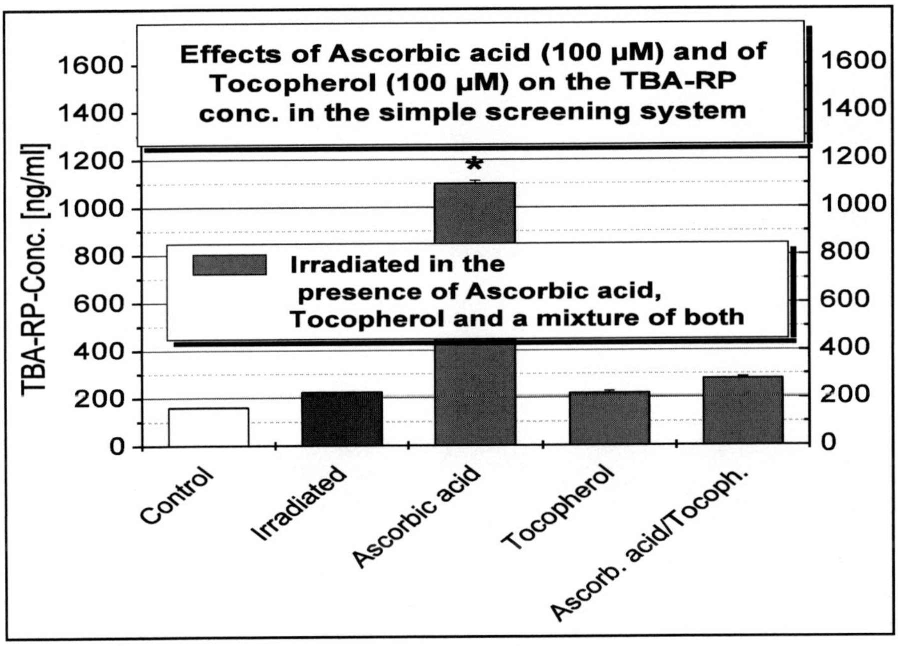

Figure 7. Concentration of the thiobarbituric acid reaction products (TBA-RP Conc.) and influences of ultraviolet irradiation, ascorbic acid and tocopherol and of a mixture of ascorbic acid and tocopherol [18].

To elucidate the mechanism of degradation of ascorbic acid at a molecular level, mass spectrometric investigations were performed using an ESI-MS device again. Figure 8A shows the negative ion mode spectrum of ascorbic acid and iron ions exposed to 0.25 J/cm^2 UV-B.

A degradation scheme is also shown (Figure 8B). In the m/z range 70 – 270, 7 main peaks were detected. The ascorbate peak at m/z = 175 disappeared completely. Dehydroascorbate, the corresponding redox partner and oxidation product could be detected at m/z = 173. However, the main peak of the irradiated system appeared at m/z = 191. This peak was assigned to the open chained compound diketogulonate as the main degradation product of ascorbic acid. However, it could also represent the monohydrate of dehydroascorbic acid. The addition of an H_2O molecule leads to a m/z of 209. This peak was identified as the dihydrate of dehydroascorbic acid or the open chained monohydrated diketogulonic acid. Another H_2O addition brings the diketogulonic acid dihydrate, the only open ring form possible.

Decarboxylation of diketogulonic acid leads to trihydroxy-keto-valeraldehyde and its tautomers. The peaks at m/z = 129 and m/z = 111 can be explained by a twice running water loss.

Using EPR spectrometry it was possible once more to elucidate the radical processes involved in the studied systems. Firstly, the ascorbic acid radical (Figure 9A) was detected as an intermediate of the corresponding redox partners ascorbic acid and dehydroascorbic acid with its typical proton hyperfine splitting (hfs) of $a^H = 0.18$ mT and a g factor of g = 2.0052 [57]. This radical was present in a freshly prepared solution of 100 μM ascorbic acid in double distilled water at room temperature.

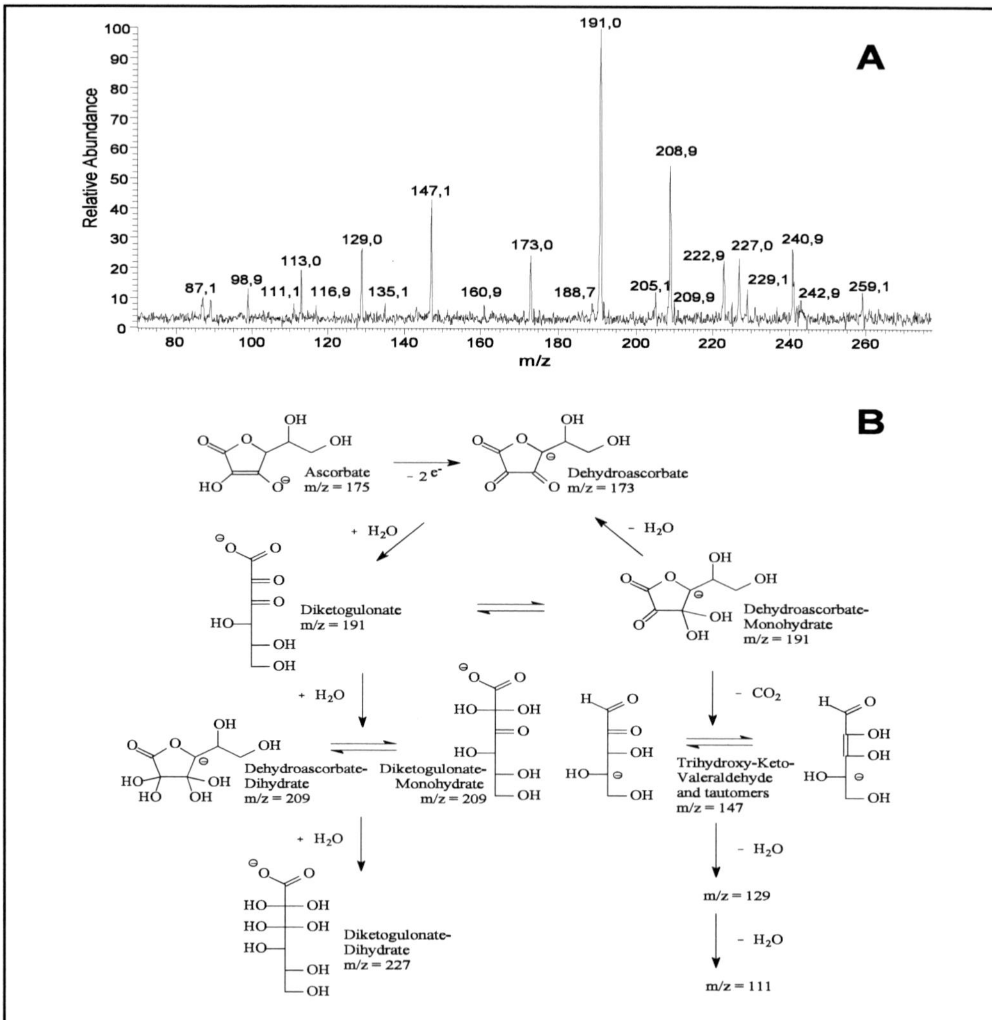

Figure 8. A) Negative ion mode ESI mass spectrum of ascorbic acid irradiated with 0.25 J/cm^2 UV-B in the presence of 10 μM Fe(II). B) Degradation scheme [18].

In the Fenton assay (Spin trapping experiments by DMPO), there were no radicals to quantify even after adding ascorbic acid in the lowest concentration. This could be due to the ability of ascorbic acid to scavenge Fenton system generated hydroxyl radicals faster than DMPO as shown for ascorbyl palmitate in various *in vitro* models [58]. In the study by Perricone et al. the lipophilic vitamin C derivate was found to be one order of magnitude faster in radical scavenging than the spin trap. Another explanation could be the reduction of the already generated paramagnetic OH-spin adduct to the corresponding hydroxylamine as concluded by Haberland et al. [59]. However, both interpretations provide evidence to the role of the vitamin as a terminal small molecule antioxidant with reducing properties in biological systems which is due to its position at the bottom of the one-electron reduction potentials list for radical couples [60].

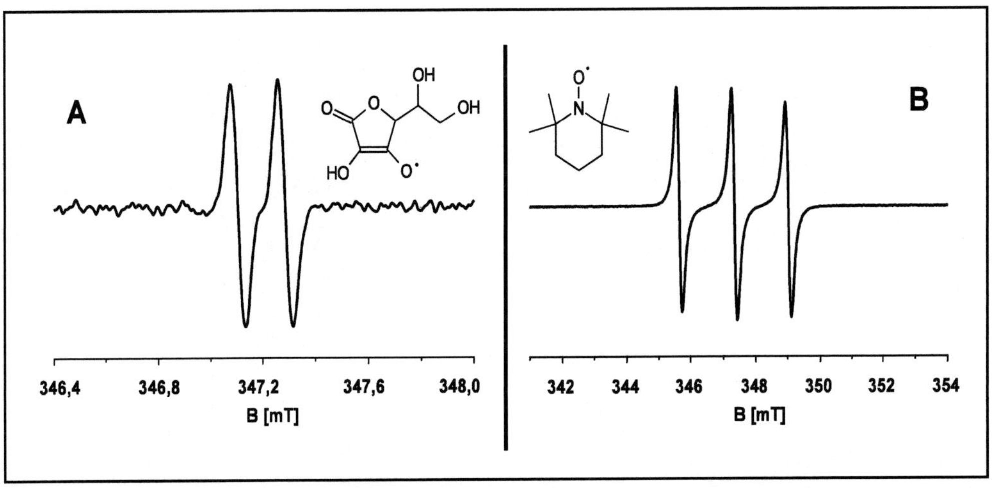

Figure 9. X-Band EPR spectra. A) The ascorbic acid radical. B) The spin probe TEMPO.

TEMPO is a stable free radical and was used as a reference specimen in the double resonator for both DMPO-OH-determinations and DPPH studies. Figure 9B illustrates the EPR spectrum of a 50 μM methanolic solution with a characteristic splitting of $a^N = 1.74$ mT.

The DPPH radical was used as an example of stable organic free radicals. The X-Band EPR spectrum of a 0.1 mM solution is shown in figure 10A. Often, the antioxidative properties of compounds are refered to their ability to reduce the concentration of the DPPH free radical. Different concentrations of ascorbic acid (a range from 1-100 μM; 2.0 ml of each specimen) were mixed with 3.0 ml of a methanolic DPPH stock solution. Spectrum recording has been started 120 s after ascorbic acid addition against TEMPO as a reference sample in the double resonator.

The results are presented in Figure 10B. By adding ascorbic acid to a DPPH solution in several concentrations a decrease of the EPR signal intensities of the stable radical in relation to the TEMPO reference could be observed.

The reducing potential of ascorbic acid could be the reason for this result. The molecule can easily provide electrons to other compounds to be oxidated itself.

The data have shown that ascorbic acid exhibits prooxidative effects on lipid model systems of differing complexity. These effects are concentration dependent and transition metal ions such as iron ions (Fe^{II}) are required. The molecular mechanism of the ascorbic acid degradation after its lipid damaging action was demonstrated by mass spectrometry.

The results of EPR investigations were useful for detailed studies regarding the redox properties of ascorbic acid.

Normally, in the human body there is an antioxidative network where several antioxidative systems influence and renew themselves. Ascorbic acid plays an import role in the collagen production and in the recycling process of these physiologically present co-antioxidants. Kitazawa et al. confirmed these relationships between skin antioxidants by EPR spectroscopy (61). The addition of hydrophilized short chain vitamin E homologues to murine skin homogenates exposed to UV irradiation prevented the oxidation of ascorbic acid.

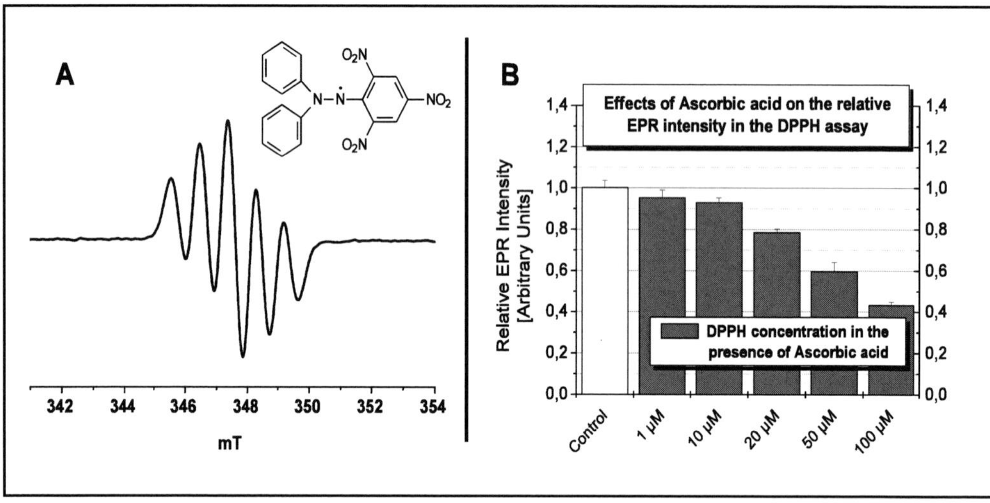

Figure 10. A) X-Band EPR spectrum of the stable organic radical DPPH. B) Effect of ascorbic acid on the concentration DPPH measured using the EPR double resonator technique in relation to the TEMPO reference [18]. The error bars represent the standard deviation (± SD) obtained by quadruple measurements (n = 4) which was always below 5 % (SD < 5%).

Under physiological conditions there is the chance for an interplay of the nonenzymatic small molecule antioxidants with the enzymatic antioxidant system of the skin (62). *In vivo* studies of topically administered vitamin C, therefore, mostly cause no harmful response but modest protective effects (63). Sunburn cell number determinations and erythema measurements by laser Doppler velocimetry after aqueous vitamin C application to animal skin of the porcine model showed protective effects of the vitamin after UV irradiation (64).

Damage of biomolecules only occurs when all antioxidative systems such as the vitamin E redox system are exhausted or reduced in function. The whole reductive potential of vitamin C would then be available for the reduction of Fe^{III} ions. This would lead to ascorbyl radicals and Fe^{II} ions as catalysts of the Haber-Weiss-reaction generating more damaging hydroxyl radicals. The represented results are evidence for the jeopardizing synergistic effects of the combination of ascorbic acid, iron ions and ultraviolet irradiation [18, 65].

Lee et al. [41] found ascorbic acid to decompose lipid hydroperoxides to endogenous genotoxins even without transition metal ion catalysis. This point is to take into consideration when discussing our results. The formation of DNA reactive bifunctional electrophiles could be an additional damaging effect of ascorbic acid in our experiments. Firstly, ascorbic acid reduces Fe^{III}. More Fe^{II} ions are available and the Fenton reaction can run on a higher level leading to more peroxidized lipids. Following the results of Lee et al., more substrate for ascorbic acid to decompose is in the system. The amount of cell toxic aldehydes is increased which could be the reason for the increased levels of the TBA assay.

Considering the presence of ascorbic acid in some cosmetical formulations and even in sunscreens our results appear to be alarming under the conditions discussed above. However, *in vivo* models are required in this case as well to confirm this assumption.

Conclusion

Several substances were screened for antioxidative effects using *in vitro* skin lipid model systems. For amantadine, melatonin, melanin, propranolol and hyaluronic acid lipid protective effects were measured using the thiobarbituric acid assay. It was shown that hyaluronan and also its degradation products with reduced molecular weight exert antioxidative effects on the skin lipid models. Mass spectrometric studies revealed that the mucopolysaccharide is degraded after acting antioxidatively.

To learn more about the radical involvement during these processes EPR experiments were applied. Hyaluronan and hyaluronic acid fragments increased the concentration of spin trapped hydroxyl radicals. This observation results from hyaluronan and its fragments acting as iron chelators which explains the results of both thiobarbituric acid assay and EPR experiments.

Prooxidative effects were found for ascorbic acid. Mass spectrometric investigations have shown that the vitamin is degraded after having acted prooxidatively as well. The degradation products of ascorbic acid were detected.

These results show new ways of skin protection by topical applicable substances with antioxidative potency on one hand and contribute to the enlightenment of the properties of ascorbic acid which are debated controversially on the other hand.

Considering human skin and its constant exposure to UV light and oxygen, combined with an increased iron ion content of the exposed skin, topical administration of some of the substances found in this study, when used in cosmetic and pharmaceutical semisolid formulations, could be protective for the lipids within the human skin. The use of substances with small molecular weights which are easy to handle or of molecules naturally occurring in the human skin could be of special advantage.

References

[1] Krutmann, J., New developments in photoprotection of human skin. *Skin Pharmacol Appl Skin Physiol*, 14:401-407, 2001.

[2] Thiele, J.J., Hsieh, S.N., Briviba, K. and Sies, H., Protein oxidation in human stratum corneum: susceptibility of keratins to oxidation in vitro and presence of a keratin oxidation gradient in vivo. *J Invest Dermatol,* 113:335-339, 1999.

[3] Ogura, R. and Sugiyama, M., Reactive oxidants in skin: UV induced lipid peroxidation, in Fuchs J: Packer L (eds), Oxidative stress in dermatology. 1st ed., *Marcel Dekker, INC*, New York, NY, pp 49-66, 1993.

[4] Samokyszyn, V.M., Miller, D.M., Reif, D.W. and Aust, S.D. Iron-catalyzed lipid peroxidation, in Vigo-Pelfrey C (ed), Membrane lipid oxidation, Volume I., 1st ed., *CRC Press*, Boca Raton, FL, pp 101-128, 1990.

[5] Herrling, T., Jung, K., Fuchs, J., UV - Generated Free Radicals (FR) in Skin and Hair – Their Formation, Action, Elimination and Prevention – A General View. *SÖFW-Journal*, 8:2-11, 2007.

[6] Fuchs, J. and Packer, L., Oxidative stress in dermatology, *Marcel Dekker*, New York, NY, USA, 1993.

[7] Betteridge, D.J., What is oxidative stress? *Metabolism*, 49:3-8, 2000.

[8] Pincemail, J., Free radicals and antioxidants in human diseases, in Favier A: Cadet J: Kalyanaraman B: Fontecave M: Pierre J-L (eds), Analysis of free radicals in biological systems, 1st ed., *Birkhäuser*, Basel, pp 83-98, 1995.

[9] Thiele, J.J., Oxidative targets in the stratum corneum. A new basis for antioxidative strategies. *Skin Pharmacol Appl Skin Physiol,* 14 Suppl 1:87-91, 2001.

[10] Cunningham, W.J., Photoaging, in Elsner P: Maibach I (eds), Cosmeceuticals: Drugs vs. Cosmetics, 1st ed., *Marcel Dekker, INC*, New York, NY, pp 13-34, 2000.

[11] Sander, C.S., Chang, H., Salzmann, S., Müller, C.S., Ekanayake-Mudiyanselage, S., Elsner, P. and Thiele, J.J., Photoaging is associated with protein oxidation in human skin in vivo. *J Invest Dermatol,* 118:618-625, 2002.

[12] Wertz, P.W., Lipids and barrier function of the skin. *Acta Derm Venereol,* Suppl 208:7-11, 2000.

[13] Shibimato, T., The role of lipid peroxidation caused by ultraviolet light in skin diseases. *J Toxicol Cut Ocular Toxicol*, 13:193-202, 1994.

[14] Guy, R.H.; Hostynek, J.J.; Hinz, R.S.; Lorence, C.R., Metals and the skin. Topical effects and systemic absorption, *Marcel Dekker,* New York, NY, 1999.

[15] Green, R., Charlton, R., Seftel, H., Bothwell, T., Mayet, F., Adams, B., Finch, C. and Layrisse, M., Body iron excretion in man. A collaborative study. *Am J Med,* 45:336-353, 1968.

[16] Buettner, G.R. and Jurkiewicz, B.A., Catalytic metals, ascorbate and free radicals: combinations to avoid. *Radiation Res,* 145:532-541, 1996.

[17] Trommer, H., Wagner, J., Graener, H. and Neubert, R.H.H., The examination of skin lipid model systems stressed by ultraviolet irradiation in the presence of transition metal ions. *Eur J Pharm Biopharm,* 51:207-214, 2001.

[18] Trommer, H., Boettcher, R., Poeppl, A., Hoentsch, J., Wartewig, S. and Neubert, R.H.H., Role of ascorbic acid in stratum corneum lipid models exposed to UV irradiation. *Pharm Res,* 19:982-990, 2002.

[19] Trommer, H., Wartewig, S., Boettcher, R., Poeppl, A., Hoentsch, J., Ozegowski, J.H. and Neubert, R.H.H., The effects of hyaluronan and its fragments on lipid models exposed to UV irradiation. *Int J Pharm,* 254:223-234, 2003.

[20] Trommer, H., Plaetzer, M., Raith, K., Podhaisky, H.P., Wohlrab, W. and Neubert, R.H.H., Examinations of the antioxidative properties of the topically administered

drug bufexamac reveal new insights into its mechanism of action. *J Pharm Pharmacol,* 55:1379-1388, 2003.

[21] Janero, D.R., Malondialdehyde and thiobarbituric acid-reactivity as diagnostic indices of lipid peroxidation and peroxidative tissue injury. *Free Radic Biol Med,* 9:515-540, 1990.

[22] Papac, D.I. and Shahrokh. Z., Mass Spectrometry Innovations in Drug Discovery and Development. *Pharm. Res.* 18:131–145, 2001.

[23] Katzhendler, I., Maeder, K., Azoury, R., and Friedman M., Investigating the structure and properties of hydrated hydroxypropyl methylcellulose and egg albumin matrices containing carbamazepine: EPR and NMR study. *Pharm. Res.* 17:1299-1308, 2000.

[24] Kroll, C., Herrmann, W., Stoesser, R., Borchert, H. H. and Maeder K., Influence of drug treatment on the microacidity in rat and human skin – an in vitro electron spin resonance imaging study. *Pharm. Res.* 18:525–530, 2001.

[25] Maeder, K., Pharmaceutical applications of in vivo EPR. *Phys. Med. Biol.* 43:1931-1935, 1998.

[26] Gunther, M.R., Tschirret-Guth, R.A., Witkowska, H.E., Fann, Y.C., Barr, D.P., Ortiz De Montellano, P.R. and Mason, R.P., Site-specific spin trapping of tyrosine radicals in the oxidation of metmyoglobin by hydrogen peroxide. *Biochem. J,* 330:1293-1299, 1998.

[27] Roberts, W.E., The Roberts skin type classification system. *J Drugs Dermatol,* 5:452-456, 2008.

[28] Buege, J.A. and Aust, S., Microsomal lipid peroxidation. *Methods Enzymol,* 52:302-310, 1978.

[29] Trommer, H., Neubert, R.H., Screening for new antioxidative compounds for topical administration using skin lipid model systems. *J Pharm Pharm Sciences* 8:494-506, 2005.

[30] Kalka, K., Mukhtar, H., Turowski-Wanke, A. and Merk, H., Biomelanin antioxidants in cosmetics: assessment based on inhibition of lipid peroxidation. *Skin Pharmacol Appl Skin Physiol,* 13:143-149, 2000.

[31] Herrling, T., Jung, K., Fuchs, J., The Important Role of Melanin as Protector against Free Radicals in Skin. *SÖFW-Journal,* 9:26-33, 2007.

[32] Aruoma, O.I., Smith, C., Cecchini, R., Evans, P.J. and Halliwell, B., Free radical scavenging and inhibition of lipid peroxidation by beta-blockers and by agents that interfere with calcium metabolism. A physiologically-significant process? *Biochem Pharmacol,* 42:735-743, 1991.

[33] Zang, L.Y., Cosma, G., Gardner, H. and Vallyathan, V., Scavenging of reactive oxygen species by melatonin. *Biochim Biophys Acta,* 1425:469-477, 1998.

[34] Fischer, T.W. and Elsner, P., The antioxidative potential of melatonin in the skin. *Curr Probl Dermatol,* 29:165-174, 2001.

[35] Dreher, F., Gabard, B., Schwindt, D.A. and Maibach, H.I., Topical melatonin in combination with vitamins E and C protects skin from ultraviolet-induced erythema: a human study in vivo. *Br J Dermatol,* 139:332-339, 1998.

[36] Albertini, R., Passi, A., Abuja, P.M. and De Luca, G., The effect of glycosaminoglycans on lipid peroxidation. *Int J Mol Med,* 6:129-136, 2000.

[37] Sipos, P., Berkesi, O., Tombacz, E., St Pierre, T.G. and Webb, J., Formation of spherical iron (III) oxyhydroxide nanoparticles sterically stabilized by chitosan in aqueous solutions. *J Inorg Biochem,* 95:55-63, 2003.

[38] Gutteridge, J.M., Richmond, R. and Halliwell, B., Inhibition of the iron-catalysed formation of hydroxyl radicals from superoxide and of lipid peroxidation by desferrioxamine. *Biochem J,* 184:469-472, 1979.

[39] Balogh, G.T., Illes, J., Szekely, Z., Forrai, E. and Gere, A., Effect of different metal ions on the oxidative damage and antioxidant capacity of hyaluronic acid. *Arch Biochem Biophys,* 410:76-82, 2003.

[40] Podmore, I.D., Griffiths, H.R., Herbert, K.E., Mistry, N., Mistry, P. and Lunec, J., Vitamin C exhibits pro-oxidant properties. *Nature,* 392:559, 1998.

[41] Chen, K., Suh, J., Carr, A.C., Morrow, J.D., Zeind, J. and Frei, B., Vitamin C suppresses oxidative lipid damage in vivo, even in the presence of iron overload. *Am J Physiol Endocrinol Metab,* 279:E1406-E1412, 2000.

[42] Lee, S.H., Oe, T. and Blair, I.A., Vitamin C-induced decomposition of lipid hydroperoxides to endogenous genotoxins. *Science,* 292:2083-2086, 2001.

[43] Albrecht-Goepfert, A., Schempp, H. and Elstner, E.F., Modulation of the production of reactive oxygen species by pre-activated neutrophils by aminoadamantane derivatives. *Biochem Pharmacol,* 56:141-152, 1998.

[44] Cantor, J.O., Nadkarni, P.P., Hyaluronan: the Jekyll and Hyde molecule. *Inflamm Allergy Drug Targets*, 5:257-260, 2006.

[45] Tan, S.W., Johns, M.R. and Greenfield, P.F., Hyaluronic acid a versatile biopolymer. *Aust J Biotechnol*, 4:38-43, 1990.

[46] Viseux N., de Hoffmann, E. and Domon, B., Structural analysis of permethylated oligosaccharides by electrospray tandem mass spectrometry. *Anal Chem,* 69:3193-3198, 1997.

[47] Takagaki, K., Munakata, H., Nakamura, W., Matsuya, H., Majima, M. and Endo, M., Ion-spray mass spectrometry for identification of the nonreducing terminal sugar of glycosaminoglycan. *Glycobiology*, 8:719-724, 1998.

[48] Price, K.N., Al Tuinman, Baker, D.C., Chisena, C. and Cysyk, R.L., Isolation and characterization by electrospray-ionization mass spectrometry and high-performance anion-exchange chromatography of oligosaccharides derived from hyaluronic acid by hyaluronate lyase digestion: observation of some heretofore unobserved oligosaccharides that contain an odd number of units. *Carbohydr Res*, 303:303-311, 1997.

[49] Mahoney, D.J., Aplin, R.T., Calabro, A., Hascall, V.C. and Day, A.J., Novel methods for the preparation and characterization of hyaluronan oligosaccharides of defined length. *Glycobiology*, 11:1025-1033, 2001.

[50] Hawkins, C.L. and Davies, M.J., Direct detection and identification of radicals generated during the hydroxyl radical-induced degradation of hyaluronic acid and related materials, *Free Radic Biol Med*, 21:275-290, 1996.

[51] Lapcik, L. Jr., Chabrecek, P. and Stasko, A., Photodegradation of hyaluronic acid: EPR and size exclusion chromatography study. *Biopolymers*, 31:1429-1435, 1991.

[52] Hadjur, C. and Jeunet, A., EPR evidence of the generation of superoxide anion radicals (O2-) by irradiation of a PDT photosensitizer: Hypericin. In: Favier, A.E., Cadet, J., Kalyanaraman, B., Fontecave, M., Pierre, J.-L. (Eds.), Analysis of Free Radicals in Biological Systems, Birkhäuser, Basel, 1995, pp. 119 126.

[53] Davies, K.J., Sevanian, A., Muakkassah-Kelly, S.F. and Hochstein, P., Uric acid-iron ion complexes. A new aspect of the antioxidant functions of uric acid. *Biochem J*, 235:747-754, 1986.

[54] Voegeli, R., Meier, J. and Doppler, S., Defence strategies against reactive oxygen species – in vitro models. *Int J Cosmet Science*, 15, 153-161, 1993.

[55] Agren, U.M., Tammi, R.H. and Tammi, M.I., Reactive oxygen species contribute to epidermal hyaluronan catabolism in human skin organ culture. *Free Radic Biol Med* 23:996-1001, 1997.

[56] Averbeck, M., Gebhardt, C.A., Voigt, S., Beilharz, S., Anderegg, U., Termeer C.C., Sleeman, J.P., Simon, J.C., Differential regulation of hyaluronan metabolism in the epidermal and dermal compartments of human skin by UVB irradiation. *J Invest Dermatol* 127:687-697, 2007.

[57] Buettner, G.R. and Jurkiewicz,. B.A., Ascorbate radical: A valuable marker of oxidative stress, In A.E. Favier, J. Cadet, B. Kalyanaraman, M. Fontecave, and J.-L. Pierre (eds.), Analysis of Free Radicals in Biological Systems, Birkhäuser, Basel, 1995, pp. 145-164

[58] Perricone, N., Nagy, K., Horvath, F., Dajko, G., Uray, I. and Zs.-Nagy, I., The hydroxyl frcc radical rcactions of ascorbyl palmitate as measured in various in vitro models. *Biochem Biophys Res Commun* 262:661-665, 1999.

[59] Haberland, A., Damerau, W., Stoesser, R., Schimke, I. and Baumann, G., Fe2+/Vitamin C – an appropriate in vitro model system to initiate lipid peroxidation. *J Inorg Biochem* 61:43-53, 1996.

[60] Buettner, G.R., The pecking order of free radicals and antioxidants: Lipid peroxidation, tocopherol and ascorbate. *Arch Biochem Biophys* 300:535-543, 1993.

[61] Kitazawa, M., Podda, M., Thiele, J., Traber, M.G., Iwasaki, K., Sakamoto, K. and Packer, L., Interactions between vitamin E homologues and ascorbate free radicals in murine skin homogenates irradiated with ultraviolet light. *Photochem Photobiol* 65:355-365, 1997.

[62] Fuchs, J., Potentials and limitations of the natural antioxidants RRR-alpha-tocopherol, L-ascorbic acid and β-carotene in cutaneous photoprotection. *Free Radic Biol Med* 25:848-873. 1998.

[63] Thiele, J.J., Dreher, F. and Packer, L., Antioxidant defense systems in skin. In P. Elsner, and H.I. Maibach (eds.), Cosmeceuticals. Drugs vs. Cosmetics, Marcel Dekker, New York, 2000, pp. 145-187.

[64] Colven, R.M. and Pinnell, S.R., Topical vitamin C in aging. *Clinics in Dermatol* 14:227-234, 1996.

[65] Trommer, H., Böttcher, R., Huschka, C., Wohlrab, W., Neubert, R.H., Further investiga-tions on the role of ascorbic acid in stratum corneum lipid models after UV exposure. *J Pharm Pharmacol* 57:963-972, 2005

In: Skin Anatomy and Physiology Research Developments
Editor: Leon F. Bukowsky
ISBN: 978-1-60741-469-8

Chapter 4

Electrodermal Measures in the Detection of Concealed Information

Eitan Elaad
Ariel University Center, Israel

The concealed information test (CIT) is a method of psychophysiological detection that identifies information a knowledgeable (guilty) person does not wish to reveal (Lykken, 1974, 1998). The rationale behind the use of CIT is based on theory and research on orienting responses (ORs) and habituation processes in humans.

Most experimental CIT studies have used electrodermal responses (e.g., skin conductance, skin resistance) as the single autonomic measure to examine various aspects of the CIT. In these studies, electrodermal measures were identified as an efficient means for detecting concealed information and for distinguishing between individuals who do or do not possess this knowledge.

Field research, however, produced large rates of false-negative outcomes and lower skin resistance detection efficiency than experimental studies. These discrepancies might have resulted from factors affecting perception and memory and from the use of a small number of CIT questions. Other explanations concern the manner in which the test was applied and possible use of countermeasures to which electrodermal responses are particularly vulnerable.

The present review describes findings from experimental and applied research studies using electrodermal measures reported in the CIT literature from a somewhat different perspective. This review highlights several concerns of CIT testing and suggests solutions based on the most recent CIT research.

The Concealed Information Test

The CIT uses a series of multiple-choice questions, each having one correct alternative (e.g., a feature of the crime under investigation) and several incorrect (control) alternatives, chosen so that an innocent person is unable to distinguish between correct and incorrect alternatives.

In a murder case, for example, the victim might have been stabbed, strangled, shot, battered, poisoned and so on. The examinees are asked, "Do you know that the victim was...?" followed by a set of alternatives: (a) stabbed, (b) strangled, (c) shot, (d) battered, and (e) poisoned. The examinees are told that if they are guilty, they will respond to the crime-related item. Typically, if the examinee's physiological responses to the correct alternative are consistently greater than his/her responses to the incorrect alternatives, knowledge about the investigated crime is inferred. As long as information about the criminal event has not been leaked, the probability that an innocent suspect would consistently show stronger responses to the correct alternative than to the controls depends only on the number of questions and the number of alternative items per question. Thus, the CIT can be designed to ensure maximal protection for the innocent.

The CIT has drawn considerable attention from researchers, but has been applied extensively only in Japan (Fukumoto, 1980; Nakayama, 2002; Yamamura & Miyata, 1990). In contrast to other psychophysiological detection methods such as the Comparison Question Technique (CQT, see Reid and Inbau, 1977), there is a general consensus that the CIT is based on solid scientific principles and proper control questions (e.g., Ben-Shakhar, Bar-Hillel, & Kremnizer, 2002; Ben-Shakhar & Elaad, 2003; Ben-Shakhar & Furedy, 1990; Lykken, 1974, 1998).

CIT Response Systems: Electrodermal and Other ANS Measures

Although several measures of the autonomic nervous system have been used to detect concealed information, (e.g., skin conductance response (SCR), heart rate (HR), and respiration line length (RLL)), Gamer, Verschuere, Crombez, and Vossel (2008) recently reported that SCR had a higher validity than HR and RLL. Similar results were obtained in earlier studies (e.g., Balloun & Holmes, 1979; Bradley & Ainsworth, 1984). Hence, electrodermal measures are considered to be the best measures of the CIT procedure. Furthermore, unlike most ANS responses, electrodermal responses provide a direct representation of sympathetic activity since the neural control of the eccrine sweat glands is entirely under the control of the sympathetic system (Dawson, Schell, & Filion, 2000). Therefore, any increase in SCR is due exclusively to an increase in sympathetic activation. Other ANS responses such as HR, pupil diameter or blood pressure, cannot be unequivocally attributed to sympathetic or parasympathetic activity. Another advantage of using electrodermal responses is that their occurrence is generally easily determined. One can easily detect an SCR response while other ANS responses are more difficult to confirm. Furthermore, electrodermal responses are influenced primarily by activation of the behavioral inhibition system that is invoked in response to punishment, passive avoidance or frustration when expected reward is denied (Dawson et al., 2000). Hence, in a situation where no active avoidance response can be made, as is the case in the CIT, the electrodermal system is the most responsive physiological system. Therefore, it is not surprising that electrodermal responses are also the most studied CIT response system and it is only reasonable to base the present review on results obtained from electrodermal responses.

Theoretical Account–The Simple Cognitive Rationale

Extensive research on orienting responses and habituation processes in humans laid the theoretical foundations for the CIT's rationale (Siddle, 1991; Sokolov, 1963). Sokolov suggested that the orienting response (OR) is a complex of physiological and behavioral reactions elicited by any change in the stimulation. When the pre-attentive mechanisms fail to identify the incoming stimulus because it does not match a neural model or a representation of the stimulus in the short-term memory, the OR is evoked due to novelty. With repetitions, a neural model of the stimulus is gradually built and the OR gradually declines in response magnitude (due to habituation). When the pre-attentive mechanisms recognize the stimulus as significant, such as is the case when the individual's own name is mentioned, enhanced OR is released as well (Bernstein, 1979; Maltzman, 1979; Sokolov, 1963). SCRs are highly sensitive to stimulus novelty and significance, and therefore strong autonomic SCRs are expected as part of the OR release.

Lykken (1974) was the first to note that the enhanced SCRs released in response to undisclosed correct information are based on the OR. He argued that, "For the guilty subject only, the 'correct' alternative will have a special significance, an added 'signal value' which will tend to produce a stronger orienting reflex than that subject will show to other alternatives" (p. 728). Hence, the correct alternative in the CIT has a special meaning and will lead to enhanced physiological responses only for suspects who possess this knowledge (i.e., guilty suspects). For persons without this particular knowledge, all items should evoke equivalent responses. In such cases, the probability of consistent responses to the crime-related details is expected to be at chance level.

Lykken's approach is a simple cognitive approach (Ben-Shakhar & Furedy, 1990) that emphasizes the individual's knowledge rather than the individual's emotions, act of deception, or motivation to deceive. This approach appealed to researchers who sought to study the basic mechanisms underlying orientation behavior such as habituation (e.g., Ben-Shakhar, 1977; Ben-Shakhar & Gati, 1987; Lieblich, Kugelmass, & Ben-Shakhar, 1970). It is agreed that the relationship between stimulus novelty and significance on the one hand, and ORs on the other hand, reflects attentional processes (e.g., Dawson, Filion, & Schell, 1989; Kahneman, 1973) and because psychophysiological differentiation in the CIT is mediated through a mechanism of attention, the enhanced electrodermal responses to the correct alternatives are not necessarily attributed to deception, motivation, or fear of punishment (Davis, 1961). Support for the simple cognitive approach can be obtained from findings that demonstrate how correct information can be detected under conditions with no involvement of deceptive verbal responses and where no motivational instructions are presented to the examinees (e.g., Ben-Shakhar, 1977; Ben-Shakhar & Lieblich, 1982; Elaad & Ben-Shakhar, 1989). The cognitive approach receives further support from indications of SCR habituation in the CIT (e.g., Elaad & Ben-Shakhar, 1997; Verschuere, Crombez, De Clercq & Koster,

2004) and from studies demonstrating OR generalization (another feature of the OR) in the CIT (see Ben-Shakhar, Frost, Gati, & Kresh, 1996).

Challenging the Simple Cognitive Approach

From a practical standpoint, the simple cognitive approach suggests that the CIT operator should guarantee that no relevant information has leaked to innocent suspects. Such information might be leaked through rumors and mass media descriptions of the crime. In addition, suspects might be exposed to some critical information during the interrogation itself. As long as innocent suspects can explain how they became aware of the critical information, they may be able to defend themselves against false-positive outcomes. However, innocent suspects who are exposed to relevant information are frequently unaware of this exposure and are unable to explain the source of their knowledge.

In fact, the predictions of the simple cognitive approach have failed to explain the results of mock crime studies where innocent participants were exposed to relevant information in an innocent context. In the first two studies (Giesen & Rollison, 1980; Stern, Breen, Watanabe, & Perry, 1981), a mock crime was used in which the same relevant information was presented to guilty participants who actually committed the mock crime and to innocent participants who received the information in a non-crime context. Thus the critical items had a special meaning for all participants. The impact of overt deception was excluded because participants in these two studies remained silent. Findings indicated that it was still possible to discriminate between guilty and innocent participants. This contradicts the simple cognitive approach because significant differences in detection were obtained between groups who shared the same information.

Subsequent studies in which innocent participants were exposed to relevant information were conducted by Bradley and his colleagues. Bradley and Warfield (1984) staged a mock crime that was committed by a group of guilty participants. Three groups of innocent participants received relevant information. One group served as witnesses, another group received details of the crime, and a third group performed innocent activities involving crime-related information (innocent associations group). A fourth group of innocents received no crime-related information. The Guilty Action Test (GAT) format was used, in which participants were asked if they actually committed the crime (e.g., "Did you murder the victim in ....?") rather than the usual CIT format, in which suspects are asked if they knew about the crime (e.g., "Did the murder take place in ...?"). When giving a verbal "no" response to GAT questions, guilty participants were reacting to recognition of the critical items and were lying about their actions as they related to that information. Innocent participants recognized the information but were not lying about the criminal act they did not commit. Results showed that the correct detection rates of guilty participants were greater than in any innocent group. Bradley and Rettinger (1992) used three groups: a group of guilty participants who committed a mock crime, a group of innocent participants who received the same information as the guilty group, and a group of innocent participants who were totally unaware of the critical information. Again, GAT questions were presented and guilty participants scored higher on the critical items than participants who merely were recipients of the information. Bradley, MacLaren, and Carle (1996) compared the standard CIT format with the GAT variation. They replicated the results of the former GAT studies for their GAT questioning format. However, they reported a very high rate of false-positive outcomes for informed innocent participants who were questioned with the usual CIT format and who were instructed to be overtly deceptive about the critical information despite their innocence.

Ben-Shakhar, Gronau and Elaad (1999) further investigated the effect on CIT accuracy of disclosing critical information to innocent participants. They used the GAT format and reported that informed innocent participants showed relatively greater electrodermal responses to the critical items than uninformed innocent participants, but not as large as the responses of guilty participants.

The state of mind of innocent suspects (e.g., Granhag & Hartwig, 2008; Kassin, 2005) may explain these results. Kassin argued that people who are falsely accused trust their interrogators and believe that truth and justice will prevail: All they have to do is to cooperate and tell the truth, which is a simple matter of "telling it like it is" (Buller & Burgoon, 1996; Miller & Stiff, 1993). In the CIT, innocent participants believe that they have to lean back, relax, and let the experienced and skilled examiner do the job, and their innocence will be confirmed. Hence, in the mind of the innocent examinee, the interest of the examiner (to make a correct decision) and that of the examinee (to yield a truthful outcome) coincide. The innocent examinee trusts the polygraph examiner and listens to his/her instructions to sit and avoid moving. Compliance with such instructions dictates a passive attitude with no attempts at countermeasures or other interferences with the test. Such an attitude seems to be beneficial when the examinee is unaware of the critical information.

The situation becomes more complicated when the innocent participant is aware of the critical information. However, informed innocent examinees still believe that they share the same interest as the examiner. Hence, the basic trust, the adoption of a passive attitude, and the lower motivation to interfere with the test, remain intact. The passive attitude decreases the attention that is directed to the critical item, makes the critical information easier to ignore and the detection of concealed information more difficult to perform. This may explain why the detection rates of informed innocent participants were lower than those of guilty participants (Ben-Shakhar, et al., 1999; Bradley & Rettinger, 1992; Bradley & Warfield, 1984). On the other hand, the recognition of the correct alternative among several neutral alternatives evokes an orienting response (Lykken, 1974). This explains why the detection rates of informed innocent participants are greater than expected by mere chance. In a re-analysis of Bradley and Warfield's (1984) data, Elaad and Ben-Shakhar (1989) demonstrated that this is actually so.

The extensive research conducted over the past four decades suggested several factors other than knowledge that might affect the validity of the CIT. Several moderators were described in a meta-analysis, which was conducted to provide estimates of CIT validity in experimental settings using electrodermal measures (Ben-Shakhar & Elaad, 2003).

CIT Validity in Experimental Settings

Studies conducted in experimental settings have implied that the CIT is a highly valid method for differentiating between guilty and innocent suspects (e.g., Ben-Shakhar &

Furedy, 1990; Elaad, 1998). More recently, Ben-Shakhar and Elaad (2003) conducted meta-analysis research on CIT experimental studies to provide an estimate for the validity of the CIT based on a large data set. Another goal was to identify factors that might moderate the validity of the CIT, such as the number of CIT questions used, the motivation to deceive, and deceptive answers to the questions. The importance of the last issue lies in the conflicting results that were obtained in various previous studies.

A total of 80 studies with 169 different conditions were identified and used in the meta-analysis. Note that conditions that involved disclosure of the correct information to innocent participants were excluded. For each experimental condition several characteristics were recorded, including the number of CIT questions; the number of repetitions of each question; the type of overt verbal response – either participants were requires to respond "no" to all the items presented to them, and consequently, a deceptive answer was given to the correct item, or no verbal response was made; the level of motivation – either motivational instructions were given or no such instructions were applied. The manipulation of motivation level was achieved either by instructions that appealed to participants' self-esteem (e.g., Gustafson & Orne, 1963), by promising a reward for a desirable outcome (e.g., Bradley & Warfield, 1984), or by imposing a punishment for an undesirable outcome (e.g., Lykken, 1959).

The 169 conditions were classified into five categories: (a) studies using card tests in which participants were requested to choose a card from a pile of several cards and hide it from the examiner. In the test, cards were presented in a random order; (b) studies using card tests and the cards were in a predetermined order known to the participants; (c) studies using code words in which participants learned a series of code words on which they were subsequently tested; (d) studies that used personal details of the participants (e.g., first name, family name) as the critical items; (e) studies that used mock crimes in which participants simulating the guilty were required to commit a mock-crime and the details of the mock-crime served later as the critical items.

Using Cohen's d as an index for effect size (Cohen, 1988), results demonstrated a high level of validity, which was reflected by an effect size of $d = 1.55$ (almost twice as large as an effect size of .80, which represents a "large effect size" according to Cohen). Considering the various categories of CIT studies, it appeared that the effect size obtained under the mock-crime paradigm, $d = 2.09$, was significantly greater ($p < .05$) than the effects obtained under all remaining paradigms (the second largest effect size was obtained for the personal items paradigm, $d = 1.58$), (for more details about the statistical procedure see Hunter & Schmidt, 1990, p. 438). Finally, when the correlation between the detection measure and the criterion of guilt versus innocence was computed, a rather large coefficient emerged for the mock crime paradigm, $r=.65$. In comparison, the respective correlation coefficient computed for the personal items paradigm was, $r=.57$.

Three factors that moderated detection efficiency were identified: (a) motivation to succeed in the CIT, where success typically translates into an innocence outcome. It appeared that high motivation conditions yielded a larger effect size ($d = 1.84$) than low motivation conditions ($d =1.36$). The difference is significant ($z = 3.12$); (b) under low motivation a deceptive verbal response to the correct item (typically a "no" answer) yielded a larger effect size ($d = 1.46$) than an absence of an answer ($d = 1.21$). The difference is significant ($z =1.89$, one tailed); and (c) the number of CIT questions. Effect sizes of ($d = 2.35$) and ($d = 1.29$)

were obtained for CIT studies with large (5 or more) and small (less than 5) items, respectively. As indicated by Ben-Shakhar and Elaad (2003, p. 144), the 95% confidence intervals computed for these two categories did not overlap, so the difference was statistically significant. This result is consistent with psychometric principles.

A subset of 10 conditions that used the mock-crime paradigm presented motivational instructions, required a deceptive verbal response, and relied on at least five CIT questions, generated impressive efficiency estimates (effect size of 3.12 or an average correlation coefficient of .79 between the detection measure and the criterion of guilt versus innocence). It was concluded that the electrodermal measure offers an efficient means for differentiating between individuals with critical information and those who do not possess this knowledge.

However, the majority of the mock crime studies reviewed by Ben-Shakhar and Elaad (2003) examined guilty participants who actively handled the critical information and lied in the test to items involving the crime-related details. Innocent participants were ignorant of the critical details of the crime and told the truth when they denied possession of the knowledge. It may be argued that the different state of knowledge and the overt deception are responsible for the close to optimal classification of the two groups in experimental settings.

However, from a practical standpoint, a situation where guilty suspects are fully aware of the critical information and innocent suspects are completely ignorant of this information, is unrealistic. To keep innocent suspects ignorant of crime-related information, measures must be taken to prevent information from leaking to anyone outside a specific investigative team. Information may be leaked through association with other people, mass media descriptions of the crime, or during the interrogation. For the latter, a bias that Birch & Bloom (2004) called the "curse of knowledge", may be an effective explanation. The curse of knowledge describes the strong tendency of people to assume that others hold the very same knowledge as they do. Due to the curse of knowledge, interrogators may overestimate the information that the suspect has on the crime and consequently may reveal too much of what they know to uninformed innocent suspects.

Additional information about the crime should be denied to guilty suspects as well. Based on the assumption that interrogators possess incomplete information of the crime, they are capable of implanting inaccurate information in guilty suspects. Research on eyewitness memory demonstrated that there is a very real danger that questioning – especially the way in which questions are worded – may distort eyewitness memory (Baddeley, 1999). Such memory distortion may also affect guilty suspects. Furthermore, it is possible to change eyewitness' recollections of the crime by subtly introducing new and incorrect information during questioning (for a review, see Loftus, 1979). When guilty suspects receive incorrect information of the crime from an authoritative interrogator they may accept it as true information and modify their memory accordingly. Some distorted information may be accidentally disclosed, while other false information may be deliberately delivered by interrogators in an attempt to intimidate the suspect to confess.

In summary, experimental CIT settings combine knowledge and deception in distinguishing guilt from innocence (i.e., comparing informed guilty examinees who are lying about crime-related information with uninformed truthful innocents). This confounding of guilt with deception and with knowledge rests on the assumption that guilty persons possess and conceal incriminating information in the test. Innocents are not expected to have been exposed to such information and therefore are truthful when denying such knowledge.

To conclude, most experimental results describe a test that is conducted under optimal and unrealistic conditions. To resemble experimental conditions, real-life tests must be conducted immediately after the occurrence of the criminal event. It is absolutely essential that the suspect is not interrogated before the test, has not discussed the crime with other people, and received no information from the mass media. Obviously, it is almost impossible to isolate a suspect from all these sources of relevant information.

To further complicate the situation, we have seen that motivation to conceal the incriminating information increases differential response to the correct items in the CIT. From a practical perspective, guilt without any motivation to conceal the critical information is meaningless, and motivation is no less integral a part of guilt than either deception or knowledge.

This last statement deserves some explanation. It may be suggested that guilt is a state of mind that encourages coping behavior. From the examinee's perspective, the polygraph examiner uses his/her skills to challenge the guilty examinee whose interest is to produce an outcome of innocence. To achieve this aim, guilty examinees must undermine the test and force the examiner to make mistakes in their favor. However, guilty examinees are well aware that they confront a skilled and well-equipped professional and that their odds of "beating" the test are low. The "illusion of transparency" that causes liars to assume that their lies are more easily detected than they actually are, enhances this feeling (Gilovich, Savitsky, & Medvec, 1998). To beat the odds, guilty examinees must remain alert and actively cope with the threats (i.e., the critical items). This may be translated to disbelief and to countermeasure attempts, in particular when the examinee recognizes the critical items. While coping behavior requires increased attention of the examinee to the critical items, which is accompanied with enhanced significance of these items, increased differential responsiveness to the critical items results in a higher level of detection (see Elaad & Ben-Shakhar, 1991).

However, in experimental settings the mere assignment of participants to guilty and innocent conditions does not create the desired motivation to "beat the test". When stakes are low, guilty participants who participated in mock crimes know perfectly well that they are participating in a game and that they are free to go after the test. Thus, the definition of guilt does not evoke the same emotions, concerns, or sense of guilt as in suspects in actual criminal interrogation experiences. This was well demonstrated by Bradley et al. (1996) who defined the state of guilt as the mere involvement in a mock crime. Results indicated that the detection rate of informed innocent participants was no different from that of guilty participants.

Additional information on the accuracy of the CIT in real-life conditions is therefore absolutely essential. Two studies assumed this challenge and made an attempt to estimate CIT validity in real-life situations. The studies were conducted in the early 1990s (Elaad 1990; Elaad, Ginton & Jungman, 1992) and are described hereafter.

The Efficiency of Skin Resistance Responses in Real-Life Criminal Investigations

A first attempt to study the efficiency of electrodermal responses (Skin Resistance Responses – SRR) in real-life criminal interrogations was made by Elaad (1990). For the purpose of the study, a random sample of 98 actual CIT criminal records was drawn from the pool of verified polygraph tests of the Israel Police Scientific Interrogation Unit. All records involved CIT examinations conducted between 1979 and 1985. Forty-eight records (with a total of 100 CIT questions) were drawn from the pool of verified deceptive examinees, and 50 records (with a total of 100 CIT questions) were drawn from a pool of examinees whose innocence had been verified by the confession of another person (for more details see Elaad, 1990).

In a follow-up study (Elaad, Ginton, & Jungman, 1992), a second sample of 80 actual GKT criminal polygraph records, taken from police investigations conducted between 1985 and 1991, was drawn from the pool of verified polygraph tests of the Israel Police Scientific Interrogation Unit. The sampling was random with the exception that one-half of the records (with a total of 76 CIT questions) were drawn from the pool of polygraph records of verified deceptive examinees and one-half (with a total of 68 CIT questions) were drawn from a similar pool of innocent examinees. Again, verification of guilt or innocence was based on the confession of the perpetrator (A more detailed description of the sample appears in Elaad et al., 1992). Since both studies were in complete agreement concerning the SRR identification rates for both guilty and innocent examinees, both studies are discussed below as a single project.

To objectively analyze the records, the largest skin resistance response amplitude (which reflects the maximal decline in skin resistance) within 10 s following the presentation of each CIT alternative, was measured in millimeters with a ruler on the pattern recorded by the polygraph SRR pen. The response to the first item in each set of items was excluded from measurement because it served as a buffer to dissipate the examinee's tendency to react strongly to the initial item. Scoring was performed by a person who had no knowledge of the guilt or innocence of the examinees or of the correct alternative.

In order to consider a wide scale of decision rules, a scoring method using standard scores was applied. Standard scores, or Z scores, refer to the relative location of each score in a frequency distribution. Thus, the mean and a measure of the distribution's variability (standard deviation) are considered. Standard scores are expressed as the deviation from the mean in standard deviation units. The use of standard scores enabled the elimination of individual differences in responsiveness and a meaningful summation of responses of different examinees. Each scored SRR amplitude was translated into a standard score, relative to the mean and standard deviation of each repetition of the CIT question. Higher standard scores represent larger SRR amplitudes. The standardized responses to correct items were averaged for each examinee across questions and repetitions, yielding one new index for each examinee. The frequency distributions of the mean Z scores were constructed separately for guilty and innocent examinees and are presented in Table 1.

Each point (Z_i) along the mean response scale generated a hit rate value and a false-positive value. The hit rate was defined as the proportion of cases from the guilty-examinee distribution that elicited a mean Z score greater than Zi. The false-positive rate was defined as the proportion of cases from the innocent-examinee distribution that elicited a Z score greater than Zi .As indicated in Table 1, the 0.7–0.8 cutoff point produced a hit rate of 40% for guilty examinees and a correct detection rate of 98% for the innocents. An alternative cutoff point set at 0.4–0.5 standard deviations yielded a hit rate of 63% (an increase of 23% over the hit rate obtained with the previous decision rule) and a correct detection rate of 91% for innocent examinees (a 7% decrease). It can be seen that as the hit rate increases, false-positive decisions also increase. In comparison, Elaad (1998) reviewed 15 mock crime studies using the CIT procedure and estimated the accuracy rates among guilty and innocent examinees as 81% and 96%, respectively. Inspection of Table 1 indicates that in order to maintain the 96% accuracy level with innocent examinees, only 47% of the guilty examinees can be detected. Hence in the field, a large false-negative error rate appears.

Table 1. Frequencies and Cumulative Relative Frequencies of Mean z Scores on the Critical Items

Mean	Guilty		Innocent	
z scale	Freq.	Cum. %	Freq.	Cum. %
1.00+	19	22	0	0
0.9 to 1.00	4	26	1	1
0.8 to 0.9	2	28	0	1
0.7 to 0.8	10	40	1	2
0.6 to 0.7	6	47	2	4
0.5 to 0.6	8	56	3	8
0.4 to 0.5	6	63	1	9
0.3 to 0.4	1	64	6	16
0.2 to 0.3	8	73	3	19
0.1 to 0.2	5	78	7	27
0.0 to 0.1	5	84	4	31
-0.1 to 0.0	4	89	9	41
-0.2 to -0.1	0	89	12	54
-0.3 to -0.2	4	93	7	62
-0.4 to -0.3	3	97	7	70
-0.5 to -0.4	0	97	7	78
-0.6 to -0.5	1	98	10	89
-0.6-	2	100	10	100
	88		90	

A receiver operating characteristic (ROC) curve was generated for the SRR by comparing the distribution of the mean Z scores computed for guilty examinees with the distribution of the mean Z scores computed for innocent examinees, across all Zi values. The computed area was 0.841.The area under the ROC curve is a statistic that assumes a value between 0 and 1. An area of 0.5 indicates that both distributions are undifferentiated. An area of 1 indicates that there is no overlap between the two distributions. The mean area computed for mock crime studies in the meta-analysis was 0.872 (Ben-Shakhar & Elaad, 2003). Bamber (1975) described a method for estimating the variance of the area statistics. According to this method, the 95% confidence interval computed for the area under the ROC curve was .783–.899. The ROC analysis indicates that SRR amplitude is a good indicator of concealed information (the area under the ROC curve is significantly better than a chance area of .50).

To further compare the present field studies with the experimental studies reviewed by Ben-Shakhar and Elaad (2003), the *d* and r values of the field studies were computed from the published results. Note that these results are based only on the electrodermal measures. Across the two field studies, $d = 1.49$ and $r = .60$. These values are similar to the *d* and r values obtained for the personal item studies, but lower than those obtained for the mock-crime studies.

Limitations of the Field Studies

In the field studies, CIT records were drawn ex post facto, and the test situation could not have been planned beforehand. Thus, factors such as time of administration (the CIT always followed a standard CQT test), or the examiner's awareness of the critical information while conducting the test, were inherent in the situation. There is, however, no evidence that these factors impaired the test's results. On the contrary, Elaad (1997) showed that participants in an experimental setting responded less to the critical information when the examiner was aware of them than when the examiner did not possess knowledge of the critical information.

Another major problem faced by field validity studies concerns the criterion for guilt or innocence. The described field studies used confessions as an external criterion. The assumption was that the confession confirmed the guilt of the confessor and exonerated other examinees from involvement in the investigated crime. The confession criterion has its shortcomings, of which vulnerability to sample selection biases is the most prominent (Iacono, 1991). The probability that a suspect will confess may depend on the CIT results, in that an outcome of guilt may encourage interrogation efforts to induce a confession. On the other hand, an outcome of innocence may convince the police interrogator to dismiss suspicions against the suspect. This may lead to an underestimation of the false-negative rate. Furthermore, one cannot exclude the possibility of false confessions. Such confessions may lead to an overestimation of the false-negative rate. Only the use of a solid criterion for truth, under highly realistic conditions, such as that used by Ginton, Daie, Elaad, and Ben-Shakhar (1982), can resolve this problem, although their procedure caused a considerable dropout of guilty participants before the test was taken.

Weaknesses of the CIT

The Problem of Formulating Proper CIT Questions

It appears that the large false-negative error rate obtained in the field studies reflects the main shortcoming of the CIT: in several cases, guilty examinees were unaware of some facts of the crime. It is possible that a person who commits a crime may disregard some relevant information, especially during great excitement, or may have subsequently forgotten crime-related details.

The assumption underlying the use of the CIT procedure requires that the guilty examinee be aware of the crime-related information. This means that guilty individuals not only notice but also remember the crime-related information during the test, which may occur long after the event. This is not a problem in experimental settings where participants are examined immediately after they commit the mock-crime. In actual interrogations, however, it is difficult to foresee whether a guilty examinee will be aware of a certain item, even when the item seems to be salient to an objective observer. To improve detection efficiency, the most salient details possible should be selected to formulate the CIT questions while taking into consideration the following factors: (a) How much time has elapsed since the commission of the crime? (b) Is the examinee interested in the subject raised by the CIT question? (c) Was the critical information actively acquired by the guilty person? (d) Were the critical items prepared in advance of the crime by the guilty person? (e) Is it likely that retroactive or proactive misdeeds of the culprit may interfere with the salience of the crime-relevant information? (Killing a man during a robbery should be very salient, whereas memories of a purse-snatching may be blurred by other thefts.); (f) Are the items in the test distinctive enough to be recognized by the guilty examinee? Using such a cautious approach may increase the probability that the critical item may not have been overlooked by the culprit.

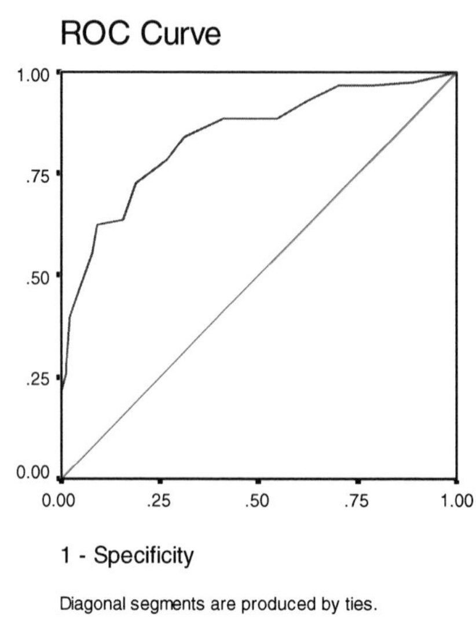

Figure 1. ROC graph generated for the mean z scores on the critical items in the field studies.

Related to the difficulty of identifying salient features of the crime, is the difficulty of gathering a sufficient number of good CIT items (features that were likely to have been noticed and remembered by guilty individuals) to be used in the test. Podlesny (1993) estimated that the CIT might have been used in only 13.1% of FBI cases for which polygraph tests were used. This estimate is based on the assumption that at least four different CIT questions are required to construct a proper CIT battery. Furthermore, the results of the meta-analysis clearly showed that the number of CIT questions contributes to the validity of the test. When the number of questions was large (five or more), the effect size (d= 2.35) was greater than in the case of fewer than five questions (d = 1.29). In the field studies, the mean number of CIT questions that were used was less than 2, supporting the notion that this might have contributed to the large false-negative error rate.

The small number of proper features of the crime that are likely to be perceived and remembered by guilty individuals was addressed by Elaad and Ben-Shakhar (1997). They showed that with a sufficient number of repetitions, a single CIT question can efficiently discriminate between guilty and innocent examinees. In this study, two experiments were conducted in which a CIT, based on four different questions, each repeated three times, was compared with a single CIT question repeated 12 times. Both experiments revealed that similar detection efficiencies were obtained in these two conditions. Naturally, this raises the question of habituation with repetitions. Results revealed, however, that the decline of SCR responsiveness to the critical items with repetitions was small and not statistically significant. Furthermore, a considerable differentiation between guilty and innocent examinees was observed even in the final block of questions (the final three questions out of 12 repetitions). In a follow-up study (Ben-Shakhar & Elaad, 2002), the effect of question repetition and variation on the efficiency of the CIT based on electrodermal measures was re-examined. This time, personal information items were used instead of details of a mock-crime procedure, and a third experimental condition (twelve different questions, each presented once) was used. In this experiment, a clear advantage for the multiple-questions conditions emerged with the electrodermal measure. The results obtained with 12 different questions were impressive and almost perfect. However, statistically significant differentiation between guilty and innocent participants was observed under all three conditions. It was suggested that an effort should be made to increase the number of CIT questions. However, if only a small number of proper questions are available, increasing the number of repetitions may to some extent compensate for the lack of question variation. Further research is required to examine this issue in a real-life context. Similar results would imply that the CIT could be more widely applied.

Leakage of Information

The results of the field studies suggest that leakage of crime-related information did not affect the results of the CIT administered to innocent examinees by the Israeli police. However, the issue of information leakage to innocent suspects is crucial to CIT implementation and must be carefully considered. The main problem is that innocent suspects might have been informed of the critical information but would not be able to indicate the source of their knowledge. One solution for this situation was proposed by Bradley and his colleagues. They showed that an alternative formulation of the CIT questions (the guilty action test) could reduce false-positive outcomes among informed innocent suspects. Ben-Shakhar et al. (1999) further showed that introducing target items that are unrelated to the event under investigation, while answering the CIT questions, may help attract the attention of innocent participants and reduce false-positive outcomes.

There is, however, another leakage problem that has been neglected to date: the leakage to guilty participants of incorrect information that might distort their perception of the crime. Techniques of deception (e.g., good cop/bad cop) are common in police interrogations (Leo, 1992), and are designed to elicit additional information from a suspect. In this context, interrogators may subtly introduce new and incorrect information about the crime to intimidate and extract a confession from suspects. This incorrect information may undermine suspects' confidence in the information they possess about the crime, and imply that the interrogator knows a lot more than they know. Note that the interrogator is in a position of authority and some guilty suspects may conform to authority and distort their knowledge accordingly. All the guilty examinees in the field studies underwent intensive interrogation before they were tested with the polygraph. Although we do not know whether or not incorrect information was implanted in them during the interrogation, we cannot exclude the possibility that some incorrect information might have been responsible for the large false-negative error rate. To deal with the interrogator's influence on the information possessed by guilty suspects, it is suggested to modify police practices by ensuring that the critical features of the event are concealed from the interrogator who conducts the interrogation. The interrogators must be aware of the fact that there is concealed information of which they were not informed. Furthermore, interrogators must be trained to be aware and avoid the potential damage in providing incorrect information about the crime to suspects.

Countermeasure Effects

It has already been indicated that guilt encourages coping behavior which may be translated into the use of countermeasures. Studies conducted in experimental settings demonstrated that the CIT is vulnerable to physical countermeasures (e.g., pressing the toes against the floor when control items are presented) as well as mental countermeasures (e.g., counting numbers each time a control item appears). This vulnerability to countermeasures might increase false-negative outcomes and impair the validity of the CIT (Ben-Shakhar & Dolev, 1996; Elaad & Ben-Shakhar, 1991; Honts, Devitt, Winbush, & Kircher, 1996). Although we have no evidence that guilty examinees used countermeasures during the tests that were included in the field studies, it is possible that countermeasure attempts were responsible for some of the false-negative outcomes that were obtained.

A recent study (Elaad & Ben-Shakhar, 2008a) re-examined the countermeasure question. Guilty examinees were trained to use either physical or mental countermeasures and apply them to distort the outcomes of the test. To combat countermeasures, two covert respiration measures, concealed in the seat and back of the examination chair (Elaad & Ben-Shakhar, 2008b), were used in addition to the standard physiological measures (SCR, FPWL, RLL).

CIT results in the countermeasure conditions were compared with results of guilty participants who did not attempt countermeasures and with results of uninformed innocents. Results indicated that the application of physical countermeasures reduced electrodermal (SCR) accuracy. In contrast, SCR was relatively resistant to mental countermeasures. The unobtrusive respiration measures were both resistant to physical, but not to the mental, countermeasures, when most participants applied them. In fact, both unobtrusive measures were more effective than SCR when physical countermeasures were actually applied. It was suggested that the two countermeasure types operate through different attentional mechanisms. Physical countermeasures may operate mainly on recognition to which SCR is relatively sensitive. Mental countermeasures may interfere with the slowly developed emotional association of the stimulus which affects SCR to a smaller degree. It was further suggested that it is essential to include physiological measures other than electrodermal measures in the CIT to compensate for the sensitivity of the SCR to physical countermeasures.

A Final Unresolved Issue: The Different Motivation of Guilty and Innocent Examinees

Previous findings in experimental situations (Ben-Shakhar & Elaad, 2003) have demonstrated that motivating participants to avoid detection leads to enhanced detection of concealed information. This implies that high levels of motivation, such as typically characterizes actual polygraph examinations in real-life settings, should contribute to better detection rates than the detection levels obtained in experimental situations. However, regarding guilty examinees, the detection efficiency reported in the field studies is considerably lower than that reported in experimental studies.

From this perspective, the field studies results are disappointing.

No attempt was made, however, to distinguish between the motivation of guilty examinees and that of innocent examinees. Based on the different states of mind that are typical to guilty and innocent examinees, it may be argued that two distinct types of motivation are involved. Hence, the motivation to deceive applies exclusively to guilty examinees who are aware of the critical information and give an overt deceptive response to these items, while being truthful to the control items. Uninformed innocent examinees are truthful concerning all items and therefore are not motivated to deceive or conceal information. On the contrary, they are motivated to cooperate and help the examiner reach the correct decision. Future research should address the different motivations of guilty and innocent participants and examine the differential effect of these motivation types on the efficiency of the CIT.

Concluding Remarks

The CIT procedure is the single psychophysiological detection technique that enjoys wide acceptance as a scientifically based technique. It is grounded in well-established electrodermal research findings and theory. The advantages and weaknesses of the CIT were discussed and it was suggested that the CIT is a highly valid procedure when properly executed. As such it has the potential to become an important aid to the criminal investigation

The CIT suffers from three major weaknesses. One is the difficulty in identifying a sufficient number of salient features of the crime. As a result, this method is not frequently used to assist the law enforcement system outside Japan. The solution for this weakness may be the use of one or two proper CIT questions with many repetitions. As earlier results indicated, this may produce relatively high levels of detection efficiency.

Second, once the features of the crime have been identified, it is difficult to keep them concealed from innocent suspects. Furthermore, an intensive interrogation might distort guilty suspects' perception of the crime and may increase false-negative outcomes. Modification of police investigation procedures may, however, minimize the possibility that critical information leaks out.

The use of countermeasures may impair CIT results and increase the rate of false-negative outcomes. A partial solution is to add physiological measures, such as unobtrusive respiration measures, which have proven to be less sensitive than SCR to physical countermeasures.

Finally, the motivation to conceal information is an integral part of the guilty suspect's state of mind. The task of future research is to clarify how this unique disposition contributes to CIT efficiency.

References

Baddeley, A. D. (1999). *Essentials of Human Memory*. Hove, UK: Psychology Press.

Balloun, K. D. & Holmes, D. S. (1979). Effects of repeated examinations on the ability to detect guilt with a polygraphic examination: A laboratory experiment with a real crime. *Journal of Applied Psychology*, *64*, 316-322.

Bamber, D. (1975). The area under the ordinal dominance graph and the area below the receiver operating characteristic graph. *Journal of Mathematical Psychology*, *12*, 378-415.

Ben-Shakhar, G. (1977). A further study of the dichotomization theory in detection of information. *Psychophysiology*, *14*, 408-413.

Ben-Shakhar, G., Bar-Hillel, M. & Kremnizer, M. (2002). Trial by polygraph: Reconsidering the use of the GKT in court. *Law and Human Behavior*, *26*, 527-541.

Ben-Shakhar, G. & Dolev, K. (1996). Psychophysiological detection through the guilty knowledge technique: Effects of mental countermeasures. *Journal of Applied Psychology*, *81*, 273-281.

Ben-Shakhar, G. & Elaad, E. (2002). Effects of questions` repetition and variation on the efficiency of the guilty knowledge test: A reexamination. *Journal of Applied Psychology*, *87*, 972-977.

Ben-Shakhar G. & Elaad, E. (2003). The validity of psychophysiological detection of information with the Guilty Knowledge Test: A meta-analytic review. *Journal of Applied Psychology*, *88*, 131-151.

Ben-Shakhar, G., Frost, R., Gati, I. & Kresh, Y. (1996). Is an apple a fruit? Semantic relatedness as reflected by psychophysiological responsivity. *Psychophysiology, 33*, 671-679.

Ben-Shakhar, G. & Furedy, J. J. (1990). *Theories and applications in the detection of deception*. Springer-Verlag, New York.

Ben-Shakhar, G. & Gati, I. (1987). Common and distinctive features of verbal and pictorial stimuli as determinants of psychophysiological responsivity. *Journal of Experimental Psychology: General, 116*, 91-105.

Ben-Shakhar, G., Gronau, N. & Elaad, E. (1999). Leakage of relevant information to innocent examinees in the GKT: An attempt to reduce false-positive outcomes by introducing target stimuli. *Journal of Applied Psychology, 84*, 651-660.

Ben-Shakhar, G. & Lieblich, I. (1982). The dichotomization theory for differential autonomic responsivity reconsidered. *Psychophysiology, 19*, 277-281.

Bernstein, A. S. (1979). The orienting response as a novelty and significance detector: Reply to O'Gorman. *Psychophysiology, 16*, 263-273.

Birch, S. A. J. & Bloom, P. (2004). Understanding children's and adults' limitations in mental state reasoning. *Trends in Cognitive Science, 8*, 255-260.

Bradley, M. T. & Ainsworth, D. (1984). Alcohol and psychophysiological detection of deception. *Psychophysiology, 21*, 63-71.

Bradley, M. T., MacLaren, V. V. & Carle, S. B. (1996). Deception and nondeception in guilty knowledge and guilty action polygraph tests. *Journal of Applied Psychology, 81*, 153-160.

Bradley, M. T. & Rettinger, J. (1992). Awareness of crime-relevant information and the guilty knowledge test. *Journal of Applied Psychology, 77*, 55-59.

Bradley, M. T. & Warfield, J.F. (1984). Innocence, information, and the guilty knowledge test in the detection of deception. *Psychophysiology, 21*, 683-689.

Buller, D. B. & Burgoon, J. K. (1996). Interpersonal deception theory. *Communication Theory, 6*, 203-242.

Cohen, J. E. (1988). *Statistical power analysis for the behavioral sciences*. Hillsdale, NJ: Lawrence Erlbaum.

Davis, R. C. (1961). Physiological responses as a means of evaluating information. In A.D. Biderman and H. Zimmer (Eds.), *The manipulation of human behavior*. New York: Wiley.

Dawson, M. E., Filion, D. L. & Schell, A. M. (1989). Is elicitation of the autonomic orientating response associated with allocation of processing resources? *Psychophysiology, 26*, 560-572.

Dawson, M. E., Schell, A. M. & Filion, D. L. (2000). The electrodermal system. In J.T. Cacioppo, L. G. Tassinary, & G. G. Berntson (Eds.) *Handbook of Psychophysiology*, Second Edition. Cambridge: Cambridge University Press.

Elaad, E. (1990). Detection of guilty knowledge in real-life criminal investigations. *Journal of Applied Psychology, 75*, 521-529.

Elaad, E. (1997). Polygraph examiner awareness of crime-relevant information and the guilty knowledge test. *Law and Human Behavior, 21*, 107-120.

Elaad, E. (1998). The challenge of the concealed knowledge polygraph test. *Expert Evidence, 6*, 161-187.

Elaad, E. & Ben-Shakhar, G. (1989). Effects of motivation and verbal response type on psychophysiological detection of information. *Psychophysiology, 26*, 442-451.

Elaad, E. & Ben-Shakhar, G. (1991). Effects of mental countermeasures on psychophysiological detection in the Guilty Knowledge Test. *International Journal of Psychophysiology, 11*, 2, 99-108.

Elaad, E. & Ben-Shakhar G. (1997). Effects of item repetitions and variations on the efficiency of the guilty knowledge test. *Psychophysiology, 34*, 587-596.

Elaad, E. & Ben-Shakhar, G. (2008a). *Countering countermeasures in the Concealed Information Test using unobtrusive respiration measures*. Unpublished Manuscript.

Elaad, E. & Ben-Shakhar, G. (2008b). Covert respiration measures for the detection of concealed information. *Biological Psychology, 77*, 284-291.

Elaad, E., Ginton, A. & Jungman, N. (1992). Detection measures in real-life criminal guilty knowledge tests. *Journal of Applied Psychology, 77*, 757-767.

Fukumoto, J. (1980). Psychophysiological detection of deception in Japan: The past and the present. *Polygraph, 11*, 234-238.

Gamer, M., Verschuere, B., Crombez, G. & Vossel, G. (2008). (in press). Combining Physiological Measures in the detection of concealed information. *Physiology and Behavior.*

Giesen, M. & Rollison, M. A. (1980). Guilty knowledge versus innocent associations: Effects of trait anxiety and stimulus context on skin conductance. *Journal of Research in Personality, 14*, 1-11.

Gilovich, T., Savitsky, K. & Medvec, V. (1998). The illusion of transparency: Biased assessments of others' ability to read one's emotional states. *Journal of Personality and Social Psychology, 75*, 332-346.

Ginton, A., Daie, N., Elaad E. & Ben-Shakhar, G. (1982). A method for evaluating the use of the polygraph in a real-life situation. *Journal of Applied Psychology, 67*, 131-137.

Granhag. P. A. & Hartwig, M. (2008). A new theoretical perspective on deception detection: On the psychology of instrumental mind-reading. *Psychology, Crime & Law, 14*, 189-200.

Gustafson, L. A. & Orne, M. T. (1963). Effects of heightened motivation on the detection of deception. *Journal of Applied Psychology, 47*, 408-411.

Honts, C. R., Devitt, M. K., Winbush, M. & Kircher, J. C. (1996). Mental and physical countermeasures reduce the accuracy of the concealed knowledge test. *Psychophysiology, 33*, 84-92.

Hunter, J. E. & Schmidt, F. L. (1990). *Methods of meta-analysis: Correcting error and bias in research findings*. Newbury Park, CA: Sage.

Iacono, W. G. (1991). Can we determine the accuracy of polygraph tests? In J.R. Jennings, P. K. Ackles, and M. G. H. Coles (Eds.), *Advances in Psychophysiology, Vol. 4*, Greenwich, Conn.: JAI Press.

Kahneman, D. (1973). *Attention and effort*. Englewood Cliffs, New Jersey: Prentice-Hall.

Kassin, S. M. 2005. On the psychology of confessions: Does innocence put innocents at risk? *American Psychology, 60*, 215-228.

Leo, R. A. (1992). From coercion to deception: the changing nature of police interrogation in America. *Crime, Law and Social Change, 18*, 35-59.

Lieblich, I., Kugelmass, S. & Ben-Shakhar, G. (1970). Efficiency of GSR detection of information as a function of stimulus set size. *Psychophysiology, 6*, 601-608.

Loftus, E. F. (1979). *Eyewitness Testimony*. Cambridge, MA: Harvard University Press.

Lykken, D. T. (1959). The GSR in the detection of guilt. *Journal of Applied Psychology, 43*, 385-388.

Lykken, D. T. (1974). Psychology and the lie detection industry. *America Psychologist, 29*, 225-239.

Lykken, D. T. (1998). *A Tremor in the blood.* Uses and abuses of the lie detector, 2nd edn., Plenum Trade, New York.

Maltzman, I. (1979). Orienting reflexes and significance: A Reply to O'Gorman. *Psychophysiology, 16*, 274-281.

Miller, G. R. & Stiff, J. B. (1993). *Deceptive communication.* Newbury Park, CA: Sage.

Nakayama, M. (2002). Practical use of the concealed information test for criminal investigation in Japan. In: Kleiner, M. (Ed.), *Handbook of Polygraph Testing*, Academic Press, San Diego, pp. 49-86.

Podlesny, J. A. (1993). Is the guilty knowledge polygraph technique applicable in criminal investigations? A review of FBI case records. *Crime Laboratory Digest, 20*, 59-63.

Reid, J. E. & Inbau, F. E. (1977). *Truth and deception: The polygraph ("lie detector") technique*, 2nd ed., Williams and Wilkins, Baltimore, MD.

Siddle, D. A. T. 1991. Orienting, habituation, and resource allocation: An associative analysis. *Psychophysiology, 28*, 245-259.

Sokolov, E. N. (1963). Perception and the conditioned reflex, Pergamon Press, New York.

Stern, R. M., Breen, J. P., Watanabe, T. & Perry, B. S. (1981). Effects of feedback of physiological information on responses to innocent association and guilty knowledge. *Journal of Applied Psychology, 66*, 677-681.

Verschuere, B., Crombez, G., De Clercq, A. & Koster, E. H. W. (2004). Autonomic and behavioral responding to concealed information: Differentiating orienting and defensive responses. *Psychophysiology, 41*, 461-466.

Yamamura, T. & Miyata, Y. (1990). Development of the polygraph technique in Japan for detection of deception. *Forensic Science International, 44*, 257-271.

In: Skin Anatomy and Physiology Research Developments ISBN: 978-1-60741-469-8
Editor: Leon F. Bukowsky

Chapter 5

Vesicles and Skin: From Surface to Systemic Effects

Gamal M. El Maghraby*

Department of Pharmaceutical Technology, College of Pharmacy, University of Tanta, Tanta, Egypt

Abstract

The use of vesicles as skin drug delivery system was introduced in the early eighties by Mezei & Gulasekharam. They reported that standard vesicles (liposomes) of dipalmitoylphosphatidylcholine (DPPC) and cholesterol (CH) increased the concentration of triamcinolone acetonide in the epidermis and dermis by 4-5 times and reduced percutaneous absorption compared with a standard ointment. This effect is known as localized effect. After this report researchers applied standard vesicles and recorded mainly localized effects and rarely targeted delivery to skin appendages or improved transdermal drug delivery. Suddenly, Cevc and coworkers introduced a new type of vesicles, *Transfersomes* in which phospholipids are the major components as liposomes but included an edge activator (surfactant) which provides the ultradeformability and flexibility of the vesicular membrane. These *Transfersomes* were reported to penetrate intact skin delivering therapeutic amounts of drugs such as insulin in efficiency similar to subcutaneous administration of the same formulation. It was difficult to conceive that large lipid vesicles could penetrate the densely packed stratum corneum in great numbers. Accordingly many workers have tested this hypothesis with controversial findings being reported regarding the mechanism of action, with the ultradeformable vesicles being better than standard liposomes. Other researchers included ethanol in liposomes to impart membrane flexibility. These vesicles were termed ethosomes. However, it is important to emphasize that, the higher the membrane flexibility and deformability of the vesicles the lower is their physical stability. Accordingly, the more stable vesicles, niosomes were studied. These vesicles comprise

* College of Pharmacy, King Saud University, Riyadh, 11451, P.O. Box 2457, Saudi Arabia.

surfactant as the major component with cholesterol and may contain minute amounts of phospholipids. Niosomes are now considered as promising transdermal delivery systems with some surfactants producing highly flexible formulations.

This chapter will critically evaluate different types of vesicles as skin drug delivery systems with respect to their functions from surface to dermal and transdermal effects. The assessment will extend to highlight the possible mechanisms of actions of vesicles before finally reporting on the feasibility of these vesicles for scaling up.

Introduction

The skin is largest single organ of the body. It provides the formulator with vast surface area for drug administration. The structure and the barrier functions of the skin have been extensively described in the literature [1-4]. Human skin comprises a series of layers penetrated by hair shafts and gland ducts which open directly into the environment (Fig.1). These layers comprise from inside to outside, the fatty subcutaneous layer (hypodermis), the dermis of connective tissue and the stratified avascular, cellular epidermis.

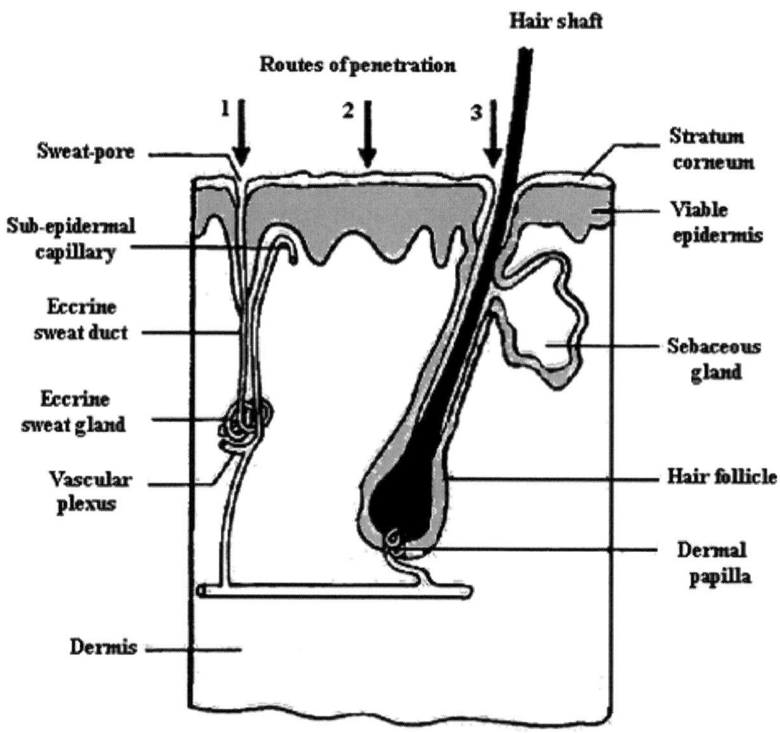

Fig. 1 Simplified diagram of skin structure and macroroutes of drug penetration: (1) via the sweat ducts; (2) across the continuous stratum corneum or (3) through the hair follicles with their associated sebaceous glands (after Barry, 1983) [3].

The dermis comprises fibrous proteins (collagen and elastin) and an interfibrillar gel of glycosaminoglycans, salts and water. Blood and lymphatic vessels, nerve endings, pilosebaceous units (hair follicles and sebaceous glands) and sweat glands are embedded within the dermis [3, 5].

The epidermis contains no blood supply and consists of five layers, which from inside to outside are the stratum germinativum (basal layer), stratum spinosum (spinous layer), stratum granulosum (granular layer), stratum lucidum and stratum corneum (SC). Because the SC cells are dead, the epidermis without the SC is usually termed the viable epidermis [3, 5]. The structure of the SC is often depicted in the so called bricks and mortar arrangement [6], in which the keratin rich corneocytes (bricks) are embedded in the intercellular lipid-rich matrix (mortar). This arrangement is illustrated in Fig. 2. Based on this packing and arrangement, the SC is considered as the rate limiting barrier in transdermal permeation of most molecules [3].

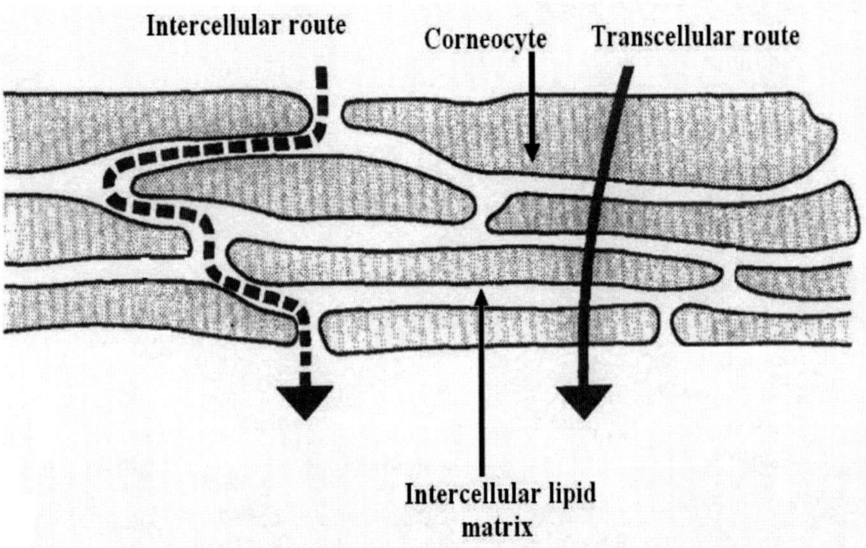

Fig. 2 Simplified diagram of the brick and mortar model of the stratum corneum with the possible drug permeation pathways through intact stratum corneum; the transcellular or the tortuous intercellular pathways (modified from Barry, 1991)[10]

For any molecules applied to the skin, two main routes of skin permeation have been defined as the transappendageal (shunt route) and transepidermal pathways [7]. The transappendageal routes include permeation through the sweat glands and across the hair follicles with their associated sebaceous glands. It was historically assumed that the follicles occupy approximately 0.1% of the surface area of human skin [8] but recent studies showed that approximately 13.7% of the surface area of the forehead is available as follicles [9]. Interestingly, the later study also showed that the historically held assumption of the follicles occupying approximately 0.1% of the surface area of the SC appears to be valid for forearm skin.

The transepidermal pathway is the main permeation route and is defined as the pathway where compounds permeate across the intact, unbroken stratum corneum. This pathway contains two micropathways including the intercellular route, which is continuous but tortuous way through the intercellular lipid domains and the transcellular pathway through the keratinocytes, then across the intercellular lipids (Fig. 2) [10].

These difficult pathways of skin drug permeation support the fact that it is difficult for many drugs to be delivered into and through the intact skin despite of the potential advantages of transdermal delivery over other routes of administration. Accordingly, researchers employed various techniques to improve transdermal delivery [11]. These include the use of chemical penetration enhancers [12], preparation of supersaturated systems [13], employing very weak electric current in iontophoresis [14], physically disrupting the skin structure as in case of electroporation or sonophoresis [15-16] or preparation of microemulsion system [17]. Vesicular drug delivery systems provided another alternative for which great claims have been made regarding their efficacy and mechanism of action. They can provide local or transdermal effects [18-19]. Accordingly, the proceeding sections will critically evaluate different types of vesicles as skin drug delivery systems with respect to their functions from surface to dermal and transdermal effects with a highlight on the possible mechanisms of action of vesicles before finally reporting on the feasibility of these vesicles for scaling up.

Types of Vesicles

Alternative terminology was reported for vesicles in literature [19]. *Liposomes* are vesicles in which one or more lipid bilayers entrap an aqueous volume. Their major components are usually phospholipids with or without cholesterol. They are the prototype of all vesicles with other vesicles developed by modifying the lipid composition with the goals of increasing the flexibility vesicular membrane, increasing the stability of the vesicles or reducing the cost. A special type of liposomes made of skin lipids with a composition similar to the lipid composition of the stratum was also developed and tested for transdermal drug delivery. These vesicles are known as *Stratum Corneum Lipid Liposomes (SCLL)*. For preparation and characterization of vesicles the reader is referred to the text book prepared by New (1990) [20]. *Transfersomes* (ultradeformable vesicles) are morphologically similar to liposomes but they differ in function (see below); phospholipids are the major components with additional surfactant being included as an edge activator to increase the elasticity of the vesicular membrane and increase the vesicle deformability. *Flexosomes* are similar to *Transfersomes* but included a surface charging agent with positively charged ones being superior. *Ethosomes* are phospholipid vesicles, in which ethanol was included in the vesicle components to increase the elasticity. N*iosomes* are vesicular systems with similar structure to liposomes but comprise surfactants as the main component with cholesterol and may include small proportions of phospholipids. These were initially produced to increase the vesicle stability and reduce the cost. *Vesosomes* are fusogenic vesicular systems which comprise a fusogenic phospholipid with a positively charged charging agent. The formulated fusogenic vesicle is incorporated in interdigitated lipid bilayer to provide vesicles within a vesicle.

Vesicles as Skin Drug Delivery Systems

Vesicles have been used as skin drug delivery systems for nearly three decades, during which alternative functions were reported. They were initially used to provide a localizing effect where they increase the drug concentration in the skin strata and reduce the systemic absorption. Alternatively they were employed for targeted drug delivery to skin appendages. Recently, numerous reports have concentrated on the enhanced transdermal drug delivery after vesicular application with systemic effects being recorded. Having these alternative functions, it is not surprising that the mechanisms of action of these vesicles as skin drug delivery systems are controversial. The following sections will thus provide a critical review of vesicular skin drug delivery with emphasis on their functions. The review will extend to cover potential mechanisms of action.

Localizing effects

The history of this effect started with the first publication on vesicular skin drug delivery in which liposomes of dipalmitoylphosphatidylcholine (DPPC) and cholesterol (CH) increased the concentration of triamcinolone acetonide in the epidermis and dermis and reduced systemic absorption compared to a standard ointment [21]. Similar findings were recorded after incorporating the same vesicles in a gel dosage form and comparing their effect to a gel containing free drug and the vesicle components at the same concentrations [22]. This finding reflected the importance of liposomal encapsulation and thus good entrapment efficiency of the drug in the vesicle for efficient skin drug delivery. The same effect was reported after topical application progesterone and econazole in DPPC-CH liposomes compared with conventional dosage forms [23]. The liposomal skin delivery of 5α-dihydrotestosterone was lower than that obtained from an acetone solution containing the same drug concentration. This was reported after monitoring the size of the flank organs of the female hamster [24]. The authors considered this as contradictory finding to Mezei and Gulasekharam's [21] early findings and attributed the discrepancy to four possible reasons. These included the use of different steroids, measuring different parameters, the use of different animals or employing different application schemes. However, the discrepancy can be explained on the basis that the biological effect on the hamster flank organs may require systemic drug delivery rather than a liposome-mediated localizing effect.

In vitro application of phosphatidylcholine (PC)/CH liposomes increased deposition of hydrocortisone into human skin compared with an emulsion ointment form. This effect was further confirmed by monitoring the blanching effect of hydrocortisone with the vesicles producing a greater effect than the ointment even when urea (a penetration enhancer) was incorporated into this base. Pharmacokinetic studies using guinea pig supported further localizing effect as evidenced by the lower serum level and urinary excretion of the drug, obtained after topical application of liposomes, compared to ointment [25].

In contrast to the previous findings which showed improved skin deposition and reduced transdermal permeation, liposomal encapsulation facilitated both the retention and permeation of triamcinolone acetonide compared with the ointment form [26]. This discrepancy could be due to the use of different membranes with permeability differences between species making direct comparisons between laboratory protocols problematic.

The improved skin deposition after liposomal encapsulation was also recorded for large molecular weight drugs with the skin delivery depending on both the vesicular composition and the method of preparation. Topical delivery of the peptide drug interferon was greater from liposomes compared to water-in-oil emulsion or aqueous solution as revealed by reduced lesion scores after topical application to a cutaneous herpes simplex virus guinea pig model. The Interferon delivery from SCLL produced greater remission of lesions compared to phospholipid liposomes. With respect to the method of liposome preparation, those produced by a dehydration rehydration (DRV) method were more effective than those prepared by mechanical shaking or extrusion [27]. The superiority of DRV liposomes was attributed to increased drug partitioning into the vesicle, but this can be explained on the basis of increased entrapment efficiency. The recorded pharmacological effect after liposomal application was due to localizing effect rather than transdermal effect. This was confirmed after determination of the skin drug deposition by tape stripping and monitoring the transdermal drug permeation after topical application to guinea pig skin in vitro. The results revealed increased interferon deposition into stratum corneum and deeper skin strata with no drug detected in the receptor after liposomal application. Again SCLL prepared by DRV were considered superior [28]. Similar findings were recorded for cyclosporin-A [29]. This series of studies reflected the localizing effects of liposomes and highlighted the dependence of deposition "efficiency" on the lipid composition and method of preparation.

The localizing effect of vesicular systems was also employed to improve topical anaesthesia. This was first tried by Gesztes & Mezei (1988) [30] who used the pin-prick assay and recorded prolonged anaesthesia from tetracaine liposomes with the cream formulation being ineffective. Using the same assay, liposomes prolonged lidocaine anaesthesia compared with a conventional cream. This effect was found to result from higher deposition in the epidermis and dermis after application of liposomes [31]. Other studies recorded both increased drug permeation through, and deposition into, human skin in vitro for liposomal tetracaine relative to an ointment containing the same drug concentration [32]. Vesicles provided even stronger and deeper anaesthesia relative to a commercial eutectic mixture of local anaesthetics (EMLA, 2.5 % lidocaine and 2.5% prilocaine) in humans [33-34].

The localizing effect was also monitored after application of *Transfersomes* which produced an improved anaesthetic effect of lidocaine and tetracaine with the ultradeformable formulation being superior compared to standard liposomes or drug solution [35]. However, it is important to note that the authors applied the tested formulations under occlusion for 25 minutes, although this application protocol is contrary to the recommended open application for *Transfersomes*. Surprisingly, topically-applied anaesthetic *Transfersomes* generated an effect equivalent to that created after subcutaneous injection of the same formulation.

Slight increase in transepidermal permeation of 5-fluorouracil was recorded after application of a finite dose of similar *Transfersomes* compared to saturated drug solution using the aqueous receptor. However, employing ethanolic receptor significantly increased drug permeation from vesicles. This was taken as indication of improved deposition of the drug in the skin as ethanol is expected to diffuse into the tissue disrupting deposited vesicles and extracting the drug [36]. However, it should be noted that drug distribution from *Transfersomes* is dose dependent [37] and the use of finite or infinite doses can affect the relative proportion of localized to transdermal drug amounts. Accordingly, optimization of the applied dose was recommended.

Elastic niosomes of Tween 61 and cholesterol have developed recently by incorporating ethanol at 25%. These vesicles combined the composition of niosomes with ethanolic components of ethosomes. They improved the delivery of diclofenac diethylammonium into and through the skin compared to non-elastic niosomes which increased the deposition of the drug only [38]. This finding is expected and can be explained on the basis that the presence of ethanol in the elastic formulation can provide a penetration enhancing effect.

Targeted delivery to skin appendages

In addition to monitoring drug deposition into the stratum corneum and viable epidermis after liposomal application, several workers have investigated the potential of vesicular systems for targeting the appendages, especially to the pilocebaceous units (hair follicles with their associated sebaceous glands) [39-40].

Selective targeting of carboxyfluorescein into the pilosebaceous units was recorded after application of liposomes of PC, CH and phosphatidylserine (PS) to the hamster ear model. The efficacy of vesicles was better than aqueous solutions even when these solutions contained 10% ethanol or 0.05% sodium lauryl sulphate or when propylene glycol was the donor vehicle [41-42]. Using similar vesicles the deposition of γ-interferon was higher in hamster skin, which possesses the highest follicular density compared to humans and hairless mice, with the vesicles improving the deposition in all species compared to drug solution. It was thus concluded that the follicular pathway could be a route for drug deposition from liposomes [43].

Measurable amounts of cimetidine were delivered into the pilosebaceous glands and other skin strata after topical application of the drug in 50% aqueous ethanol, nosomes, or in liposomes. It should be noted that the later formulation was pharmacologically inactive with respect to the reduction in the size of sebaceous glands (anti-androgenic effect). This was attributed to formation of inactive ion pair between the drug and the negatively charged lipids of liposomes [44].

In contrast to the previous findings, neither liposomes nor mixed micelles showed any advantage over the ethanolic gel with respect to follicular delivery. This finding was attributed to the highly lipophilic nature of the drug which would intrinsically target the sebaceous gland [45]. However, the presence of ethanol in the control can add some enhancement for the follicular delivery by partial solubilization of the sebum or softening of the material in the duct. Other formulations were thus shown to be equivalent to the control. Whilst this explanation could suggest a positive effect of liposomes and mixed micelles, we can only suggest that they were as effective as the ethanolic gel.

Efficient treatment of acne vulgaris was recorded after vesicular drug delivery compared with conventional preparations including alcoholic lotions [46-47]. This efficacy can be taken as strong evidence that vesicles can effectively target drug delivery to skin appendages.

Recently, successful delivery of finasteride to the pilosebaceous unit of the hamster ears was recorded in vitro and in vivo after application of either liquid-state liposomes or niosomes [48].

Improved transdermal delivery

The improved vesicular transdermal drug delivery was reported in early publications. Greater permeation of lipophilic drugs was reported after topical application of finite doses of liposomes to hairless mouse skin in vitro [49]. Formulations containing unilamellar standard liposomes enhanced the transdermal absorption of methyl nicotinate compared with aqueous solution or gel formulations [50]. Fluid liposomes made of Epikuron 200, a phospholipid with unsaturated alkyl side chains were able to increase percutaneous absorption and tissue distribution rather than skin accumulation of drug. This was confirmed further by increased renal elimination of inulin after application of such vesicles compared to aqueous solution [51].

The introduction of *Transfersomes* was accompanied with great claims on transdermal drug delivery from vesicular systems. They were thought to penetrate intact to the deep layers of the skin and may progress far enough to reach the systemic circulation [52]. For efficient systemic effect after topical application, the authors recommended that, *Transfersomes* must be applied under non-occlusive conditions, although a deviation from this protocol can be found [35], where an improved anaesthetic effect was reported after occlusive application of anaesthetic *Transfersomes*. However, the later effect may require only improved skin deposition, an effect which might have been achieved under occlusion. *Transfersomes* encapsulated corticosteroids provided suppression of arachidonic acid-induced oedema with an efficiency equivalent to a lotion containing 5-times the drug concentration of that in deformable vesicles, after 0.5 hour. Subsequently, after 2 hours, the *Transfersome* formulation was more efficacious than the lotion [37].

In addition, the arachidonic acid-induced oedema suppression test was used to evaluate the antiinflammatory effect of Cu, Zn-superoxide dismutase after topical application in *Transfersomes,* mixed micelles or liposomes. Of all the tested carriers only *Transfersomes* significantly reduced the oedema [53].

Employing estradiol as a model drug the skin delivery from various vesicular formulations was compared. The tested formulations included ultradeformable and standard vesicles [54]. The ultradeformable formulations included PC with sodium cholate, PC with Span 80 and PC with Tween 80 at the previously optimized proportions [55]. The standard vesicles comprised pure PC vesicles (non rigid), PC with CH (membrane stabilized), and two rigid liposomes of DPPC and DPPC/CH. The results revealed that all types of liposomes improved both estradiol deposition into and permeation through the epidermis compared with the saturated aqueous control. The ultradeformable vesicles were the best with respect to transepidermal drug flux with all vesicular formulations being equivalent with regard to estradiol accumulation in the skin. As for liposomes, flexible niosomes showed higher efficiency compared to rigid niosomes [56-57].

The transdermal delivering capacity of vesicular systems was extended to deliver large molecular weight drugs including peptides and vaccines. Few reports are available for standard liposomes with the majority of authors utilizing flexible vesicles. Qualitative immunohistochemical examination revealed that liposome-encapsulated antibodies distributed rapidly into the deep cutaneous regions of piglet skin in vivo, compared with no penetration after application of aqueous solution or empty vesicles. Subsequent studies revealed not only improved skin deposition but also a significant increase in transdermal delivery from vesicles [58-59].

Successful transdermal input of insulin has been achieved by *Transfersomes* as reported from in vivo mice and human studies which showed a reduction in the blood glucose level after topical application of insulin in *Transfersomes*. Surprisingly, the efficiency of the topical applied vesicles was comparable to that obtained after S.C. injection of the same preparation but with a longer lag time. The recorded lag time may be required for vesicle skin penetration. Both mixed micelles and standard liposome formulations of insulin failed to reduce blood glucose. It was thus concluded that *Transfersomes* provide non-invasive transdermal delivery of therapeutic agents, including insulin [60-61].

The skin delivery of low molecular weight heparin was reported after application of surface charged flexible vesicles made of lipids with Tween 80. These vesicles were termed flexosomes with the cationic ones being the most efficient [62].

Topical immunization using Gap junction proteins (GJP) was recorded using *Transfersomes* which provided marginally higher antibody level compared to those elicited by subcutaneous injections of GJP in *Transfersomes*, mixed lipid micelles or liposomes. The latter two systems did not give significant biological response after topical administration [63]. In a more recent investigation the potential of non invasive topical immunization using vesicular systems loaded with tetanus toxoid (TT) was evaluated with *Transfersomes*, niosomes (Span 85 and cholesterol, 1:1) and liposomes (PC and CH, 7:3) being compared. The results revealed that topically given TT containing *Transfersomes*, could produce an immune response equivalent to that obtained after intramuscular injection of alum-adsorbed TT, with niosomes and liposomes producing weaker immune response [64]. In another study, span 85 and cholesterol niosomes, encapsulating DNA hepatitis B vaccine and prepared by reversed phase evaporation technique were tried for topical immunization. Topical application of niosomes produced comparable serum antibody titer and endogenous cytokines levels as compared to intramuscular administration of the same DNA vaccine and topical liposomes. This was taken as an indication of the potential of niosomes as DNA vaccine carriers for effective topical immunization [65].

Topical application of DNA loaded cationic *Transfersomes* made of dioleoyl trimethyl ammonium propane (DOTAP) and sodium deoxycholate elicited a comparable immune response as produced after intramuscular recombinant hepatitis B surface antigen (HBsAg) administration [66]. The Span 80 based ultradeformable vesicles which were initially optimized by El Maghraby et al (2000) [55], have been recently employed for topical immunization. The results suggested that hepatitis B loaded ultradeformable vesicles are able to provide protective immune response [67].

Ethosomes were also tried for topical immunization. Transcutaneous delivery potential of the HBsAG-loaded ethosomes using human cadaver skin revealed a significantly higher skin permeation of the antigen in comparison to conventional liposomes and soluble antigen formulation. Ethosomal application to experimental mice showed a stronger systemic and mucosal humoral immune response compared to intramuscularly administered alum adsorbed HBsAg suspension, topically applied plain HBsAg solution and hydroalcoholic solution of HBsAg. This suggested a potential for transdermal immunization using ethosomes [68].

The potential of fusogenic liposomes for transdermal delivery was also tested by introduction of vesosomes. In this study, the tetanus toxoid was incorporated into cataionic liposomes made of PC, dioleoyl phosphatidylethanolamine (DOPE) and DOTAP. These vesicles were subsequently entrapped in an interdigitated lipid bilayer to provide vesicles within a vesicle (vesosomes). These liposomes have been claimed to provide a promising system for transcutaneous immunization [69].

Mechanisms Of Action Of Vesicles As Skin Drug Delivery Systems

The mechanisms of vesicular skin delivery have been extensively reviewed with different mechanisms being suggested [18-19]. The reported mechanisms (Fig. 3) included five mechanisms. The first mechanism is the free drug process in which the drug has to be released from the vesicle before independent permeation into and through the skin. According to this process the vesicles can be considered only as a carrier which may control the drug release. The second mechanism is the penetration enhancing mechanism in which the vesicular components produce disruption of the packing characteristic of the SC, thus reducing the barrier nature of the skin. The third mechanism depends on the possibility that vesicles can be adsorbed into or fused with the skin surface before subsequently transferring their contents to the skin. The fourth process is the intact vesicular skin penetration in which the intact vesicles are thought to penetrate into the intact skin carrying their payload. The last possibility depends on vesicular penetration into and through the skin appendages. These mechanisms will be covered in the subsequent sections, illustrating some examples for both supportive and negative findings.

Free drug mechanism (see Fig. 3 at A)

The impact of this process was suggested by only one report [49]. The role of this process in transdermal delivery was considered negligible for different vesicular systems after comparing the transepidermal flux plots with the in vitro drug release profile obtained from the same formulation and reporting that the peak estradiol flux through skin appeared at a time during which drug release was negligible [54].

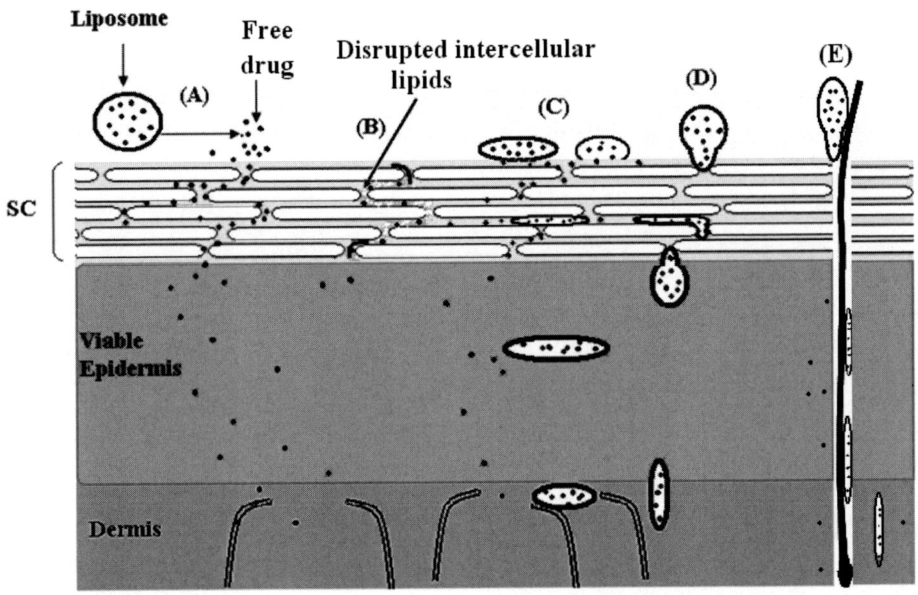

Fig. 3 Possible mechanisms of action of liposomes as skin drug delivery systems. (A) is the free drug mechanism, (B) is the penetration enhancing process of liposome components, (C) indicates vesicle adsorption to and/or fusion with the stratum corneum (SC) and (D) illustrates intact vesicle penetration into or into and through the intact skin (not to scale) (modified from El Maghraby et al., 2008) [19].

Penetration enhancing mechanism (see Fig. 3 at B)

Ultra-structural changes in the intercellular lipids were recorded after application of the vesicles suggesting a penetration enhancing effect. It was concluded that vesicles containing relatively smaller hydrophilic head groups can interact with human SC lipids in vitro [70]. Differential scanning calorimetric investigations suggested that the lipid components of liposomes can diffuse into the SC and change the enthalpy of the lipid-related transitions of the SC [71]. It was also shown that, depending on composition, liposomes can produce an enhancing effect (shown by skin pre-treatment) or may fuse and mix with skin lipids perturbing their arrangement. Liposomes containing DOPE or lyso-PC produced the greatest effect with the conical shape of DOPE being essential for this effect.

Enhanced skin drug delivery and short lag time values were recorded after skin pre-treatment with phospholipids. This effect was absent on repeating the same study using silastic membrane instead of skin. In addition, the phospholipids did not show any significant affect on the percutaneous absorption of indomethacin through skin lacking stratum corneum. These findings clearly indicated that phospholipids act directly on the permeability barrier of SC [72].

Negative findings concerning the penetration enhancing process were also recorded. No penetration enhancement can be recorded after coapplication of empty SCLL with free interferon [27]. Also skin pretreatment with empty vesicles was not as efficient as liposomes encapsulated drugs [73]. It was thus concluded that the hypothesis that liposomes interact with SC is invalid.

To verify the controversy obtained from different authors the penetration enhancing effect of a variety of vesicular systems was evaluated by treating the skin with empty vesicles before evaluating the transdermal permeation parameters of estradiol from saturated aqueous solution. The tested systems included vesicles with different membrane elasticity. The ultradeformable formulations included PC with sodium cholate, PC with Span 80 and PC with Tween 80. The standard vesicles comprised pure PC vesicles (non rigid), PC with CH (membrane stabilized), and two rigid liposomes of DPPC and DPPC/CH. The results revealed a possible penetration enhancing effect only for the non-rigid PC vesicles with the rest of the tested formulations showing negative effect. However, comparing enhancing effect of PC vesicles (4-fold) with the relative flux obtained after application of estradiol loaded in the same liposomes (8-fold) it was concluded that penetration enhancement is not the main mechanism operating [54]. This process was further investigated by probing the importance of liposome structure for transdermal delivery [74]. This was conducted by comparing estradiol skin delivery from standard and ultradeformable vesicles with that obtained from propylene glycol solutions containing the same vesicular components. The results indicated the importance of the colloidal structure, excluding a major role for the penetration enhancing mechanism in improved skin delivery from such liposomes.

It was also reported that drug molecules must be applied together with and entrapped within niosomes themselves, suggesting that elastic niosomes act as drug carrier systems and not as penetration enhancers [56]

Vesicle adsorption to and/or fusion with the stratum corneum (see Fig. 3 at C)

Vesicles can inter into but not through intact healthy SC; instead, they dissolve and form a unit membrane structures. This conclusion was reported after reviewing the interaction of liposomes with human skin [75]. The processes of adhesion onto the skin surface and fusion or mixing with the lipid matrix of the SC have been suggested for liposome lipids [76]. It was also hypothesized that the phospholipids of liposomes can inter the skin increasing the continuity of the lipid matrix of the skin and thus facilitating the movement of lipophilic molecules [77]. Based on the previous reports increased drug uptake should be obtained from aqueous solutions after skin pre-treatment with empty vesicles. This attracted researchers to conduct uptake studies in which SC membranes were dipped into the liposomes or aqueous solution for a short time (10 minutes). Only medicated vesicular systems were able to improve drug uptake compared to aqueous drug solution. The uptake ratios (UR) between the vesicles and solution ranged from 23 to 29 with no significant differences between deformable and standard vesicles. Correlating this finding with superiority of deformable vesicles over traditional liposomes in increasing transepidermal flux it was suggested that deformable vesicles either improved the diffusion or penetrated deeper in the epidermis, thus allowing more efficient drug clearance [54].

Intact vesicular skin penetration mechanism (see Fig. 3 at D)

This mechanism was suggested early in the first articles on vesicular skin drug delivery [21-22]. It was difficult to believe that large aggregates like liposomes could penetrate through the densely packed SC in significant amounts. Accordingly many researchers have tested this hypothesis. The presence of intact vesicles in the dermis was shown after application of the rigid DPPC-CH vesicles. The authors suggested that liposomes can penetrate the epidermis carrying the drug [31]. In contrast to this, liposomes showed greater efficiency than traditional gel in the treatment of eczema but not for psoriasis [78]. It was thus concluded that liposomes can penetrate diseased skin with its ruptured SC (as in eczema) but cannot invade skin with hyperkeratosis, as in psoriasis.

The ratio of [^{3}H] DPPC (liposomes component) to [^{14}C] tretinoin (encapsulated drug) deposited into various skin strata was constant throughout the SC but not in the viable epidermis and dermis. It was thus suggested that liposomes and tretinoin co-transport into SC was accompanied by independent penetration of free drug, which could have escaped from liposomes on the skin surface [79]. This report suggests that vesicles can penetrate only into the SC.

The introduction of *Transfersomes* into this field was associated with strong claim suggesting that vesicles can invade the skin intact and go deep enough to be absorbed by the systemic circulation. The transdermal hydration gradient is said to produce a force sufficient to drive *Transfersomes* through the intact SC and into the epidermis. Phospholipid being hydrophilic leads to vesicle xerophobia (tendency to avoid dry surrounding). Vesicles will thus try to follow the local hydration gradient, moving into deeper skin strata to escape from the dry conditions on the skin surface [52, 60]. Occlusion which is believed to prevent surface dryness and maintain excessive SC hydration with loss of the physiologic hydration gradient can thus inhibit *Transfersome* skin penetration. The fact that both standard liposomes and the *Transfersomes* contain phospholipids which are responsible for the xerophobia as integral component suggests that both types of vesicles can similarly penetrate the intact skin. This suggestion was not accepted by the proponents of *Transfersomes* who reported that the process of vesicle skin penetration requires high degree of deformability so that the vesicles can permeate through the narrow tortuous intercellular pathway (Fig. 4). This deformability is only available in case of *Transfersomes* and was attributed to the presence of edge activator molecules (e.g surfactants) which tend to accumulate at the site of high stress due to their high propensity for highly curved structures. This rearrangement reduces the energy required for deformation. The stress is reportedly produced upon drying of the vesicles which, being flexible, can follow the transdermal hydration gradient [60, 80].

To test this hypothesis the effect of vesicle size on the transepidermal permeation of estradiol was monitored. This study was conducted to investigate the possibility that intact vesicles penetrate through skin, assuming that this penetration is a function of the vesicle size [54]. The small unilamellar vesicles were as effective as the large mulilamellar vesicles, a finding which suggests that intact vesicles do not permeate *through* human epidermal membrane in vitro [54]. In more recent studies, reduction of vesicle size improved both drug deposition into deeper strata and penetration through skin, with large structures improving deposition only [81].

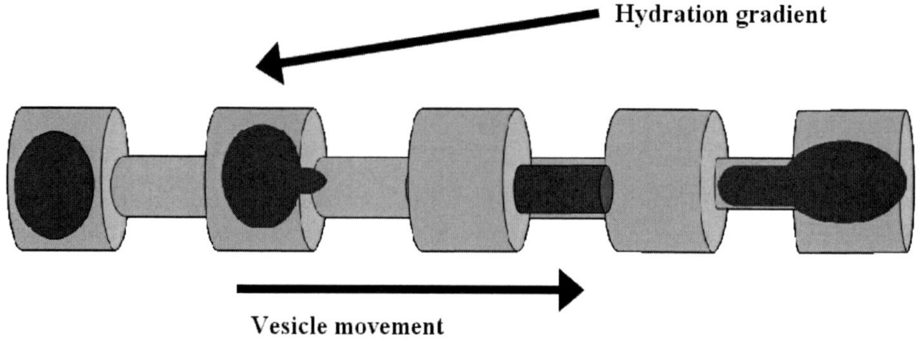

Fig. 4 Hydration gradient and deformability-driven movement of *Transfersomes* through small pores (after Cevc et al 1996) [80].

The amphiphilic anti-inflammatory drug dipotassium glycyrrhizinate (DG) was incorporated into liposomes. This agent was reported to increase the elasticity of the vesicles. The vesicle elasticity was confirmed by measuring the vesicle size before and after extrusion through a microporous filter, which revealed that they were capable of penetrating a pore with a diameter three times smaller than their own span. Despite of being elastic these liposomes showed only improved skin deposition of DG [82]. This finding may support the possibility that vesicles can penetrate *into* but not *through* skin. In similar studies the size of *Transfersomes* did not change after extrusion through semi-permeable membrane barriers. The authors reported the presence of the vesicles in mice blood after topical application of fluorescent labeled *Transfersomes*. Surprisingly, the size of these vesicles was similar to that of the starting liposome suspension. This was taken as a clear evidence for vesicle invasion into and through skin [83-84].

The transport of niosomes components and a model drug into human skin was monitored in vivo. Only elastic vesicle materials were able to enter the SC reaching almost the SC-viable epidermal junction but the distribution profile of the drug in the lower SC layers was different from that of the vesicle component. This finding indicates possible drug release after partitioning of the vesicles into the SC [56].

In light of the above findings, it appears that some vesicles particularly the flexible ones may penetrate intact to some extent into healthy skin. However, it is not clear if the intact vesicles will penetrate deep enough to pass through the entire tissue carrying their payload to the systemic circulation.

Trans-appendageal penetration (see Fig. 3 at E)

Excessive hydration of the skin and occlusive application of vesicles was found to reduce the transdermal delivery from *Transfersomes*. This was explained on the bases of inhibiting the transdermal hydration gradient, which is considered as the driving force for vesicle-skin penetration [60]. Another possible explanation is that excessive skin hydration may lead to swelling of the corneocytes and thus closing or at least minimizing the size of shunts that may play a role in liposomal skin delivery. The role of this pathway will be reviewed in this section.

The drug deposition into and permeation through skin was monitored after liposomal application. The skin deposition was higher in hairy guinea pigs. However, with regard to penetration though skin, no difference could be found between hairless and hairy guinea pigs. Despite this it was concluded that invasion is mainly along the hair sheath [85]. This conclusion is not valid as the previous findings can reflect only delivery into, rather than through, the hair follicles. The shunt pathway for vesicular delivery was excluded after recording similar transfersomal insulin delivery through different animals or humans with diverse densities of hair follicles [61].

The role of appendageal transport in liposomal skin delivery of estradiol was investigated using a novel in vitro technique employing human abdominal skin. This technique monitored vesicular delivery through epidermis and compared this with penetration through a sandwich of SC and epidermis. The concept of this study was based on the fact that the orifices of shunts occupy only a small surface area of the skin. Accordingly, there will be a negligible chance that the shunts in the two membranes of the skin sandwich can superimpose. The authors thus assumed that the top layer of SC will block most of the shunts available in the bottom membrane [86]. The results of this study revealed no significant role for the shunt route in liposomal trandermal delivery of estradiol. More recently, the enhanced transfollicular vesicular delivery was only achieved after combination with iontophoresis [87].

In the light of the above reports, it could be concluded that the shunt routes play no major role in liposomal transdermal delivery. However, it is important to emphasize that vesicle penetration into but not necessarily through hair follicles (i.e. targeting) can not be excluded.

Conclusion

Vesicular systems are promising candidates for skin drug delivery improving both dermal and transdermal delivery. The flexible and ultradeformable vesicles are superior with respect to transdermal drug delivery. However, their mechanisms of action as skin delivery systems remain controversial. The controversy results from the use of vesicles with variable composition and characteristics or employing skin from different sources with different experimental design. A combination of different mechanisms of action is the most probable in many situations.

The recent findings especially concerning the vesicular transdermal delivery of large molecular weight compounds such as insulin and various vaccines are encouraging but it should be noted that the studies used the vesicles in the form of simple dispersion. Accordingly, it could be concluded that long time is still necessary before commercialization of such systems, during which authors should investigate the feasibility of these systems for scaling up. These studies should incorporate the vesicular systems in a pharmaceutically acceptable dosage forms before studying the effect of this incorporation on the transdermal delivery potential of the vesicular systems.

References

[1] Scheuplein, R.J. & Blank, I.H. (1971). Permeability of the skin. *Physiol. Rev., 51*, 702-747.

[2] Orland, G.F. (1983). Structure of the skin. In L.A. Goldsmith (Ed.), *Biochemistry and physiology of the skin* (Vol. 1, pp 3-63), Oxford University Press.

[3] Barry, B.W. (1983). *Dermatological Formulations: Percutaneous Absorption.* New York and Basel: Marcel Dekker.

[4] Bouwstra, J.A. & Ponec, M. (2006). The skin barrier in healthy and diseased state. *Biochim. Biophys. Acta, 1758,* 2080–2095.

[5] Bissett, D.L., (1987). Anatomy and biochemistry of the skin. In A.F. Kydonieus & B. Berner (Eds.), *Trandermal Delivery of Drugs* (Vol. 1, pp 29-42). Boca Raton: CRC Press.

[6] Elias, P.M. (1983). Epidermal lipids; barrier functions and desquamation. *J. Invest. Dermatol., 80*, 44-49(S).

[7] Scheuplein, R.J. (1965). Mechanisms of percutaneous absorption. I. Routes of penetration and the influence of solubility. *J. Invest. Dermatol., 45,* 334-346.

[8] Scheuplein, R.J. (1967). Mechanisms of percutaneous absorption. II. Transient diffusion and the relative importance of various routes of skin penetration. *J. Invest. Dermatol., 48*, 79-88.

[9] Otberg, N., Richter, H., Schaefer, H., Blume-Peytavi, U., Sterry, W. & Lademann, J. (2004). Variations of Hair Follicle Size and Distribution in Different Body Sites. *J. Invest. Dermatol., 122,* 14–19.

[10] Barry, B.W. (1991). Lipid protein partitioning theory of skin penetration enhancement. *J. Control. Rel. 15*, 237-248.

[11] Williams, A.C. (2003). Transdermal and Topical Drug Delivery; from theory to clinical practice. London: Pharmaceutical Press.

[12] Goodman, M. & Barry, B.W. (1988). Action of penetration enhancers on human skin as assessed by permeation of model drugs 5-fluorouracil and estradiol. I. Infinite dose technique. *J. Invest. Dermatol., 91(4)*, 323-327.

[13] Megrab, N.A., Williams, A.C. & Barry, B.W. (1995) Oestradiol permeation across human skin and silastic membranes: effects of propylene glycol and supersaturation. *J. Control. Rel. 36*, 277-294.

[14] Miller, L.L., Kolaskie, C.J., Smith, G.A. & Rivier, J. (1990). Transdermal iontophoresis of gonadotropin releasing hormone and two analogues. *J. Pharm. Sci., 79*, 490–493.

[15] Prausnitz, M.R., Gimm, J.A., Guy, R.H., Langer, R., Weaver, J.C. & Cullander, C. (1996). Imaging of transport pathways across human stratum corneum during high-voltage and low-voltage electrical exposures. *J. Pharm. Sci., 85*, 1363–1370.

[16] Kost, J., Pliquett, U., Mitragotri, S., Yamamoto, A., Langer R. & Weaver, J. (1996). Synergistic effect of electric field and ultrasound on transdermal transport. *Pharm. Res., 13*, 633–638.

[17] El Maghraby, G.M. (2008). Transdermal delivery of hydrocortisone from eucalyptus oil microemulsion: Effects of cosurfactants. *Int. J. Pharm., 355*, 285-292.

[18] El Maghraby, G.M., Williams, A.C. & Barry, B.W., (2006). Can drug bearing liposomes penetrate intact skin? *J. Pharm Pharmacol., 58*, 415-429.

[19] El Maghraby, G.M., Williams, A.C. & Barry, B.W. (2008). Liposomes and skin. From drug delivery to model membranes. *Eur. J. Pharm Sci., 34*, 203-222.

[20] New, R.R.C. (1990). *Liposomes: A Practical Approach*. Oxford: Oxford University Press.

[21] Mezei, M. & Gulasekharam, V. (1980). Liposomes-a selective drug delivery system for topical route of administration. 1. lotion dosage form. *Life Sci. 26*, 1473-1477.

[22] Mezei, M. & Gulasekharam, V. (1982). Liposomes-a selective drug delivery system for topical route of administration: gel dosage form. *J. Pharm. Pharmacol. 34*, 473-474.

[23] Mezei, M. (1985). Liposomes as a skin drug delivery system. In D.D. Breimer & P. Speiser (Eds.), *Topics in Pharmaceutical Sciences,* (pp. 345-358). Amsterdam, New York, Oxford: Elsevier.

[24] Vermorken, A.J.M., Hukkelhoven, M.W.A.C., Vermeesch-Marksiag, A.M.G., Goos, C.M.A.A., Wirtz, P. & Ziegenmeyer, J. (1984). The use of liposomes in topical application of steroids. *J. Pharm. Pharmacol., 36*, 334-336.

[25] Wohlrab, W., Lasch, J., Laub, R., Taube, C.M. & Wellner, K. (1992). Distribution of liposome-encapsulated ingredients in human skin ex vivo. In O.B. Falco, H.C., Korting & H.I., Maibach, (Eds), *Liposome Dermatics*, (pp. 217-225). Berlin: Springer-Verlag.

[26] Yu, H.Y. & Liao, H.M. (1996). Triamcinolone permeation from different liposome formulations through rat skin in vitro. *Int. J. Pharm. 127*, 1-7.

[27] Weiner, N., Williams, N., Birch, G., Ramachandran, C., Shipman, C. JR. & Flynn, G. (1989). Topical delivery of liposomally encapsulated interferon evaluated in cutaneous herpes guinea pig model. *Antimicrob. Agents Chemother., 33(8)*, 1217 1221.

[28] Egbaria, K., Ramachandran, C. Kittayanond, D. & Weiner, N. (1990). Topical delivery of liposomally encapsulated interferon evaluated by in vitro diffusion studies. *Antimicrob. Agents Chemother. 34(1)*, 107-110.

[29] Egbaria, K., Ramachandran, C. & Weiner, N. (1990) Topical delivery of cyclosporin: evaluation of various formulations using in vitro diffusion studies in hairless mouse skin. *Skin Pharmacol. 3*, 21-28.

[30] Gesztes, A. & Mezei, M. (1988). Topical anaesthesia of skin by liposome-encapsulated tetracaine. *Aneth. Analg. 67*, 1079-1081.

[31] Foldvari, M., Gesztes, A. & Mezei, M. (1990). Dermal drug delivery by liposome encapsulation: Clinical and electron microscopic studies. *J. Microencaps. 7(4)*, 479-489.

[32] Foldvari, M. (1994). In vitro cutaneous and percutaneous delivery and in vivo effecacy of tetracaine from liposomal and conventional vehicles. *Pharm. Res. 11(11)*, 1593-1598.

[33] Hung, O.R., Comeau, L., Riley, M.R., Tan, S., Whynot, S. & Mezei, M. (1997) Comparative topical anaesthesia of EMLA and liposome-encapsulated tetracaine. *Can. J. Anaesth. 44*, 707-711.

[34] Fisher, R., Hung, O., Mezei, M. & Stewart, R. (1998). Topical anaesthesia of intact skin: Liposome-encapsulated tetracaine vs EMLA. *Br. J. Anaesth. 81*, 972-973.

[35] Planas, M.E., Gonzalez, P.,Rodriguez, L., Sanchez, S. & Cevc, G.(1992). Noninvasive percutaneous induction of topical analgesia by a new type of drug carrier, and prolongation of local pain insensitivity by anesthetic liposomes. *Aneth. Analg. 75*, 615-621.

[36] El Maghraby, G.M., Williams, A.C. & Barry, B.W. (2001). Skin delivery of 5-fluorouracil from ultradeformable and standard liposomes in vitro. *J. Pharm. Pharmacol. 53*, 1069-1077.

[37] Cevc, G., Blume, G. & Schätzlein, A. (1997). *Transfersomes*-mediated transepidermal delivery improves the regio-specificity and biological activity of corticosteroids in vivo. *J. Control. Rel. 45*, 211-226.

[38] Manosroi, A., Jantrawut, P. & Manosroi, J. (2008). Anti-inflammatory activity of gel containing novel elastic niosomes entrapped with diclofenac diethylammonium *Int. J. Pharm. 360*, 156–163.

[39] Lauer, A.C., Ramachandran, C., Leib, L.M., Niemiec, S. & Weiner, N.D. (1996). Targeted delivery to pilosebaceous unit via liposomes. *Adv. Drug Deliv. Rev. 18*, 311-324.

[40] Lauer, A.C. (1999). Percutaneous drug delivery to the hair follicle. In R.L., Bronaugh & H.I., Maibach, (Eds.), *Percutaneous Absorption Drugs-Cosmetics-Mechanisms-Methodology*, (3rd Edition, pp. 427-449). New York. Basel: Marcel Dekker, Inc.

[41] Lieb, L.M., Ramachandran, C., Egbaria, K. & Weiner, N. (1992). Liposomally encapsulated active ingredients penetrate through the hair follicle. In O.B., Falco, H.C., Korting, & H.I., Maibach (Eds.), *Liposome Dermatics*, (pp. 200-205). Berlin: Springer-Verlag.

[42] Lieb, L.M., Ramachandran, C., Egbaria, K. & Weiner, N. (1992). Topical delivery enhancement with multilamellar liposomes into pliosebaceous units: I. In vitro evaluation using fluorescent techniques with hamster ear model. *J. Invest. Dermatol. 99(1)*, 108-113.

[43] Du Plessis, J., Egbaria, K., Ramachandran, C. & Weiner, N.D. (1992). Topical delivery of liposomally encapsulated gamma-interferon. *Antiviral Res. 18*, 259-265.

[44] Lieb, L.M., Flynn, G., & Weiner, N. (1994). Follicular (pilosebaceous unit) deposition and pharmacological behavior of cimetidine as a function of formulation. *Pharm. Res. 11(10)*, 1419-1423.

[45] Tschan, T., Steffen, H. & Supersaxo, A. (1997). Sebaceous-gland deposition of isotretinoin after topical application: an in vitro study using human facial skin. *Skin Pharmacol. 10*, 126-134.

[46] Skalko, N., Cajkovac, M. & Jalsenjak, I. (1992). Liposomes with clindamycin hydrochloride in therapy of acne vulgaris. *Int. J. Pharm. 85*, 97-101.

[47] Meybeck, A. (1992). Comedolytic activity of liposomal antiacne drug in an experimental model. In O.B., Falco, H.C., Korting & H. I., Maibach, (Eds), *Liposome Dermatics*, (pp. 235-241). Berlin: Springer-Verlag.

[48] Tabbakhian, M., Tavakoli, N., Jaafari, M.R. & Daneshamouz, S, (2006). Enhancement of follicular delivery of finasteride by liposomes and niosomes. 1. In vitro permeation and in vivo deposition studies using hamster flank and ear models. *Int. J. Pharm. 323*, 1–10.

[49] Ganesan, M. G., Weiner, N.D., Flynn, G. L. & Ho, N. F. H. (1984). Influence of liposomal drug entrapment on percutaneous absorption. *Int. J. Pharm. 20*, 139-154.

[50] Bonina, F.B., Montenegro, L., Scrofani, N., Esposito, E., Cortesi, R., Menegatti, E. & Nastruzzi, C. (1995). Effects of phospholipid based formulations on in vitro and in vivo percutaneous absorption of methyl nicotinate. *J. Control. Rel. 34*, 53-63.

[51] Fresta, M. & Puglisi, G. (1996). Application of liposomes as potential cutaneous drug delivery systems. In vitro and in vivo investigation with radioactivity labelled vesicles. *J. Drug. Target. 4*, 95-101.

[52] Cevc, G. & Blume, G. (1992). Lipid vesicles penetrate into intact skin owing to the transdermal osmotic gradients and hydration force. *Biochim. Biophys. Acta 1104*, 226-232.

[53] Simoes, S.I., Martins, M.B.F., Cruz, M.E.M. & Cevc, G. (1998). Anti-inflammatory effects of Cu, Zn-superoxide dismutase in liposomes, Transfersomes or micelles, in the acute murine ear edema model. In K.R. Brain, & K.A., Walters (Eds.), *Perspectives in Percutaneous Penetration, sixth International Conference* (Vol. 6a, p. 50). Cardiff: STS Publishing.

[54] El Maghraby, G.M., Williams, A.C. & Barry, B.W. (1999). Skin delivery of oestradiol from deformable and traditional liposomes: Mechanistic studies. *J. Pharm. Pharmacol. 51*, 1123-1134.

[55] El Maghraby, G.M., Williams, A.C. & Barry, B.W. (2000). Oestradiol skin delivery from ultradeformable liposomes: refinement of surfactant concentration. *Int. J. Pharm. 196*, 63-74.

[56] Honeywell-Nguyen, P.L., Arenja, S. & Bouwstra, J.A. (2003). Skin penetration and mechanisms of action in the delivery of the D2-agonist rotigotine from surfactant-based elastic vesicle formulations. *Pharm. Res. 20(10)*, 1619-1625.

[57] Honeywell-Nguyen, P.L., Gooris, G.S. & Bouwstra, J.A. (2004). Quantitative assessment of the transport of elastic and rigid vesicle components and a model drug from these vesicle formulations into human skin in vivo. *J. Invest. Dermatol. 123(5)*, 902-910.

[58] Artman, C., Roding, J.,Ghyczy, M. & Prazel, H.G. (1990) Liposomes from soya phospholipids as percutaneous drug carriers: Qualitative in vivo investigations with antibody-loaded liposomes. *Arzneium. Forsch. Drug. Res., 40(II)*, 1363-1365.

[59] Artman, C., Roding, J.,Ghyczy, M. & Prazel, H.G. (1990). Liposomes from soya phospholipids as percutaneous drug carriers: Quantitative in vivo investigations with radioactivity labelled liposomes. *Arzneium. Forsch. Drug. Res., 40(II)*, 1365-1368.

[60] Cevc, G., Schätzlein, A., Blume, G. (1995). Transdermal drug carriers: basic properties, optimization and transfer efficiency in the case of epicutaneously applied peptides. *J. Control. Rel. 36*, 3-16.

[61] Cevc, G., Gebauer, D., Stieber, J., Schätzlein, A. & Blume, G. (1998). Ultraflexible vesicles, Transfersomes, have an extremely low pore penetration resistance and transport therapeutic amounts of insulin across the intact mammalian skin. *Biochim. Biophys. Acta 1368*, 201-215.

[62] Song, Y.K. & Kim, C.K. (2006). Topical delivery of low-molecular-weight heparinwith surface-charged flexible liposomes. *Biomaterials, 27*, 271-280.

[63] Paul, A., Cevc, G. & Bachhawat, B.K. (1995). Transdermal immunization with large proteins by means of ultradeformable drug carriers. *Eur. J. Immunol. 25*, 3521-3524.

[64] Gupta, P.N., Mishra, V, Rawat, A., Dubey, P, Mahor, S., Jain, S., Chatterji, D.P. & Vyas, S.P. (2005). Non-invasive vaccine delivery in transfersomes, niosomes and liposomes: a comparative study. *Int. J. Pharm. 293*, 73–82.

[65] Vyas, S.P., Singh, R.P., Jain, S., Mishra, V., Mahor,S., Singh, P, Gupta, PN., Rawat, A. & Dubey, P. (2005). Non-ionic surfactant based vesicles (niosomes) for non-invasive topical genetic immunization against hepatitis B. *Int. J. Pharm. 296*, 80–86.

[66] Mahor, S., Rawat, A., Dubey, P.K., Gupta, P.N., Khatri, K., Goyal, A.K. & Vyas, S.P. (2007). Cationic transfersomes based topical genetic vaccine against hepatitis B. *Int. J. Pharm., 340*, 13–19.

[67] Mishra, D., Dubey, V., Asthana, A., Saraf, D.K. & Jain, N.K., (2006). Elastic liposomes mediated transcutaneous immunization against Hepatitis B. *Vaccine, 24*, 4847-4855.

[68] Mishra, D., Mishra, P.K., Dubey, V., Nahar, N., Dabadghao, S. & Jain, N.K. (2008). Systemic and mucosal immune response induced by transcutaneous immunization using Hepatitis B surface antigen-loaded modified liposomes. *Eur. J. Pharm. Sci., 33*, 424-433.

[69] Mishra, V., Mahor, S., Rawat, A., Dubey, P., Gupta, P. N., Singh, P. & Vyas, S.P. (2006). Development of novel fusogenic vesosomes for transcutaneous immunization. *Vaccine, 24*, 5559-5570.

[70] Hofland, H. E. J., Bouwstra, J. A., Bodde, H. E., Spies, F. & Junginger, H. E. (1995). Interaction between liposomes and human stratum corneum in vitro: freeze fracture electron microscopical visualization and small angle X-ray scattering studies. *Br. J. Dermatol. 132*, 853-866.

[71] Zellmer, S., Pfeil, W. & Lasch, J. (1995). Interaction of phosphatidylcholine liposomes with the human stratum corneum. *Biochim. Biophys. Acta 1237*, 176-182.

[72] Yokomizo, Y. & Sagitani, H. (1996). Effects of phospholipids on the percutaneous penetration of indomethacin through the dorsal skin of the guinea pig, in vitro. *J. Control. Rel. 38*, 267-274.

[73] Du Plessis, J., Weiner, N. & Muller, D.G. (1994a). The influence of in vivo treatment of skin with liposomes on the topical absorption of a hydrophilic and a hydrophobic drug in vitro. *Int. J. Pharm., 103*, R_1-R_5.

[74] El Maghraby, G.M., Williams, A.C. & Barry, B.W. (2000) Skin delivery of oestradiol from lipid vesicles: importance of liposome structure. *Int. J. Pharm.* **204:** 159-169.

[75] Schaller, M. & Korting, H.C. (1996). Interaction of liposomes with human skin: the role of the stratum corneum. *Adv. Drug Deliv. Rev. 18*, 303-309.

[76] Kirjavainen, M., Urtti, A., Jaaskelainen, I., Suhonen, T. M., Paronen, P., Koskela, R. V., Kiesvaara, J. & Monkkonen, J. (1996). Interaction of liposomes with human skin in vitro - the influence of lipid composition and structure. *Biochim. Biophys. Acta. 1304*, 179-189.

[77] Keith, A.D. & Snipes, W. (1982). Phospholipids as moisturizing agents. In P., Frost & S., Horovitz (Eds.), P*rinciples of Cosmetics for the Dermatologist,* (pp. 59-69). St. Louis: The C.V. Mosby Company.

[78] Korting, H.C., Zeinicke, H., Schafer, K.M. & Falco, O.B. (1990). Liposome encapsulation improves efficacy of betamethasone dipropionate in atopic eczema but not in psoriasis vulgaris. *Eur. J. Clin. Pharmacol. 39*, 349-351.

[79] Masini, V., Bonte, F., Meybeck, A. & Wepierre, J. (1993). Cutaneous bioavailability in hairless rats of tretinoin liposomes or gel. *J. Pharm. Sci. 82(1)*, 17-21.

[80] Cevc, G., Blume, G., Schätzlein, A., Gebauer, D. & Paul, A. (1996). The skin: a pathway for systemic treatment with patches and lipid-based agent carriers. *Adv. Drug Deliv. Rev. 18*, 349-378.

[81] Verma, D.D., Verma, S., Blume, G. & Fahr, A. (2003). Particle size of liposomes influences dermal delivery of substance into skin. *Int. J. Pharm. 258*, 141-151.

[82] Trotta, M., Peira, E., Debernardi, F. & Gallarate, M. (2002). Elastic liposomes for skin delivery of dipotassium glycyrrhizinate. Int. J. Pharm. *241*, 319-327.

[83] Cevc, G., Schätzlein, A. & Richardsen, H. (2002). Ultradeformable lipid vesicles can penetrate skin and other semi-permeable membrane barriers unfragmented. Evidence from double label CLSM experiments and direct size measurement. *Biochim. Biophys. Acta 1564*, 21-30.

[84] Cevc, G. & Gebauer, D. (2003). Hydration-driven transport of deformable lipid vesicles through fine pores and skin barrier. *Biophys. J. 84*, 1010-1024.

[85] Schramlova, J., Blazek, K., Bartackova, M., Otova, B., Mardesicova, L., Zizkovsky, V. & Hulinska, D. (1997). Electron microscopic demonstration of the penetration of liposomes through skin. *Folia Biol. 43(4)*, 165-169.

[86] El Maghraby, G.M., Williams, A.C. & Barry, B.W. (2001). Skin hydration and possible shunt route penetration in controlled skin delivery of estradiol from ultradeformable and standard liposomes in vitro. *J. Pharm. Pharmacol. 53*, 1311-1322.

[87] Han, I., Kim, M. & Kim, J. (2004). Enhanced transfollicular delivery of adriamycin with a liposome and iontophoresis. *Exp Dermatol. 13(2)*, 86-92.

In: Skin Anatomy and Physiology Research Developments ISBN: 978-1-60741-469-8
Editor: Leon F. Bukowsky

Chapter 6

Experimental Physiology in Anti-Skin Aging

*Neena Philips**
School of Natural Sciences, Fairleigh Dickinson University, Teaneck, NJ 07666, USA

Abstract

Skin contains a network of extracellular matrix (ECM) proteins, including collagen and elastin. Collagen provides structure whereas elastin gives skin firmness and elasticity. The ECM proteins can be degraded or remodelled by the matrixmetalloproteinases (MMPs) and elastase. The MMPs are inhibited by tissue inhibitors of matrixmetalloproteinases (TIMPs). The dermal fibroblasts are primarily responsible for the ECM maintenance. However, there is cross talk between the epidermis and dermis via growth factors and cytokines; which regulate signaling pathways, transcription factors and gene expression. Transforming growth factor (TGF-β) released by epidermal keratinocytes stimulates ECM expression in fibroblasts.

With chronological aging there is fine wrinkling and loss/atrophy of collagen and elastin/fibrillin. Ultraviolet (UV) radiation and environmental pollutants, that can be metabolized in skin, cause direct or indirect DNA damage, formation of reactive oxygen species (ROS), and damage to the extracellular matrix. In photoaged skin there is degeneration of collagen and elastin; enhanced MMPs and elastase; and elastin accumulation as solar elastosis. The manifestations are wrinkles, diminished structural integrity, impaired wound healing, and cancer.

The experimental physiology in skin anti-aging is the identification of actives, and their mechanisms of action, by investigating effects of potential agents on various targets including (i) the regulation of gene expression (at protein, mRNA and transcription levels) of elastin, collagen, heat shock proteins, MMPs, and TIMPs in dermal fibroblasts; and growth factors, cytokines, MMPs and TIMPs in keratinocytes, (ii) cellular effects such as viability, metabolism and lipid peroxidation, (iii) keratinocyte-fibroblast

* Fairleigh Dickinson University, H-DH4-03, Teaneck, NJ 07666, USA; Ph no: 201 692 6494; Fax: 201 692 7349
Email: nphilips@fdu.edu; neenaphilips@optonline.net

modulation via soluble factors (conditioned media) and skin equivalents; and (iv) actives' direct inhibitory effect on MMPs, elastase and reactive oxygen species. These experiments are simultaneously performed in UV irradiated cells to determine photo protective effects.

Several actives have been identified that beneficially regulate the ECM for skin health, the predominant being *Polypodium leucotomos*, lutein, and xanthohumol. The effects of these plant extracts are similar to hormones and TGF-β. In addition, these actives counteract the damaging effects of ultraviolet radiation and environmental pollutants.

Keywords: Skin, Extracellular matrix, Matrixmetalloproteinases, Collagen, Elastin, Skin aging, Cancer, Wound healing, Transforming growth facotr-beta, Experimental design

Skin and Extracellular Matrix

The skin is the body's envelope and the first line of defense. It consists of two layers: the epidermis (cornified, stratified squamous epithelium) and the dermis (a dense connective tissue lamina propria) [1]. The epidermis is composed of an outermost layer of cornified cells filled with keratin, a layer of granular cells, melanocytes and keratinocytes. The dermal cells include fibroblasts and macrophages, embedded in an extracellular matrix (ECM) synthesized predominantly by fibroblasts [2]. The structural ECM are primarily fibrillar collagens, in order of predominance types I, III, and V that provide structure, and elastin which forms fibers with fibrillin to gives skin firmness and elasticity. The ECM is largely responsible for skin integrity.

The ECM is remodeled or degraded by matrix metalloproteinases (MMPs), Zn^{2+} dependent endopeptidases [3-8]. MMPs are classified into three major classes: the collagenases, stromelysins, and gelatinases [5]. The collagenases that include MMP-1 degrade collagen and the gelatinases that include MMP-2 degrade the basement membrane. MMP-2 is also considered a collagenase for its activity on denatured structural collagen [6]. MMP function is primarily regulated at three levels: expression, activation, and inhibition. The regulation of MMP expression is by cytokines and growth factors in a cell specific manner [7]. MMPs are secreted as inactive zymogens, activated only on the cleavage of the enzymes' prodomains [8]. Additionally, MMP activity is inhibited by tissue inhibitors of matrix metalloproteinases (TIMPs) [9-10].

A primary regulator of the ECM is transforming growth factor-β (TGF-β). It has differential effects in different cell types [11-15]. TGF-β enhances collagen formation and inhibits MMP expression in fibroblasts, without altering cell growth [15]. In epithelial cells, it inhibits growth and stimulates the expression of MMPs [11, 14]. Cancer metastasis is associated with enhanced MMPs and TGF-β expression [12, 13].

Skin Aging

Skin aging occurs with chronological (intrinsic) aging and exposure to environmental factors, including ultraviolet (UV) radiation. It manifests as wrinkles, sagging, diminished structural integrity and delayed wound healing. Alterations in collagen and elastin, which form the extracellular matrix (ECM), are responsible for the clinical manifestations of skin aging [16-21]. There is decrease in structural collagen and elastin [22-26]. The atrophy of collagen and elastin fibers is from reduced synthesis and the increased expression of their degradative enzymes, especially MMP-1 (collagenases), MMP-2 /-9 (gelatinases) and elastases [16-21, 27-34]. The ECM damaging enzymes are produced by epidermal keratinocytes, dermal fibroblasts and neutrophils, which are the predominant source for photoaged skin [29-34].

In photoaged skin with coarse wrinkling, in addition to reduced levels of collagen from increased MMPs, there are elastotic deposits [35-44]. Photoaging is from the ultraviolet (UV) spectrum of solar radiation and includes the long wavelength UVA rays (320-400 nm) and the short wavelength UVB rays (290-320 nm). UVA and UVB radiation are involved in the degenerative changes in skin. Solar radiation contains 10-20 fold more UVA radiation that is deeper penetrating and UVB radiation has greater energy and thereby damaging to cells [36].

Environmental xenobiotics have effects similar to UV radiation. Environmental toxins include benzene and its metabolites [45-50]. Benzene is metabolized in-vivo to phenolic metabolites such as phenol, catechol, hydroquinone and 1,2,4-benzenetriol [51, 52]. Benzene and its metabolites (catechol, hydroquninone, phenol, and toluene) compose cigarette smoke and cause skin aging [53-55]. The phenolic metabolites cause cell loss and lipid peroxidation [56]. Skin is active in the absorption of xenobiotics; benzene and its metabolites can be absorbed through the skin and metabolized by phase I and phase II reactions [57-71]. The dermal fibroblasts metabolize benzene to non-phenolic metabolites that damage the ECM [56, 72, 73].

Skin Aging and Cellular Effects

Intrinsic aging, photoaging and xenobiotic-facilitated aging is associated with DNA mutations and generation of reactive oxygen species (ROS), which lead to cell loss, apoptosis, membrane damage and lipid peroxidation [35-44,56]. Intrinsic aging is often associated with diminished levels of hormones, such as estrogen. Environmental aging is accentuated by DNA damage, excessive generation of ROS, oxidative stress and inflammation [35-44]. ROS alters signal transduction pathways and thereby cell differentiation or senescence, membrane damage and extracellular matrix (ECM) alterations [38-40]. The ECM alterations are reduced structural collagen and elastin, with elastosis in environmental aging, and increased expression or activities of MMPs and elastases. Skin aging is associated with inhibition of TGF-β expression whereas in cancer TGF-β is over expressed.

Antioxidants in Counteracting Skin Aging

Oxidative stress is an established factor in skin aging and so is prevention with antioxidants. Extracts from several plants exhibit antioxidant, anti-inflammatory and anticarcinogenic properties. Some examples of anti-skin aging compounds researched in our laboratory are lutein, a non-vitamin carotenoid, *Polypodium leucotomos*, a fern extract, and xanthohumol, a flavonoid from *Humulus lupulus* plant.

Lutein: Lutein is a compound with superior antioxidant anti-aging and anti-carcinogenic properties. It accumulates in the macula of the eye, where it prevents macular degeneration [74-76]. It accumulates in the skin to provide anti-oxidant and anti-inflammatory protection from acute UVB exposure [77, 78]. Lutein has anticarcinogenic properties in hepatoma, breast and colon cancer [79-82]. There is an inverse correlation between lutein in diet and melanoma risk [84].The mechanism of lutein's anti-aging and anti-carcinogenic effects is via the regulation the extracellular matrix (ECM) degrading enzymes, matrix metalloproteinases (MMP) or their inhibitors (tissue inhibitor of metalloproteinases, TIMP) in intrinsic skin aging, cancer and photoaging [84]. Lutein inhibits MMP-1 and MMP-2 while stimulating TIMP-1 and TIMP-2 in dermal fibroblasts or melanoma cells; reduces elastin expression in UV irradiated fibroblasts and enhances cell viability and membrane integrity in UVA or UVB exposed fibroblasts [84]. The effects of lutein in fibroblasts are similar to superoxide dismutase indicating inhibition of cellular ROS. In vivo, lutein reduces photoaging and photocarcinogenesis in acute and chronically UVB irradiated mice by reducing inflammation, associated with oxidative stress [85].

Polypodium leucotomos (PL): PL is a tropical fern plant belonging to a natural order Polypodianceae. It has potent antioxidant and anti-inflammatory properties [85-91]. Its extract can prevent sunburn reaction, inhibit the photosensitized generation/reactions of ROS and is effective in the reduction of UV induced tumors [85-91].The cellular and molecular mechanisms for the antagonism of UV radiation effects in skin cells by PL are inhibition of apoptosis, membrane damage, lipid peroxidation, inflammatory cytokine (tumor necrosis factor-α), nitric oxide, transcription factors AP-1 and NF-κB known to be induced by ROS following activation of MAPK (mitogen activated protein kinase) or PKA (protein kinase A) pathways [92, 93]. In skin cells, PL inhibits the expression of MMP-1 and MMP-2 and simultaneously stimulates TIMPs [92]. In melanoma cells, PL preferentially inhibits MMP-1, indicating prevention of interstitial collagen degradation, and stimulates TIMP-2, implicating inhibition of basement membrane remodeling. The inhibition of MMP-1 promoter in melanoma cells by PL is via the AP-1 sequence, suggesting involvement of the AP-1 transcription factor [94]. The effects of PL on MMPs and TIMPs expression in melanoma cells mirror that of lutein [84].

PL mediates its effects on fibroblasts via the stimulation of TGF-β and its anti-oxidant properties, and in melanoma cells by inhibiting TGF-β. TGF- β reciprocally regulates MMPs (except MMP-2) and TIMPs in dermal fibroblasts to reduce the MMPs/TIMPs balance and strengthen the ECM [92, data not shown]. The reciprocal regulation of MMPs and TIMPs by TGF-β is by different mechanisms [21, 95]. While the stimulation of TIMPs by *P. leucotomos* in dermal fibroblasts may be via TGF- β stimulation, its inhibition of MMP-2 was similar to the effect of ascorbate and suggests an antioxidant mechanism [data not shown]. In cancer, TGF- β contributes to tumor pathogenesis by inducing MMPs, angiogenesis, and modification of the extracellular matrix [12, 13, 84, 96]. PL was inhibitory to TGF- β expression in melanoma cells, which in turn may be responsible PL inhibition of MMP-1 expression in these cells [data not shown].

Xanthohumol: Xanthohumol is the major prenylated flavonoid isolated from the hop plant *Humulus lupulus L.* (Cannabinaceae) (Hops), and its metabolites include isoxanthohumol, and 8-prenylnaringenin (8-PN) [97]. From among the Hops components, xanthohumol is the most potent anti-cancer, anti-inflammatory and antioxidant compound [97-106]. Xanthohumol inhibits the ECM degrading enzymes, MMPs and elastase, and stimulates the structural ECM proteins (types I, III, and V collagens) [data not shown].

The anti-inflammatory effects of xanthohumol include inhibition of cycloxygenases/prostaglandins [105,106]. A major mechanism of xanthohumol effect is via the inhibition of NF-κB transcription factor that is associated with pro-oxidant, inflammatory, angiogenic and carcinogenic genes' expression [107-110]. Further, xanthohumol inhibits nitric oxide production by inflammatory cytokines/mediators, with nitric oxide being associated with proinflammatory and carcinogenic effects [111]. The hops flavonoids regulate estrogen regulated pathways and genes, with the xanthohumol metabolite 8-PN being a strong phytoestrogen [112-115].

Xanthohumol is effective in preventing the initiation (chemopreventive) and progression of cancer (anti-carcinogenic). It's chemopreventive property is primarily from its anti-genotoxic mechanisms, including the inhibition of cytochrome P450 enzymes that activate xenobiotics for DNA/cell damage, the induction of detoxification enzymes such as quinine reductase, and the activation of antioxidant response element (ARE) in genes via Nrf2 transcription factor release from its cytoplasmic inhibitor Keap on alkylation [116-122]. Xanthohumol inhibits cancer progression by inhibiting cell proliferation/inducing apoptosis, upregulating E-cadherin/catenin (ant invasiveness), inhibiting topoisomerase I and preventing drug resistance by inhibiting drug efflux transporters [123].

Hormones and Growth Factors in Counteracting Skin Aging

Hormones: With aging there is decrease in several hormones, especially estrogen that leads to reduced ECM structure and delayed wound healing. Skin is an important target for estrogen and progesterone, and the receptors for these hormones have been localized to skin fibroblasts and keratinocytes [124]. Topical application of estrogen stimulates epidermal reepithelilization, TGF- β activity and collagen deposition and thereby accelerates the wound healing process in aged skin [125-128]. The mechanisms by which the hormones improve skin quality and wound healing are increased TGF- β activity, scavenging of superoxides and an altered inflammatory response [125-128]. Estrogen and progesterone stimulate extracellular matrix deposition via TGF- β [129].

Transforming Growth Factor-beta (TGF-β): An important physiological regulator of skin aging, photoaging, cancer and wound healing is transforming growth factor-β (TGF-β). There are three isoforms of TGF-β (1,2, and 3), with TGF-β1 being the predominant isoform.

TGF-β is secreted in an inactive form, non-covalently bound to a dimer of latency associated peptide (LAP) [12]. Activation of TGF- β involves dissociation of mature TGF-β from LAP [12]. Signal transduction is via a complex of transmembrane serine/threonine kinase receptors. Although there are three types of receptors that specifically bind TGF-β, only Type I (TβRI) and Type II (TβRII) have intrinsic serine/threonine kinase activity. Type III (TβRIII) facilitates TGF-β binding to T β RII. On TGF-β binding, TβRI and TβRII form a heteromeric complex leading to phosphorylation of TβRI and transduction of signal to the nucleus via Smads [15, 130, 131].

In intrinsic aging, there is reduction of TGF-β and thereby ECM integrity. TGF-β is the primary regulator of the expression of the structural ECM genes as well as the remodeling enzymes [15, 130, 131]. TGF-β's role has especially been studies in wound healing [132-141]. Fetal wounds heal without scars, and this has been attributed largely to the lower transforming growth factor-β (TGF-β) activity in fetal wounds, relative to neonatal or adult wounds [133-134]. TGF-β is an auto-regulator of its own expression, positively or negatively. TGF-β amplifies its expression in peritoneal wounds, scleroderma and pancreatic regeneration, while exogenous TGF- β is reported to induce scars in a fetal wound repair model [135-140]. The anti TGF-β antibodies can neutralize or prevent the effects of enhanced TGF-β expression on the ECM [138, 141]. In our laboratory, a polyclonal anti TGF-β antibody [AT] that neutralizes the activities of TGF-β 1-3,5 (all isoforms) (AB–100–NA, R&D Systems), stimulates further release of TGF-β in dermal fibroblasts, epidermal keratinocytes, and a renal adenocarcinoma cell line [12, 14, 41]. Also, the AT antibody causes TGF-β like regulation of ECM expression in the skin cells, with the stimulation of elastin and inhibition of MMP-1 proteins in fibroblasts, and the stimulation of elastin protein in keratinocytes [14, 41]. Further, the antibody is antagonistic to UV radiation effects by predominant stimulation of TIMPs in non-irradiated and UV radiated fibroblasts [143]. The antibody is therefore beneficial to counteracting skin aging, though plant extracts or micronutrients (lutein, PL, xanthohumol, ascorbic acid) may be safer alternatives.

Experimental Goal and Methodology

The experimental goal is the identification of actives or chemopreventive agents and their mechanisms of action such as: (i) Direct inhibition of elastase and MMPs and ROS; (ii) Inhibition of cellular oxidative effects – cell loss, membrane damage, lipid peroxidation; (iii) Inhibition of expression (protein, mRNA, and/or promoter levels) of MMPs; (iv) Stimulation of expression of TIMPs, collagen, elastin and TGF-β to manage skin physiology or pathology by incorporation into skin care products.

The methodology is chemical, direct inhibition of MMPs, elastases or ROS, and cellular employing skin cultures, keratinocytes, fibroblasts or skin equivalents. The experimental design is the exposure of non-irradiated or UV radiated cells to different concentrations of potential chemo-preventive agents and examining various cellular and molecular targets that mediate anti-skin aging and cancer or facilitate wound helaing. The cellular assays are based on the conversion of specific target substrates to products - Cell Viability/Proliferation: MTS assay (Promega), Apoptosis: Caspases activities; DNA fragmentation (Roche, Clontech),

Membrane Damage: LDH assay (Sigma), Lipid peroxidation: K-assay (Kamiya Biomedical). The molecular assays for gene expression and regulation are at the protein (ELISA, Western, immunohistochemistry), mRNA analysis (Northern blotting, RT-PCR or reverse transcriptase polymerase chain reaction, Real time-PCR) and transcriptional levels (transient and permanent transfections with recombinant DNA).

Conclusion

In skin aging, impaired wound healing and cancer there is cell/bimolecular damage, excess MMPs to TIMPs ratio, reduction of structural collagen, and altered expression of TGF-β. The goal of experimental research is the identification of actives with predominant beneficial skin effects: (i) Direct inhibition of elastase and MMPs and ROS, (ii) Inhibition of cellular oxidative effects – cell loss (except in cancer), membrane damage, lipid peroxidation, (iii) Inhibition of expression (protein, mRNA, and/or promoter levels) of MMPs, (iv) Stimulation of expression of TIMPs, collagen, elastin and TGF-β (except in cancer) for management of skin physiology or pathology by incorporation of these actives or chemo preventive agents into skin care products

Acknowledgment

February 20, 2009. Marvin Tuason and Tiffany Chang for editing or reference collation

References

[1] Patroi I; Annessi G; Girolomoni G. Mid-dermal elastolysis: a clinical, histologic, and immunohistochemical study of 11 patients. Journal of American Academy of Dermatology (2003) 48: 846-851.

[2] Wang JF; Olson ME; Reno CR; Kulyk W; Wright JB; Hart DA. Molecular and cell biology of skin wound healing in a pig model. Connec Tissue (2000) 41: 195-211.

[3] Tenaud I; Sainte-Marie I; Jumbou O; Litoux P; Dreno B. In vitro modulation of keratinocyte wound healing integrins by zinc, copper and manganese. British Journal of Dermatology (1999) 140: 26-34.

[4] MacDougall JR; Bani MR; Lin Y. 'Proteolytic switching': opposite patterns of regulation of gelatinase B and its inhibitor TIMP-1 during human melanoma progression and consequences of gelatinase B overexpression. Br J Cancer (1999) 80: 504-512.

[5] Westermarck J; Kahari VM. Regulation of matrix metalloproteinase expression in tumor invasion. FASEB J (1999) 13: 781-792.

[6] Aimes RT; Quigley JP. Matrix metalloproteinase-2 is an interstitial collagenase. Inhibitor-free enzyme catalyzes the cleavage of collagen fibrils and soluble native type

I collagen generating the specific 3/4 – and 1/4 – length fragments. J Biol Chem (1995) 270: 5872-5876.

[7] Matrisian LM. The matrix-degrading metalloproteinases. Bioessays (1992) 14: 455-463.

[8] Nagase H; Woessner JF. Matrix metalloproteinases. J Biol Chem (1999) 274: 21491-21494.

[9] Birkedal-Hansen H; Moore WG; Bodden MK; Windsor LJ; Birkedal-Hansen B; DeCarlo A; Engler JA. Matrix metalloproteinases: a review. Crit Rev Oral Biol Med (1993) 4:197-250.

[10] Kazuki N; Teruhiko I; Yoshiya S; Tetsuro S. Matrix metalloproteinases in tumor invasion: Role for cell migration. Path Int. (2002) 52: 255-264.

[11] Merryman JI; Nielsen N; Staton DD. Transforming growth factor-beta enhances the ultraviolet-mediated stress response in p53-/- keratinocytes. Int. J. Oncol (1998) 13: 781-789.

[12] Philips N; Onwubalili N. Anti transforming growth factor-beta (TGF-β) increases the expressions of matrix metalloproteinase-1 (MMP-1) and growth factors in a renal adenocarcinoma cell line. Bios (2002) 73: 86-90.

[13] Philips N; McFadden K. Inhibition of transforming growth factor-beta and matrix metalloproteinases by estrogen and prolactin in breast cancer cells. Cancer Letters (2004) 206: 63-68.

[14] Philips N. An anti TGF-β increased the expression of transforming growth factor-β, matrix metallproteinase-1, and elastin, and its effects were antagonized by ultraviolet radiation in epidermal keratinocytes. J Dermatological Science (2003) 33: 177-179.

[15] Chen SJ; Yuan W; Mori Y; Levenson A; Trojanowaska M; Varga J. Stimulation of type I collagen transcription in human skin fibroblasts by TGF-beta: involvement of Smad 3. J Invest Dermatol (1999) 112: 49-57.

[16] Shin MH; Rhie GE; Park CH; Kim KH; Cho KH; Eun HC; Chung JH. Modulation of collagen metabolism by the topical application of dehydroepiandrosterone to human skin. J. Invest Dermatol (2005) 124: 315-323.

[17] Uitto J; Fazio MJ; Olsen D. Molecular mechanisms of cutaneous aging. J. Am Acad (1989) 21: 614-622.

[18] Varani J; Warner RL; Gharaee-Kermani M. Vitamin A antagonizes decreased cell growth and elevated collagen-degrading matrix metalloproteinases and stimulates collagen accumulation in naturally aged human skin. J. Invest Dermatol (2000) 114: 480-486.

[19] Lee C; Choi H; Kim H; Kim D; Chang I; Moon HT; Lee S; Oh WK; Woo E. Biflavonoids isolated from Selaginella tamariscina regulate the expression of matrix metalloproteinase in human skin fibroblasts. Bioorg Med Chem (2008) 16: 732-738.

[20] Khorramizadeh MR; Tredget EE; Telasky C; Shen Q; Ghahary A. Aging differentially modulates the expression of collagen and collagenase in dermal fibroblasts. Mol Cell Biochem (1999) 194: 99-108.

[21] Millis AJ; Hoyle M; McCue HM; Martini H. Differential expression of metalloproteinase and tissue inhibitor of metalloproteinase genes in aged human fibroblasts. Exp Cell Res (1992) 201: 373-379.

[22] Koh JS; Kang H; Choi SW; Kim HO. Cigarette smoking associated with premature facial wrinkling: image analysis of facial skin replicas. Int J Dermatol (2002) 41:21-27.

[23] Kadunce DP; Burr R; Gress R; Kanner R; Lyon JL; Zone JJ. Cigarette smoking: risk factor for premature facial wrinkling. Ann Intern Med (1991) 114: 840-844.

[24] Giacomoni PU; Rein G. Factors of skin ageing share common mechanisms. Biogerontology (2001) 2: 219-229.

[25] Seba BA. Dermatological manifestations of smoking. Harefuah (2002) 141: 736-740.

[26] Pasquali-Ronchetti I; Baccarani-Contri M. Elastic fiber during development and aging. Microsc Res Tech (1997) 38: 428-435.

[27] Berton A; Godeau G; Emonard H; Baba K; Bellon P; Hornebeck W; Bellon G. Analysis of the ex vivo specificity of human gelatinases A and B towards skin collagen and elastic fibers by computerized morphometry. Matrix Biology (2000) 19: 139-148.

[28] Brennan M; Bhatti H; Nerusu KC; Bhagavathula N; Kang S; Fisher GJ; Varani J; Voorhees JJ. Matrix metalloproteinase-1 is the major collagenolytic enzyme responsible for collagen damage in UV-irradiated human skin. Photochem Photobiol (2003) 78: 43-48.

[29] Tsuji N; Moriwaki S; Suzuki Y; Takema Y; Imokawa G. The role of elastases secreted by fibroblasts in wrinkle formation: implication through selective inhibition of elastase activity. Photochem Photobiol. (2001) 71: 283-290.

[30] Rijken F; Kiekens RC; van den Worm E; Lee PL; van Weelden H; Bruijnzeek PL. Pathophysiology of photoaging of human skin: focus on neutrophils. Photochem Photobiol Sci (2006) 5: 184-189.

[31] Rijken F; Kiekens RC; Bruijnzeek PL. Skin-infiltrating neutrophils following exposure to solar-simulated radiation could play an important role in photoageing of human skin. Br J Dermatol (2005) 152: 321-328.

[32] Jung E; Lee J; Baek J; Jung K; Lee J; Huh S; Kim S; Koh J; Park D. Effect of Camellia japonica oil on human type I procollagen production and skin barrier function. J Ethnopharmacol (2007) 112: 127-131.

[33] Cho HS; Lee MH; Lee JW; No KO; Park SK; Lee HS; Kang S; Cho WG; Park; HJ; Oh KW; Hong JT. Anti-wrinkling effects of the mixture of vitamin C; vitamin E; pycnogenol and evening primrose oil; and molecular mechanisms on hairless mouse skin caused by chronic ultraviolet B irradiation. Photodermatol Photoimmunol Photomed (2007) 23: 155-162.

[34] Labat-Robert J; Fourtanier A; Boyer-Lafargue B; Robert L. Age dependent increase of elastase type protease activity in mouse skin. Effect of UV-irradiation. J Photochem Photobiol B (2000) 57: 113-118.

[35] Francz PI; Conrad J; Biesalski HK. Modulation of UVA-induced lipid peroxidation and suppression of UVB-induced ornithine decarboxylase response by all-trans-retinoic acid in human skin fibroblasts in vitro. Biol Chem (1998) 379: 1263-1269.

[36] Marrot L; Meunier J. Skin DNA photodamage and its biological consequences. Journal of the American Academy of Dermatology (2008) 58: S139-S148.

[37] Moysan A; Marquis I; Gaboriau F; Santus R; Dubertret L; Morliere P. Ultraviolet A-induced lipid peroxidation and antioxidant defense systems in cultured human skin fibroblasts. Journal of Investigative Dermatology (1999) 100: 692-698.

[38] Scharffetter-Kochanek K; Brenneisen P; Wenk J; Herrmann G; Ma W; Kuhr L; Meewes C; Wlaschek M. Photoaging of the skin from phenotype to mechanisms. Experimental Gerontology (2000) 35: 307-316.

[39] Perez S; Sergent O; Morel P; Chevanne M; Dubos MP; Cillard P; Cillard J. Kinetics of lipid peroxidation induced by UV beta rays in human keratinocyte and fibroblast cultures. C R Seances Soc Biol Fil (1995) 189: 453-465.

[40] Tupet A; Lebreton-De Coster C; Dubertret L; Bernard C. Low doses of ultraviolet A Irradiation stimulate adhesion of human dermal fibroblasts by integrins in a protein kinase C-dependent pathway. J. Photochem Photobiol (1999) 49: 150-155.

[41] Petersen MJ; Hansen C; Craig S. Ultraviolet A irradiation stimulates collagenase production in cultured human fibroblasts. Journal of Investigative Dermatology (1992) 99: 440-444.

[42] Scharffetter K; Wlaschek M; Hogg A; Bolsen K; Schothorst A; Goerz G; Krieg T; Plewig G. UVA irradiation induces collagenase in human dermal fibroblasts in vitro and in vivo. Archives of Dermatological Research (1991) 283: 506-511.

[43] Quan T; He T; Kang S; Voorhees JJ; Fisher GJ. Ultraviolet irradiation alters transforming growth factor beta/smad pathway in human skin in vivo. Journal of Investigative Dermatology (2002) 119: 499-506.

[44] Wang H; Kochevar IE. Involvement of UVB-induced reactive oxygen species in TGF-beta biosynthesis and activation in keratinocytes. Free Radic Biol Med (2005) 38: 890-897.

[45] Vojdani A; Mordechai E; Brautbar N. Abnormal apoptosis and cell cycle progression in humans exposed to methyl tertiary-butyl ether and benzene contaminated water. Hum Exp Toxicol (1997) 16: 485-494.

[46] Paustenbach DJ; Bass RD; Price P. Benzene Toxicity and Risk Assessment; 1972-1992: Implications for Future Regulation. Environ Health Perspect (1993) 101: 117-200.

[47] Gist GL; Burg JR. Benzene-a review of the literature from a health effects perspective. Toxicology and Industrial Health (1997) 13: 661-713.

[48] Hiraku Y; Kawanishi S. Oxidative DNA damage and apoptosis induced by benzene metabolites. Cancer Res (1996) 56: 5172-5178.

[49] Lewis JG; Stewart W; Adams DO. Role of oxygen radicals in induction of DNA damage by metabolites of benzene. Cancer Res (1988) 48: 4762-4765.

[50] Joseph P; Klein-Szanto AJP; Jaiswal AK. Hydroquinones cause specific mutations and lead to cellular transformation and in vivo tumorigenesis. Br J Cancer Res (1998) 78: 312-320.

[51] Seaton MJ; Schlosser PM; Bond JA; Medinsky MA. Benzene metabolism by human liver microsomes in relation to cytochrome P450 2E1 activity. Carcinogenesis (1994) 15: 1799-1806.

[52] Gut I; Nedelcheva V; Soucek P; Stopka P; Tichavska B. Cytochromes P450 in benzene metabolism and involvement of their metabolites and reactive oxygen species in toxicity. Environ Health Perspect (1996) 104: 1211-1218.

[53] Li Q; Aubrey MT; Christian T; Freed BM. Differential inhibition of DNA synthesis in human T cells by the cigarette tar components hydroquinone and catechol. Fundam Appl Toxicol (1997) 38: 158-165.

[54] Rubin H. Synergistic mechanisms in carcinogenesis by polycyclic aromatic hydrocarbons and by tobacco smoke: a bio-historic perspective with updates. Carcinogenesis (2001) 22: 1903-1930.

[55] Moran JL; Siegel D; Sun X; Ross D. Induction of apoptosis by benzene metabolites in HL60 and CD34+ human bone marrow progenitor cells. Mol Pharmacol (1996) 50: 610-615.

[56] Philips N; Burchill D; O'Donoghue D; Keller T; Gonzalez S. Identification of benzene metabolites in dermal fibroblasts: Regulation of cell viability; apoptosis; lipid peroxidation; and expression of MMP-1 and elastin by benzene metabolites. Skin Pharmacol and Physiol (2004) 17: 147-152.

[57] Susten AS; Niemeier RW; Simon SD. In vivo percutaneous absorption studies of volatile organic solvents in hairless mice. II. Toluene; ethylbenzene and aniline. J Appl Toxicol (1990) 10:217-225.

[58] Blank IH; McAuliffe DJ. Penetration of benzene through human skin. J Invest Dermatol (1985) 85: 522-526.

[59] McDougal JN; Jepson GW; Clewell HJ; Gargas ML; Andersen ME. Dermal absorption of organic chemical vapours in rats and humans. Fundam Appl Toxicol (1990) 14: 299-308.

[60] Morgan DL; Cooper SW; Carlock DL; Sykora JJ; Sutton B; Mattie DR; McDougal JN. Dermal absorption of neat and aqueous volatile organic chemicals in the Fisher 344 rat. Environ Res (1991) 55: 51-63.

[61] Moody RP; Nadeau B. An automated in vitro dermal absorption procedure: III. In vivo and in vitro comparison with the insect repellent N;N-diethyl-m-toluamide in mouse; rat; guinea pig; pig; human and tissue-cultured skin. Toxicol In Vitro (1993) 7: 167-176.

[62] Nakai JS; Chu I; Li-Muller A; Aucoin R. Effect of environmental conditions on the penetration of benzene through human skin. J Toxicol Environ Health (1997) 51: 447-462.

[63] Kalnas J; Teitelbaum DT. Dermal absorption of benzene: implications for work practices and regulations. Int J Occup Environ Health (2000) 6: 114-121.

[64] Hanke J; Dutkiewicz T; Piotrowski J. The absorption of benzene through human skin. Int J Occup Environ Health (2000) 6: 104-111.

[65] Franz TJ. Percutaneous absorption on the relevance of in vitro data. J Invest Dermatol (1975) 64: 190-195.

[66] Kao J; Carver MP. Cutaneous metabolism of xenobiotics. Drug Met Rev (1990) 22: 363-410.

[67] Pannatier A; Jenner P; Testa B; Etter JC. The skin as a drug-metabolizing organ. Drug Met Rev (1978) 8: 319-343.

[68] Merk H; Jugert F; Bonnekoh B; Mahrle G Induction and inhibition of NAD(P)H: quinone reductase in murine and human skin. Skin Pharmacology (1991) 4: 183-190.

[69] Jugert FK; Agarwal R; Kuhn A; Bickers DR; Merk HF; Mukhtar H. Multiple cytochrome P450 isozymes in murine skin: induction of P450 1A; 2B; 2E; and 3A by dexamethasone. J Invest Dermatol (1994) 102: 970-975

[70] Ahmad N; Agarwal R; Mukhtar H. Cytochrome P-450 and drug development for skin diseases. Skin Pharmacol (1996) 9:231-241.

[71] Lehmann B; Tiebel O; Meurer M. Expression of vitamin D3 25-hydroxylase (CYP27) mRNA after induction by vitamin D3 or UVB radiation in keratinocytes of human skin equivalents—a preliminary study. Arch Dermatol Res (1999) 291: 507-510.

[72] Braier L. Anti-benzene compounds. Conversion of Benzene to Toluene by Methyl Donors; in Man. Rev Bras Pesqui Med Biol (1977) 10: 319-323.

[73] Braier L. Conversion of Benzene to Toluene by Methyl Donors in Man. Nouv Rev Fr Hematol (1978) 20: 63-66.

[74] Beatty S; Boulton M; Henson D; Koh HH; Murray IJ. Macular pigment and age related macular degeneration. Br J Ophthalmol (1999) 83: 867-877.

[75] Broekmans WMR; Berendschot TTJM; Klöpping-Ketelaars IAA; de Vries AJ; Goldbohm RA; Tjiburg BM. Macular pigment density in relation to serum and adipose tissue concentrations of lutein and serum concentrations of zeaxanthin. Am J Clin Nutr (2002) 76: 595-603.

[76] Pratt S. Dietary prevention of age-related macular degeneration. J Am Optom Assoc (1990) 70: 39-47.

[77] Gonzalez S; Astner S; An W; Goukassian D; Pathak MA. Dietary lutein/zeaxanthin decreases ultraviolet B-induced epidermal hyperproliferation and acute inflammation in hairless mice. J Invest Dermatol (2003) 121: 399-405.

[78] Wingerath T; Sies H; Stahl W. Xanthophyll esters in human skin. Arch Biochem Biophys (1998) 355: 271-274.

[79] Khachik F; Beecher GR; Smith JC. Lutein; lycopene; and their oxidative metabolites in chemoprevention of cancer. J Cell Biochem (1995) 22: 236-246.

[80] Kozuki Y; Miura Y; Yagasaki K. Inhibitory effects of carotenoids on the invasion of rat ascites hepatoma cells in culture. Cancer Letters (2000) 151: 111-115.

[81] Narisawa T; Fukaura Y; Hasebe M; Michiko I; Aizawa R; Murakoshi M; Uemura S; Khachik F; Nishino H. Inhibitory effects of natural carotenoids, ol-carotene, B-carotene, lycopene and lutein on colonic aberrant crypt foci formation in rats. Cancer Letters (1996) 106: 137-142.

[82] Slattery ML; Benson J; Curtin K; Khe-NI M; Schaeffer D; Potter JD. Carotenoids and colon cancer1-4. Am J Clin Nutr (2000) 71: 575-582.

[83] Millen AE; Tucker MA; Hartge P; Halpern A; Elder DE; Guerry D 4th; Holly EA; Sagebiel RW; Potischman N. Diet and melanoma in a case-control study. Cancer Epidemiol Biomarkers Prev. (2004) 13: 1042-1051.

[84] Philips N; Keller T; Hendrix C; Hamilton S; Arena R; Tuason M; Gonzalez S. Regulation of the Extracellular Matrix Remodeling by Lutein in Dermal Fibroblasts; Melanoma cells; and Ultraviolet Radiation Exposed Fibroblasts. Arch Dermatol Res (2007) 299: 373-379.

[85] Astner S; Wu A; Chen J; Philips N; Rius-Diaz F; Parrado C; Mihm MC; Goukassian DA; Pathak MA; González; S. Dietary lutein/zeaxanthin reduces photoaging and

photocarcinogenesis in chronically UVB irradiated SKH -1 hairless mice. Skin Pharmacol and Physiol (2007) 20:281-283

[86] Alcaraz MV; Pathak MA; Rius F; Kollias Nl; Gonzalez S. An extract of polypodium leucotomos appears to minimize certain photoaging changes in a hairless albino mouse animal model. Photodermatol Photoimmunol Photomed (1999) 15: 120-126.

[87] Gonzalez S; Alcaraz MV; Cuevas J; Perez M; Jaen P; Alvarex-Mon M; Villarrubia VG. An extract of the fern polypodium leucotomos (Difur®) modulates Th1/Th2 cytokines balance in vitro and appears to exhibit anti-angiogenic activities in vivo: pathogenic relationships and therapeutic implications. Anticancer Research (2000) 20: 1567-1576.

[88] Gonzalez S; Pathak MA; Cuevas J; Villarrubia VG; Fitzpatrick TB. Topical or oral administration with an extract of polypodium leucotomos prevents acute sunburn and psoralen induced phototoxic reactions as well as depletion of Langerhans cells in human skin. Photodermatol Photoimmunol Photomed (1997) 13: 50-60.

[89] Fernandez-Novoa L; Alvarex XA; Dempere JM; Miguel-Hidalgo JJ; Diaz J; Franco-Maside A; Cacabelos R. Effects of anapsos on the activity of the enzyme cu-zn-superoxide dismutase in an animal model of neuronal degeneration. Exp Clin Parmacol (1997) 19: 99-106.

[90] Bernd A; Ramirez-Bosca A; Huber H; Diaz-Alperi J; Thaci D; Sewell A Auintanilla-Almagro E; Holzmann H. In vitro studies on the immunomodulating effects of poloypodium leucotomos extract on human leukocyte fractions. Arzneim-Forsch Drug Res (1995) 45: 901-904.

[91] Gonzalez S; Pathak MS. Inhibition of ultraviolet-induced formation of reactive oxygen species, lipid peroxidation, erythema and skin photosensitization by Polypodium leucotomos. Photodermatol Photoimmunol Photomed (1996) 12: 45-56.

[92] Philips N; Smith J; Keller T; Gonzalez S. Predominant effects of Polypodium leucotomos on membrane integrity; lipid peroxidation; and expression of elastin and matrixmetalloproteinase-1 in ultraviolet radiation exposed fibroblasts; and keratinocytes. J Dermatol Sci (2003) 32: 1-9.

[93] Janczyk A; Garcia-Lopez MA; Penas P; Alonso-Lebrero JL; Benedicto I; Lopez-Cabrera; Gonzalez S. A Polypodium leucotomos extract (PL) inhibits solar-simulated radiation-induced TNF-α and iNOS expression; transcriptional activation and apoptosis. Expt Dermatol. (2007) In press.

[94] Doyle GA; Pierce RA; and Parks WC. Transcriptional Induction of Collagenase-1 in Differentiated Monocyte-like (U937) Cells is Regulated by AP-1 and an Upstream C/EBP-β Site. J Biol Chem (1997) 272: 11840-11849.

[95] Edwards DR; Leco KJ; Beaudry PP; Atadja PW; Veillette C; and Riabowol KT. Differential effects of transforming growth factor-beta 1 on the expression of matrix metalloproteinases and tissue inhibitors of metalloproteinases in young and old human fibroblasts. Exp Gerantol (1996) 31: 207-223.

[96] Kaminska B; Wesolowska A; Danilkiewicz M. TGF beta signalling and its role in tumour pathogenesis. Acta Biochim Pol (2005) 329-337.

[97] Nikolic D; Li Y; Chadwick LR; Pauli GF; van Breemen RB. Metabolism of xanthohumol and isoxanthohumol; prenylated flavonoids from hops (Humulus lupulus L.); by human liver microsomes. J Mass Spectrom (2005) 40: 289-299.

[98] Delmulle L; Bellahcène A; Dhooge W; Comhaire F; Roelens F; Huvaere K; Heyerick A; Castronovo V; De Keukeleire D. Anti-proliferative properties of prenylated flavonoids from hops (Humulus lupulus L.) in human prostate cancer cell lines. Phytomedicine (2006) 13:732-734.

[99] Lust S; Vanhoecke B; Janssens A; Philippe J; Bracke M; Offner F. Xanthohumol kills B-chronic lymphocytic leukemia cells by an apoptotic mechanism. Mol Nutr Food Res (2005) 49: 844-850.

[100] Yang JY; Della-Fera MA; Rayalam S; Baile CA. Effect of xanthohumol and isoxanthohumol on 3T3-L1 cell apoptosis and adipogenesis. Apoptosis (2007) 12: 1953-1963.

[101] Delmulle L; Berghe TV; Keukeleire DD; Vandenabeele P. Treatment of PC-3 and DU145 prostate cancer cells by prenylflavonoids from hop (Humulus lupulus L.) induces a caspase-independent form of cell death. Phytother Res (2007).

[102] Monteiro R; Faria A; Azevedo I; Calhau C. Modulation of breast cancer cell survival by aromatase inhibiting hop (Humulus lupulus L.) flavonoids. J Steroid Biochem Mol Biol (2007) 105: 124-130.

[103] Vanhoecke B; Derycke L; Van Marck V; Depypere H; De Keukeleire D; Bracke M. Antiinvasive effect of xanthohumol; a prenylated chalcone present in hops (Humulus lupulus L.) and beer. Int J Cancer (2005) 117: 889-895.

[104] Lemay M; Murray MA; Davies A; Roh-Schmidt H; Randolph R. In vitro and ex vivo cyclooxygenase inhibition by a hops extract. Asia Pac J Clin Nutr (2004) 13: S110.

[105] Tripp M; Darland G; Lerman R; Lukaczer D; Bland J; Babish J. Hop and Modified Hop Extracts have potent in vitro anti-inflammatory properties. Acta Hort (2005) 668: 217-228.

[106] Gerhauser C; Alt A; Heiss E; Gamal-Eldeen A; Klimo K; Knauft J; Neumann I; Scherf HR; Frank N; Bartsch H; Becker H. Cancer chemopreventive activity of Xanthohumol; a natural product derived from hop. Mol Cancer Ther (2002) 1: 959-969.

[107] Noonan M; Benelli R; Albini A. Angiogenesis and cancer prevention: a vision.Recent Results Cancer Res (2007) 174: 219-224.

[108] Colgte EC; Miranda CL; Stevens JF; Bray TM; Ho E. Xanthohumol; a prenylflavonoid derived from hops induces apoptosis and inhibits NF-kappaB activation in prostate epithelial cells. Cancer Letters (2007) 246: 201-209.

[109] Albini A; Dell'Eva R; Vené R; Ferrari N; Buhler DR; Noonan DM; Fassina G. Mechanisms of the antiangiogenic activity by the hop flavonoid xanthohumol: NF-kappaB and Akt as targets. FASEB J (2006) 20: 527-529.

[110] Zhao F; Nozawa H; Daikonnya A; Kondo K; Kitanaka S. Inhibitors of nitric oxide production from hops (Humulus lupulus L.). Biol Pharm Bull (2003) 26: 61-65.

[111] Overk CR; Yao P; Chadwick LR; Nikolic D; Sun Y; Cuendet MA; Deng Y; Hedayat AS; Pauli GF; Farnsworth NR; van Breemen RB; Bolton JL. Comparison of the in vitro estrogenic activities of compounds from hops (Humulus lupulus) and red clover (Trifolium pratense). J Agric Food Chem (2005) 53: 6246-6253.

[112] Effenberger KE; Johnsen SA; Monroe DG; Spelsberg TC; Westendorf JJ. Regulation of osteoblastic phenotype and gene expression by hop-derived phytoestrogens. J Steroid Biochem Mol Biol (2005) 96: 387-399.

[113] Monteiro R; Becker H; Azevedo I; Calhau C. Effect of hop (Humulus lupulus L.) flavonoids on aromatase (estrogen synthase) activity. J Agric Food Chem (2006) 54: 2938-2943.

[114] Guerreiro S; Monteiro R; Martins MJ; Calhau C; Azevedo I; Soares R. Distinct modulation of alkaline phosphatase isoenzymes by 17beta-estradiol and xanthohumol in breast cancer MCF-7 cells. Clin Biochem (2007) 40:268-273.

[115] Plazar J; Filipič M; Groothuis GM. Antigenotoxic effect of Xanthohumol in rat liver slices. Toxicol In Vitro (2007).

[116] Luo Y; Eggler AL; Liu D; Liu G; Mesecar AD; van Breemen RB. Sites of alkylation of human keap1 by natural chemoprevention agents. J Am Soc Mass Spectrom (2007) 18: 2226-2232.

[117] Plazar J; Zegura B; Lah TT; Filipic M. Protective effects of xanthohumol against the genotoxicity of benzo(a)pyrene (BaP); 2-amino-3-methylimidazo[4;5-f]quinoline (IQ) and tert-butyl hydroperoxide (t-BOOH) in HepG2 human hepatoma cells. Mutat Res (2007) 632: 1-8.

[118] Liu G; Eggler AL; Dietz BM; Mesecar AD; Bolton JL; Pezzuto JM; van Breemen RB. Screening method for the discovery of potential cancer chemoprevention agents based on mass spectrometric detection of alkylated Keap1. Anal Chem (2005) 77: 6407-6414.

[119] Dietz BM; Kang YH; Liu G; Eggler AL; Yao P; Chadwick LR; Pauli GF; Farnsworth NR; Mesecar AD; van Breemen RB; Bolton JL. Xanthohumol isolated from Humulus lupulus Inhibits menadione-induced DNA damage through induction of quinone reductase. Chem Res Toxicol (2005) 18: 1296-1305.

[120] Miranda CL; Yang YH; Henderson MC; Stevens JF; Santana-Rios G; Deinzer ML; Buhler DR. Prenylflavonoids from hops inhibit the metabolic activation of the carcinogenic heterocyclic amine 2-amino-3-methylimidazo[4; 5-f]quinoline; mediated by cDNA-expressed human CYP1A2. Drug Metab Dispos (2000) 28: 1297-1302.

[121] Miranda CL; Aponso GL; Stevens JF; Deinzer ML; Buhler DR. Prenylated chalcones and flavanones as inducers of quinone reductase in mouse Hepa 1c1c7 cells. Cancer Letters (2000) 149: 21-29.

[122] Henderson MC; Miranda CL; Stevens JF; Deinzer ML; Buhler DR. In vitro inhibition of human P450 enzymes by prenylated flavonoids from hops; Humulus lupulus. Xenobiotica (2000) 30:235-251.

[123] Lee SH; Kim HJ; Lee JS; Lee IS; Kang BY. Inhibition of topoisomerase I activity and efflux drug transporters' expression by xanthohumol from hops. Arch Pharm Res (2007) 30: 1435-1439.

[124] Im; S; Lee; E; Kim; W; Song; J; Kim; J; Lee; M; Kang; W. Expression of Progersterone Receptor in Human Keratinocytes. J Korean Med Sci (2000) 15: 647-654.

[125] Ikeda T; Shigeno C; Kasai R; Kohno H; Ohta S; Okumura H; Konishi J; Yamamuro T. Ovariectomy Decreases the mRNA Levels of Transforming Growth Factor-Beta 1 and Increases the mRNA levels of Osteocalcin in Rat Bone in Vivo. Biochem Biophys Res Commun (1993) 194: 1228-1233.

[126] Tranquilli A; Mazzanti L; Cugini A; Cester N; Garzetti G; Romanini C. Transdermal Estradiol and Medroxyprogesterone Acetate in Hormone Replacement Therapy are Both Antioxidants. Gynecol Endocrinol (1995) 9: 137-141.

[127] Leal M; Diaz J; Serrano E; Abellan J; Carbonell L. Hormone Replacement Therapy for Oxidative Stress in Postmenopausal Women with Hot Flushes. Obstet Gynecol (2000) 95: 804-809.

[128] Ayres S; Abplanalp W; Liu J; Subbiah M. Mechanisms Involved in the Protective effect of Estradiol-17 Beta on lipid Peroxidation and DNA damage. Am J Physiol (1998) 274: E1002-E1008.

[129] Philips N; Devaney J. Beneficial Regulation of Type I Collagen and Matrixmetalloproteinase–1 Expression by Estrogen; Progesterone; and its Combination in Skin Fibroblasts J Am Aging Association (2004) 26: 59-62.

[130] Yuan W; Varga J. Transforming Growth Factor – beta Repression of Matrix Metalloproteinase–1 in dermal fibroblasts involve Smad3. J Biol Chem (2001) 276: 38302-38310.

[131] Overall CM; Wrana JL; Sodek J. Transcriptional and post-transcriptional regulation of 72-kDa gelatinase/typeIV collagenase by transforming growth factor-beta 1 in human fibroblasts. Comparison with collagenase and tissue inhibitor of matrix metalloproteinase gene expression. J Biol Chem (1991) 266: 14064-14071.

[132] Chegini N. The role of growth factors in peritoneal healing: transforming growth factor beta (TGF-beta). Eur J Surg Suppl (1997) 577: 17-23.

[133] Ellis IR; Schor SL. Differential Effects of TGF-b1 on Hyaluronan Synthesis by fetal and Adult Skin Fibroblasts: Implications for Cell Migration and Wound Healing. Experiment Cell Res (1996) 228: 326-333.

[134] Gosiewska A; Yi CF; Brown LJ; Cullen B; Silcock D; Geesin JC. Differential expression and regulation of extracellular matrix associated genes in fetal and neonatal fibroblasts. Wound Repair Regen (2001) 9: 213-224.

[135] Kawakami T; Ihn H; Xu W; Smith E; LeRoy C; Trojanowaska M. Increased expression of TGF –beta receptors by scleroderma fibroblasts: evidence for contribution autocrine TGF –beta signaling to scleroderma phenotype. J Invest Dermatol (1998) 110: 47-51.

[136] Lin RY; Sullivan KM; Argenta PA; Meuli M; Lorenz HP; Adzick NS. Exogenous transforming growth factor beta amplifies its own expression and induces scar formation in a model of a human fetal skin repair. Ann Surg (1995) 222: 146-154.

[137] Menke A; Geerling I; Giehl K; Vogelmann R; Reinshagen M; Adler G. Transforming growth factor beta induced up regulation of transforming growth factor beta receptor expression in pancreatic regeneration. Biochim Biophys Acta (1999) 1449: 178-185.

[138] Chodon T; Sugihara T; Igawa HH; Funayama E; Furukawa H. Keloid-derived fibroblasts are refractory to Fas-mediated apoptosis and neutralization of autocrine transforming growth factor-beta1 can abrogate this resistance. Am J Pathol (2000) 157: 1661-1669.

[139] Brahmatewari J; Serafini A; Serralta V; Mertz PM; and Eaglstein WH. The effects of topical transforming growth factor beta 2,3 on scarring in pigs. J Cutan Med Surg J (2000): 126-131.

[140] Wang X; Smith P; Pu LLQ; Kim YJ; Ko F; and Robson MC. Exogenous transforming growth factor b2 modulates collagen I and collagen III synthesis in proliferative scar xenografts in nude rats. J Surg Res (1999) 87:194-200.

[141] Philips N; Keller T; Gonzalez S. TGF-β like regulation of matrix mettalloproteinases by anti transforming growth factor-β and anti transforming growth factor-β1 antibodies in dermal fibroblasts: implications to wound healing. Wound Rep Reg (2004) 12: 53-59.

[142] Philips N; Arena R; and Yarlagadda S. Inhibition of Ultraviolet Radiation mediated Extracellular Matrix Remodeling in Fibroblasts by Transforming Growth Factor-β. Bios (2008) : in press

In: Skin Anatomy and Physiology Research Developments
Editor: Leon F. Bukowsky
ISBN: 978-1-60741-469-8

Chapter 7

Comparative *in Vitro-In Vivo* Skin Permeation of Cosmetic Ingredients

V. Iannuccelli[a*], G. Coppi[a] and S. Scalia[b]

[a]Department of Pharmaceutical Sciences, University of Modena and Reggio Emilia, Italy

[b]Department of Pharmaceutical Sciences, University of Ferrara, Italy

Abstract

The potential EU ban on the use of animals in the testing of cosmetic products and their ingredients from 2009 together with the ethical reasons for avoiding tests on humans have recently prompted the development of guidelines on *in vitro* alternative methods and an extensive search for novel validated *in vitro* permeation models. The prediction of the percutaneous absorption by means of *in vitro* methodologies requires good *in vitro-in vivo* correlation. Moreover, due to differences in the type of vehicle (conventional vehicles or particulate carriers) and in the physicochemical properties of a substance such as its solubility, the selection of appropriate *in vitro* conditions is crucial. In particular, the validation of an *in vitro* skin penetration model appears quite difficult for highly lipophilic substances because of their limited rate of transfer between the stratum corneum and the viable epidermis due to their low solubility in most physiological receptor fluids.

This chapter focuses on comparative *in vitro-in vivo* skin permeation of butyl methoxydibenzoylmethane, a highly lipophilic UV-A absorber (log $P_{o/w}$ = 5.6); methylbenzylidene camphor (log $P_{o/w}$ = 4.8), a less lipophilic sunscreen agent; and glycolic acid, a hydrophilic active substance (log $P_{o/w} < 0$). Special attention is paid to the influence of the *in vitro* receptor medium on the *in vitro-in vivo* correlation. Skin absorption of micro- and nanoparticulate carriers and their suitability for cosmetic formulations are also reviewed.

[*] Corresponding Author: e-mail: valentina.iannuccelli@unimore.it

Introduction

Percutaneous absorption is strongly affected by the physicochemical properties of the active substance, such as molecular weight (MW) and liposolubility (octanol/water partition coefficient, log $P_{o/w}$) as well as by the nature and properties of the vehicle in which it is applied. Lien and Tong have shown an increasing flux through the skin as a function of increasing octanol/water partition coefficient over a very wide range for two different homologous series of compounds: alcohols and steroids. It should be noted that the fluxes of alcohols were about two or three orders of magnitude higher than those of steroids at equal partition coefficients [1]. A relationship between the permeability coefficient K_p and log $P_{o/w}$ and MW of the permeant was demonstrated from *in vitro* data [2]:

$$\log K_p = -2.7 + 0.71 \log P_{o/w} - 0.0061 \text{ MW}$$

However, this equation doesn't consider tissue distribution, affinity of the compound with available binding site in the skin, metabolism in the viable tissue and excretion. Generally, for substances with log $P_{o/w}$ above 4, the rate of penetration may be limited by the rate of transfer between the stratum corneum (SC) and the viable epidermis. For example, the SC could represent not only a barrier but also a reservoir for clobetasol proprionate which was located in the upper part of the SC after a topical application on human skin [3]. Values between 1 and 4 favour dermal and hence systemic absorption, particularly if the substance is more lipid soluble than water soluble. For substances with log $P_{o/w}$ values below 0, hydrophilicity will limit penetration into the SC. In fact, removal of the SC by tape-stripping resulted in a 1300 fold increase in penciclovir (log $P_{o/w}$ = -2.03) absorption and a 440-fold increase in aciclovir (log $P_{o/w}$ = -1.76) absorption, confirming that the SC is the major barrier to hydrophilic drug absorption [4].

The nature of the vehicle is known to affect greatly the skin penetration of active substances owing to its role in their solubility and release as well as in the Trans Epidermal Water Loss (TEWL). More precisely, the thermodynamic activity of the penetrant (chemical potential) in the vehicle determines the rate of transfer more than its concentration in the vehicle. The human skin permeability of nonsteroidal antiinflammatory drugs (NSAIDs) applied in a lipophilic vehicle is a function of their vehicle solubilities, decreasing with increasing NSAIDs' lipophilicity [5]. In these lipophilic formulations the viable epidermis, not the SC, is the rate-limiting barrier for the transport of NSAIDs. Moreover, the nature of the vehicle could determine occlusion-induced enhancement in the penetration of the active compound. It appears that the relationship linking TEWL and percutaneous absorption is independent of the physicochemical properties of the applied compound [6]. Percutaneous absorption could be strongly affected by micro- or nanoparticulate systems. For solid particulate microcarriers, a penetration into the stratum corneum of the intact particles could be excluded owing to the micrometer size [7]. However, they can deliver active substances into the hair follicles or they can act as follicle blockers to stop the penetration of topically applied substances [8]. In fact, microparticles with a diameter <1.5 μm were found in hair follicles up to a depth >2 mm with a maximum penetration depth for 1 μm diameter particles [9]. Similarly, larger microparticles (3–10 μm) topically applied to human skin clustered at the hair follicle (Figure 1) [10].

As far as nanoparticles are concerned, some authors have stated that they do not penetrate intracellularly, nor between corneocytes of the SC, but that they diffuse into the hair follicles [11, 12]. Polystirene nanoparticles (20–200 nm) accumulated preferentially in the follicular openings of porcine skin and no evidence for uptake of the vectors away from the follicles was observed [12]. Contrary to this, metallic nanoparticles smaller than 10 nm were observed to penetrate the hair follicle and SC through the lipidic matrix, occasionally reaching the viable epidermis [13]. Kreligaard argued that very small titanium dioxide particles (5–20 nm) penetrate into the skin and can interact with the immune system [14]. Moreover, the comparison between the penetration of coenzyme Q10 from lipid microparticles and lipid nanoparticles showed an increased penetration of the active substance when applying the nanoparticles, owing to their greater occlusive effect [15]. Because of the controversial results, several international organizations are focusing on precautionary principles to avoid the risk associated with nanoparticles, specifically with insoluble nanomaterials presently used in sunscreens [16-18]. With regard to liposomes, they mix with skin lipids providing either localized effects, reduced percutaneous absorption, targeted delivery to skin appendages or improved transdermal delivery [19]. Micro-sized and even submicron-sized liposomes did not easily penetrate into the viable epidermis, while liposomes with an average diameter of 272 nm can reach the viable epidermis, and some are found in the dermis. Smaller-sized liposomes (71–116 nm) were found in higher concentration in the dermis [20].

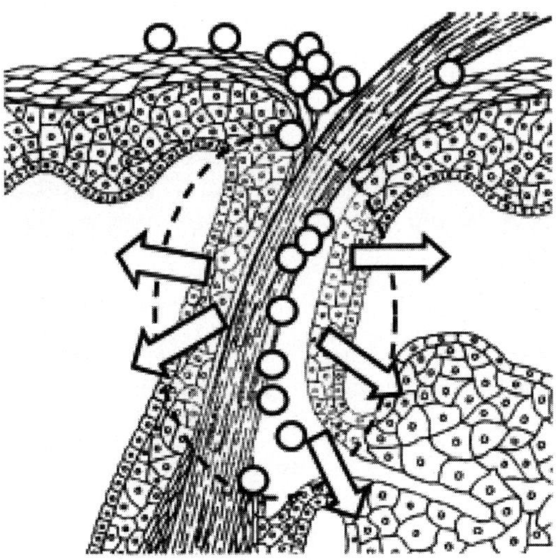

Figure 1. Microparticles enter selectively into the hair follicle and may yield high local concentrations of the active compound. The controlled destabilization of the microspheres may allow a controlled release of the compounds. The penetration depth depends on the size of the particles and the size of the target (from ref. n. 10 with permission from Nature Publishing Group).

To measure percutaneous absorption, human volunteer studies by means of tape-stripping together with blood, urine and faeces collection represent the best method. However, many *in vivo* experiments take into account only the data obtained by means of the tape-stripping technique on humans. The underlying basis of the method is the correlation between short-term uptake and steady-state permeability. It is hypothesized that if a compound is applied to the skin for a limited time (for example, for 30 min) the amount of chemical in the upper layers of the SC will equal the fraction that ultimately reaches the systemic circulation [21]. Tape-stripping, involving a gradual removal of SC cells which transfer the corneocyte aggregates as well as the topically applied substances to the tape strips, is a simple, inexpensive and non invasive method to measure *in vivo* skin penetration into the SC. It has been proposed by the American Association of Pharmaceutical Scientists/Food and Drug Administration (AAPS/FDA) as part of a standard method to evaluate bioequivalence of topical dermatological dosage forms [22]. For a range of compounds (mostly low molecular weight, low lipophilicity) the amount of active in the SC after 30 min application and subsequent removal of the vehicle, was determined by tape-stripping [23]. The same 30 min application was carried out to quantify the penetration of chemical by its urinary excretion over the next four days. Good correlation between the two measurements was observed suggesting the suitability of the tape-stripping approach in the evaluation of the absorption extent.

Alternatively, many animal species and strains have been used for studying skin absorption with the rat being used most frequently. However, animal studies will typically overestimate the human systemic levels of chemicals following dermal exposure since the animal skin is often more permeable than human skin [21]. Moreover, there is increasing pressure for industry to reduce the numbers of animals in safety testing.

In the cosmetic field, by considering the potential EU ban on the use of animals in the testing of cosmetic products and their ingredients from 2009 and the ethical reasons for avoiding tests on human beings, an extensive search for novel validated *in vitro* penetration models is recommended by several scientific organizations, such as the Scientific Committee on Cosmetic Products and Non-Food Products Intended for Consumers (SCCNFP) [24], the Scientific Committee on Consumer Products (SCCP) [25], the European Cosmetic Toiletry and Perfumery Association (COLIPA) [26], the European Centre for the Validation of Alternative Methods (ECVAM) [21] and the Organization for Economic Cooperation and Development (OECD) [27], which have prepared recently guidelines on alternative methods. However, as it was noticed by OECD, it is especially difficult to examine very lipophilic substances *in vitro* and, consequently, to find good *in vitro-in vivo* correlations because of their low solubility in most physiological receptors fluids as well as their binding to skin components.

Basic criteria for the *in vitro* assessment of percutaneous absorption adopted by the current guidelines identify the SC as the principal diffusion barrier. The viability of the skin is not a pre-requisite for penetration testing, since the process depends on passive diffusion. Excised human or animal skin are recommended, though the scarcity of human tissue and the high intra- and interindividual variability of both human and animal skin are disadvantages [28, 29]. The concentration of the active in the receptor fluid should be less than 10% of its saturation level, in order to prevent underestimation of absorption [25, 26]. While there is a general agreement for hydrophilic substances, for which a saline or buffered saline solution is recommended, it is not yet possible to define the optimal receiving fluid for lipophilic compounds. There is a tendency for the use of solubilizers (serum albumin, non-ionic surfactants, PEG 20) [26, 29] even if an overestimation of absorption is described [29], or of aqueous-ethanolic phases [21, 29] which are not physiologically realistic and can provide overestimations, too [30]. *In vitro* methods have been widely used for studying the relative percutaneous absorption of compounds from different vehicles. Typically, the results of these *in vitro* experiments accurately reflect the vehicle effects seen *in vivo* [21].

In Vitro-In Vivo Skin Permeation of Butyl Methoxydibenzoylmethane (BMDBM)

Australia, Canada and the USA regulate sunscreen products as drugs, whereas the EU classifies sunscreens in the cosmetic category. Notwithstanding this, EU authorities acknowledge the role of anti-UV products in preventing skin damage and, recently, they have been focused on UV-A absorbers recommending that sunscreen products should provide a sufficient protection not only against UV-B (290–320 nm) but also against UV-A (320–400 nm) radiation [31]. Another important characteristic that sunscreens should have is minimal percutaneous penetration as they exert their effect on the skin surface or within the uppermost layers of the SC. Among the authorized UV-A absorbers, butyl methoxydibenzoylmethane (BMDBM) is the most efficient and widely used compound even if it decomposes under sunlight exposure. In earlier investigations, it was shown that the light-induced decomposition of BMDBM was significantly reduced by loading the sunscreen in lipid microparticles [32]. Lipospheres, lipoparticles consisting of a solid fat core stabilized by a layer of phospholipid molecules at the surface, utilize naturally occurring lipids having chemical affinity with cutaneous components. On the basis of these remarks and by considering the known difficulty to examine very lipophilic substances, BMDBM *in vitro* skin permeation was evaluated by using a nylon membrane soaked in a lipophilic medium (dodecyl alcohol), as a skin model. A synthetic membrane could represent a useful model for the human skin barrier owing to stability, interbatch uniformity, ease of usage and commercial availability. Although it could not be considered a physiological and realistic skin, it was shown to replicate the barrier properties of skin [33] and it could represent an appropriate model for permeants which exhibit high lipophilicity (log $P_{o/w} > 4$) and diffuse through the SC *via* the lamellar lipid domains (intercellular route). The lipophilic membrane was assembled in a static diffusion cell placed horizontally and connected with a receptor compartment. The static cell, in accordance with the procedures described in SCCP guideline for the *in vitro* permeation study [25], can be considered as an appropriate diffusion design for highly lipophilic permeants (log $P_{o/w} > 4$) having slow rate of transfer between the SC and the viable epidermis. An O/W emulsion, containing 2% of BMDBM alone or loaded in lipospheres, represented the donor compartment. The experimentation involved two different receptor media, a mixture of ethanol 96%/Mygliol (9:1) in which BMDBM is highly soluble (11%, w/v), and a phosphate buffer solution at pH 7.4 containing 1.5% bovine serum albumin, in which BMDBM is poorly soluble (0.01%, w/v). Both the media ensured, at any time of the experimentation, BMDBM amounts in the receptor fluid less than 10% of the saturation level. The sunscreen alone, dissolved in the oil phase of the emulsion, showed a short lag-time related to the unfavourable partitioning from the oil emulsion droplets to the water phase of the emulsion. Following the emulsion water evaporation, BMDBM diffused quickly through the membrane into the lipophilic medium and the amount of sunscreen permeated reached a plateau at about 80% of the applied dose after 4 h. By loading the sunscreen into the lipid microparticle crystalline matrix, a significant declining in the penetrated levels of BMDBM combined with a longer lag-time was obtained owing to the modulating effect provided by the lipospheres on the sunscreen release (Figure 2a) [34].

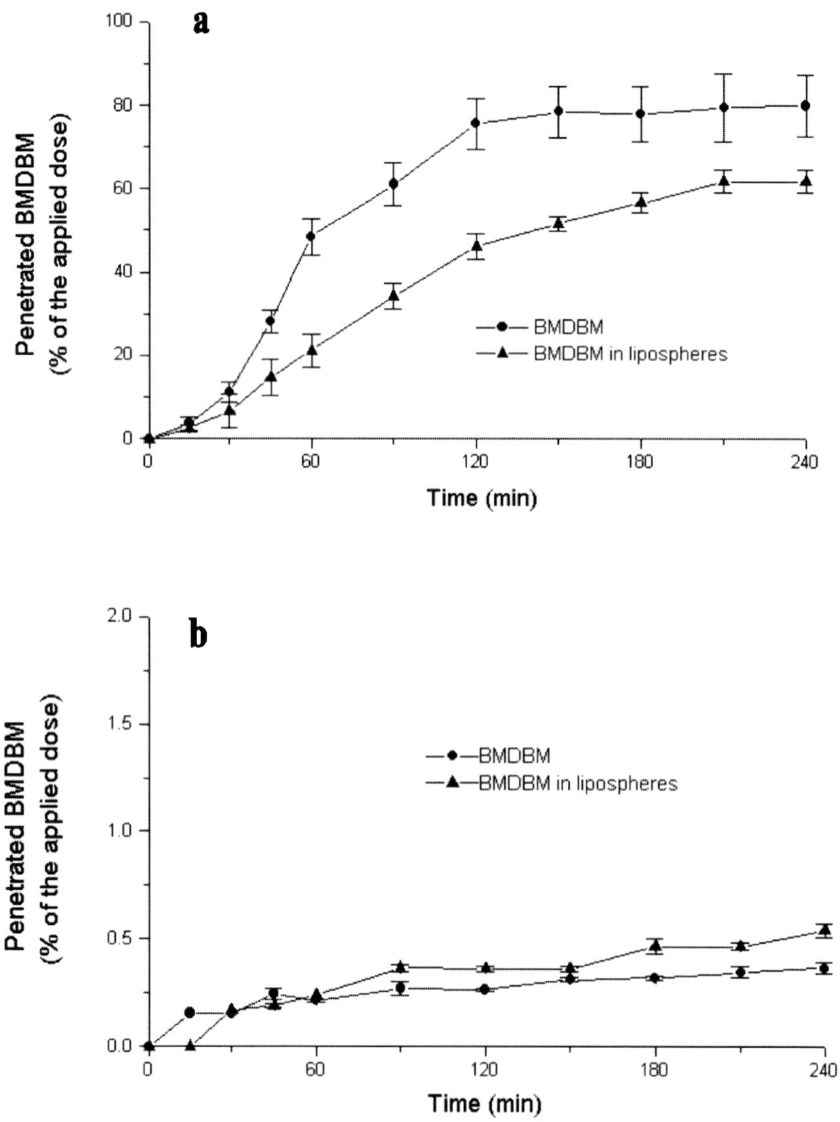

Figure 2. (a) BMDBM in vitro permeation into a lipophilic receptor medium: BMDBM alone (●) and BMDBM loaded in lipospheres (▲). Values are means ± S.D. (n = 3); (b) BMDBM in vitro permeation into a hydrophilic receptor medium: BMDBM alone (●) and BMDBM loaded in lipospheres (▲). Values are means ± S.D. (n = 3) (from ref. n. 34, with permission from Karger AG, Basel).

The cumulative sunscreen permeation through the membrane into the hydrophilic receptor phase was significantly lower than the values obtained by using the lipophilic receptor medium, regardless the formulation (Figure 2b). Since BMDBM concentrations in the receptor medium were less than 10% of its solubility, the permeation process would be reasonably controlled by the unfavourable partitioning of the highly lipophilic sunscreen which prevails on the liposphere modulating effect and represents the rate-limiting step of the process.

The *in vivo* skin permation study was carried out by applying to human volunteers the same O/W emulsion used for the *in vitro* experiments and containing BMDBM (2%) alone or loaded in lipospheres. In order to evaluate the sunscreen skin permeation, in terms of BMDBM concentration and distribution inside SC, the tape-stripping method was carried out. In this study, SC was stripped 10 times as proposed by FDA bioequivalence guidelines. The average penetrated percentage of the sunscreen was approximately 10% and 17% of the applied dose, for unencapsulated and encapsulated BMDBM, respectively. Moreover, the UV filter concentration decreased with SC depth for both formulations, as shown by BMDBM average penetrated percentage values in the combined tapes (Tables I and II). By considering that a relative SC thickness of about 40% could presumably be removed by 10 tape strips [35], it could be argued that BMDBM accumulated in the outermost part of the SC, up to a relative depth of approximately 40% of the SC.

In view of a possible *in vitro-in vivo* correlation, the *in vivo* permeation data were overestimated by the *in vitro* study carried out by a lipophilic receptor medium. Moreover, the *in vivo* data did not reveal the hampering effect of the microparticulate system on the permeation. Therefore, an *in vitro-in vivo* correlation could not be provided by the lipophilic receptor medium. On the other hand, the poor *in vitro* BMDBM skin permeation into the hydrophilic receptor could better reflect the *in vivo* skin penetration values. Furthermore, more similar effects provided by the microencapsulation on the sunscreen skin permeation were observed. This is probably duc to thc fact that thc unfavourablc BMDBM partitioning represents the rate-limiting step in both *in vitro* and *in vivo* methods.Therefore, by considering that the high lipophilicity of BMDBM (log $P_{o/w}$ = 5.6) could induce a great affinity for the SC which can act as a "reservoir" for the sunscreen, the *in vivo* BMDBM values determined by the tape-stripping technique could be considered as not systemically absorbed. According to this, a good *in vitro-in vivo* correlation could be obtained.

Table I. *In vivo* BMDBM permeation data: cumulative recovery in the SC (% of the applied dose ± S.D) and analysis of variance ANOVA (from ref. n. 34, with permission from Karger AG, Basel)

	BMDBM alone	BMDBM in lipospheres	P value
Unabsorbed	81.30 ± 12.34	85.27 ± 8.26	< 0.05
Recovery in SC (tapes 2–10)	9.68 ± 1.51	16.65 ± 2.99	< 0.05
Total recovery	90.98 ± 5.67	101.92 ± 4.77	< 0.05

Table II. *In vivo* BMDBM permeation data: sunscreen distribution in the SC (% of the applied dose ± S.D) and analysis of variance ANOVA (From Ref. n. 32, with permission from Karger AG, Basel)

Combined tapes	BMDBM alone	BMDBM in lipospheres	P value
Tapes 2–4	6.30 ± 2.58	8.03 ± 2.76	> 0.05
Tapes 5–7	1.75 ± 0.35	4.92 ± 0.58	< 0.05
Tapes 8–10	1.63 ± 0.61	3.70 ± 1.30	< 0.05

In Vitro-In Vivo Skin Permeation of 4-Methilbenzylidene Camphor (4-MBC)

4-MBC is a common sunscreen agent which is included in the list of authorized UV filters in Europe and Australia and has been submitted for approval in the United States [36]. MBC provides excellent protection against UV-B radiation (290–320 nm) and, in addition, it has been shown to exert a photostabilizing effect on butyl methoxydibenzoylmethane, the most frequently used and efficient UV-A (320-400 nm) filter [37]. However, recent investigations in rats as well as in humans have reported systemic absorption of MBC after topical application [38, 39] which reduces its concentration at the skin surface, where the UV filter action is most desirable. In addition, the percutaneous penetration of MBC poses further reasons for concern since *in vitro* and animal studies have raised the issue that MBC can acts as endocrine disruptor [40, 41]. Therefore, there is a need for new systems able to minimize the skin penetration of MBC. Lipid microparticles loaded with MBC were prepared and their influence on the sunscreen percutaneous penetration was examined after incorporation in a cream (O/W emulsion) as model formulation. *In vitro* measurements [42], performed in Franz cells, indicated that the 4-MBC diffusion into the receptor fluid (pH 7.4 phosphate buffer containing randomly methylated-β-cyclodextrin to ensure sink conditions) was significantly decrease when the UV filter was incorporated into the microparticles (Figure 3a). *In vivo* human skin penetration was investigated by tape stripping on the same formulations subjected to the *in vitro* experiment. The obtained results (Figure 3b) indicated that the amount of sunscreen penetrated into the SC was greater for the emulsion containing non-encapsulated MBC (36.55% of the applied dose) compared to the formulation with the sunscreen-loaded microparticles (24.57% of the applied dose). However, the differences between the two formulations were statistically significant only in the first (2–4) horny layer strips [42]. The results of the *in vivo* investigation (Figure n.3b) show a certain degree of correlation with the *in vitro* study (Figure 3a), although the effect of the lipid microparticles in the Franz test was greater (the sunscreen diffusion was decreased by 66.7–77.3 % in the *in vitro* Franz test compared to 27.3–46.9 % in the stripping test). This difference can be ascribed to the fact that human skin represents a more efficient barrier than the synthetic membrane. Moreover, the interaction of the microparticle excipients (lipid and surfactant) with the horny layer constituents represents an additional factor which could affect the degree of cutaneous permeation [43].

In Vitro-In Vivo Skin Permeation of Glycolic Acid

Alpha hydroxy acids (AHA) such as glycolic acid (GA) are used extensively in cosmetic and dermatological products to facilitate progressive wakening of cohesion of the intercellular material of the SC resulting in exfoliation of its outmost layers. They are thus useful in treating hypercheratosis and seems to have an "antiaging" activity as well. Although the mechanism is poorly understood, an enhance breakdown of corneodesmosomes is believed to be involved [44]. The Cosmetic Ingredient Review (CIR) Expert Panel and FDA's AHA Review Committee reviewed the safety of topically applied AHAs in cosmetic products. A total of 107 adverse dermatologic experience reports on AHA-containing skin care products between 1992 and 2000, with the maximum number in 1994 were found. The reported adverse experiences include burning, dermatitis or rash, swelling, pigmentary changes, blisters or welts, skin peeling, itching, irritation or tenderness, chemical burns, and increased sunburn. In 2005 FDA announced the availability of a guidance document entitled "Guidance for Industry: Labeling for Topically Applied Cosmetic Products Containing Alpha Hydroxy Acids as Ingredients". The guidance recommends content for a labeling statement for cosmetic products containing AHAs as ingredients. Moreover, concentrations of AHA up to 10% with pH down to 3.5 are considered safe by U.S. Cosmetic Ingredient Review for leave on products [45, 46].

Percutaneous absorption studies suggest that topically applied AHAs in cosmetic products may be absorbed by the skin to some extent, depending on product formulation, pH, and contact time [47, 48]. The studies measured absorption of glycolic acid, lactic acid, and other AHAs by human skin at pH 3 and pH 7 using various product formulations. Although much greater absorption was observed at pH 3, substantial absorption was observed at pH 7.

In vitro skin permeation studies of GA from two different skin formulations (petrolatum jelly and O/W emulsion) were performed to compare the *in vitro* data with those obtained *in vivo* by means of tape-stripping technique on humans. GA *in vitro* skin penetration was assayed through a modified diffusion chamber by applying two different formulations containing 10% GA, in a finite dose of 1.44 mg/cm^2, on a synthetic membrane lipophilized by cetyl alcohol and monitoring GA concentration in the receptor fluid based on pH 7.4 phosphate buffer solution mimicing the aqueous viable epidermis. GA *in vivo* skin permeation was carried out by the tape-stripping technique on both forearms of volunteers reaching a SC depth of approximately 40%. After an application time of 30 min, GA amounts in combined strips were analysed by HPLC. GA ($\log P_{o/w}$= -1.11) diffuses *in vitro* quickly from petrolatum jelly and gradually from the O/W emulsion (Figure n. 4), owing to the different GA partitioning from the vehicle to the membrane. Notwithstanding this, about 50% of the applied dose was detected in the receptor fluid at 30 min after application, regardless the vehicle, suggesting that the higher GA solubility in the water phase of the emulsion compensates for the effect of favourable GA partitioning from petrolatum jelly.

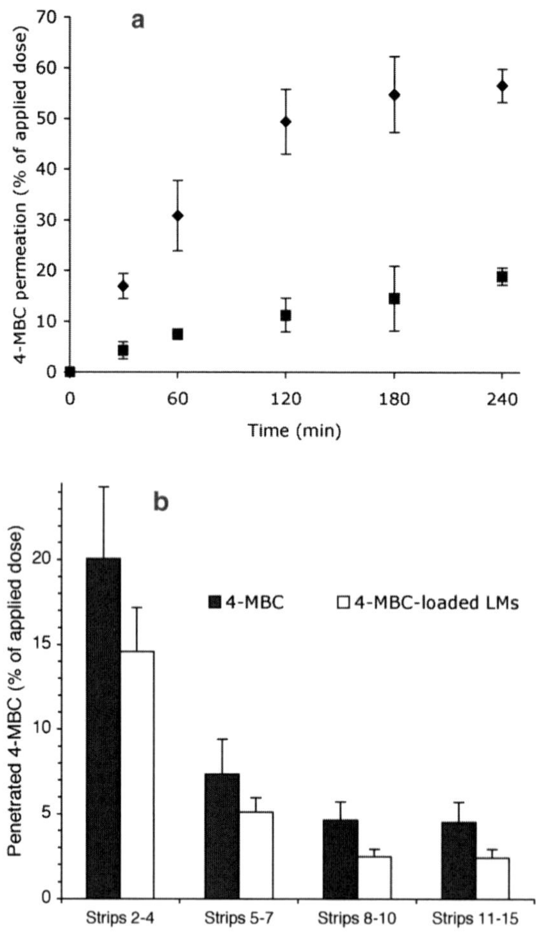

Figure 3. (a) Franz diffusion cells permeation profiles of 4-MBC from o/w emulsion (◆) and LMs in o/w emulsion (■).Values are means ± SD (n=5); (b) Concentration profiles of 4-MBC in the stratum corneum in vivo after application of emulsions containing free 4-MBC or sunscreen-loaded lipoparticles. The UV filter amounts in strips 2–4, 5–7, 8–10 and 11–15 of the stratum corneum are shown (mean ± SD, n=6) (from ref. n. 42, with permission from Pharmaceutical Press).

Table III. *In vivo* GA permeation data: cumulative recovery in the SC (% of the applied dose ± S.D) and analysis of variance ANOVA

	Petrolatum jelly	O/W emulsion	P value
Tapes 2–5	12.50 ± 6.30	29.80 ± 11.60	< 0.05
Tapes 6–10	13.00 ± 5.70	5.70 ± 2.30	< 0.05
Total recovery	25.50 ± 8.70	35.50 ± 13.50	> 0.05

Likewise, no significant differences in total GA recovery in the SC were observed *in vivo* between petrolatum jelly (25.5±13.5% of the applied dose) and O/W emulsion (35.5±8.7% of the applied dose). However, petrolatum jelly provided a higher GA amount in the deeper SC layers compared with the O/W emulsion, probably owing to the greater occlusive effect of petrolatum (Table III). Therefore, with relation to the vehicle influence, *in vivo* GA skin permeation extent was predicted by the *in vitro* data. On the contrary, the *in vitro* assay provided an overestimation of the *in vivo* absorption. This difference probably can be traced to GA penetration into the unremoved SC layers.

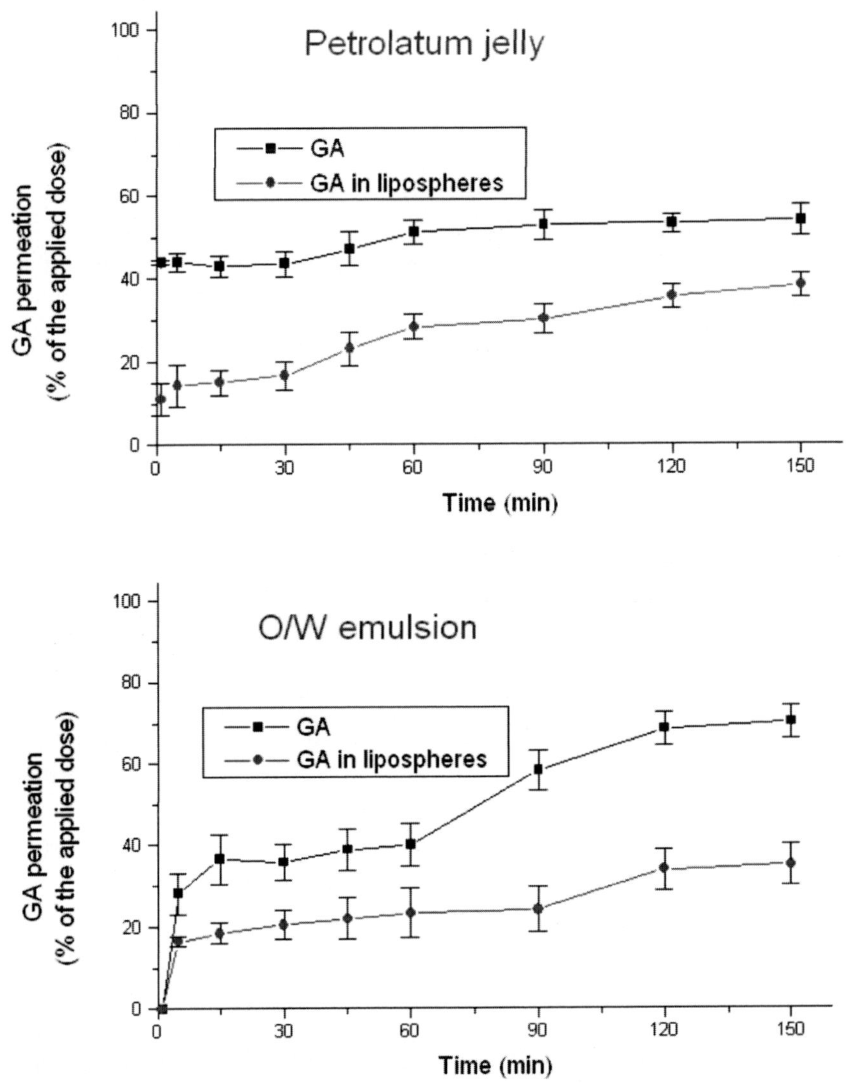

Figure 4. *In vitro* skin permeation of GA (alone or loaded into lipospheres) from a petrolatuim jelly or an O/W emulsion through a lipophilized sinthetic membrane.

Conclusion

An *in vitro* diffusion method through a lipophilized synthetic membrane simulating the SC into an aqueous phase, which mimics the viable epidermis, predicts the *in vivo* behaviour when the limiting step for skin permeation is the partitioning of the active substance from the SC to the viable epidermis (lipophilic substances having a great affinity for the SC). However, an overestimation was provided when the partitioning of the substance from the vehicle to the SC (hydrophilic substances) represented the limiting step of the process. In any case, the above-reported data indicate that the effect of the vehicle on skin permeation could be properly estimated by such *in vitro* experimentation.

References

[1] Lien, EJ; Tong, GL. Physicochemical properties and percutaneous absorption of drugs. *J. Soc. Cosmet. Chem.*, 1973, 24, 371-384.

[2] Yamashita, F; Hashida, M. Mechanistic and empirical modeling of skin permeation of drugs. *Adv. Drug Del. Rev.*, 2003, 55, 1185-1199.

[3] Pelchrzim, RV; Weigmann, HJ; Schaefer, H; Hagemeister, T; Linscheid, M; Shah, VP; Sterry, W; Lademann, J. Determination of the formation of the stratum corneum reservoir for two different corticosteroid formulations using tape stripping combined with UV/VIS spectroscopy. *J. Dtsch. Dermatol. Ges.*, 2004, 2, 914-919.

[4] Morgan, CJ; Renwick, AG; Friedmann, PS. The role of stratum corneum and dermal microvascular perfusion in penetration and tissue levels of water-soluble drugs investigated by microdialysis. *Br. J. Dermatol.*, 2003, 148, 434-443.

[5] Wenkers, BP; Lippold, BC. Skin penetration of nonsteroidal antiinflammatory drugs out of a lipophilic vehicle: influence of the viable epidermis. *J. Pharm. Sci.*, 1999, 88, 1326-1331.

[6] Rougier, A; Lotte, C; Maibach, HI. *In vivo* relationship between percutaneous absorption and transepidermal water loss. In: Bronaugh, RL; Maibach, HI, editors. *Percutaneous absorption: drugs – cosmetics – mechanisms – methodology.* Boca Raton, FL: Taylor & Francis Group; 2005, 95-106.

[7] Lademann, J; Weigmann, HJ; Rickmeyer, C; Barthlmes, H; Schaefer, H; Mueller, G; Sterry, W. Penetration of titanium dioxide microparticles in a sunscreen formulation into the horny layer and the follicular orifice. *Skin Pharmacol. Appl. Skin Physiol.*, 1999, 12, 247-256.

[8] Teichmann, A; Ossadnik, M; Richter, H; Sterry, W; Lademann, J. Semiquantitative determination of the penetration of a fluorescent hydrogel formulation into the hair follicle with and without follicular closure by microparticles by means of differential stripping. *Skin. Pharmacol. Physiol.*, 2006, 19, 101-105.

[9] Lademann, J; Schaefer, H; Otberg, N; Teichmann, A; Blume-Peytavi, U; Sterry, W. Penetration of microparticles into human skin. *Hautarzt*, 2004, 55, 1117-1119.

[10] Vogt, A; Mandt, N; Lademann, J; Schaefer, H; Blume-Peytavi, U. Follicular targeting – a promising tool in selective dermatotherapy. *J. Inv. Derm. Symp. Proc.*, 2005, 10, 252-255.

[11] Lademann, J; Richter, H; Teichmann, A; Otberg, N; Blume-Peytavi, U; Luengo, J; Weiss, B; Schaefer, UF; Lehr, CM; Wepf, R; Sterry, W. Nanoparticles: an efficient carrier for drug delivery into the hair follicles. *Eur. J. Pharm. Biopharm.*, 2007, 66, 159-164.

[12] Alvarez-Roman, R; Nalk, A; Kalia, YN; Guy, RH; Fessi, H. Skin penetration and distribution of polymeric nanoparticles. *J. Control. Release*, 2004, 99, 53-62.

[13] Baroli, B; Ennas, MG; Loffredo, F; Isola, M; Pinna, R; Lopez-Quintela, MA. Penetration of metallic nanoparticles in human full-thickness skin. *J. Invest. Dermatol.*, 2007, 127, 1701-1712.

[14] Kreilgaard, M. Influence of microemulsions on cutaneous drug delivery. *Adv. Drug Del. Rev.*, 2002, 54, S77-S98.

[15] Müller, RH; Mehnert, W; Souto, EB. Solid lipid nanoparticles (SLN) and nanostructured lipid carriers (NLC) for dermal delivery. In: Bronaugh, RL; Maibach, HI, editors. *Percutaneous absorption: drugs – cosmetics – mechanisms – methodology.* Boca Raton, FL: Taylor & Francis Group; 2005, 719-738.

[16] U.S. Food and Drug Administration. Nanotechnology – a report of the U.S. food and drug administration nanotechnology task force. FDA, Washington DC, 2007.

[17] European Commission - Scientific Committee on Consumer Products. Opinion on safety of nanomaterials in cosmetic products. SCCP/1147/07. Brussels, 2007.

[18] Faunce, T; Murray, K; Nasu, H; Bowman, D. Sunscreen safety: the precautionary principle, the Australian Therapeutic Goods Administration and nanoparticles in sunscreens. *Nanoethics*, 2008, 2, 231-240.

[19] El Maghraby, GM; Barry, BW; Williams, AC. Liposomes and skin: from drug delivery to model membranes. *Eur. J. Pharm. Sci.*, 2008, 34, 203-222.

[20] Hoet, PHM; Bruske-Hohlfeld, I; Salata, OV. Nanoparticles – known and unknown health risks. *J. Nanobiotechnology*, 2004, 2, 12-27.

[21] Howes, D; Guy, R; Hadgraft, J; Heylings, J; Hoeck, U; Kemper, F; Maibach, H; Marty, JP; Merk, H; Parra, J; Rekkas, D; Rondelli, I; Schaefer, H; Täuber, U; Verbiese, N. Methods for assessing percutaneous absorption. *The Report and Recommendations of ECVAM Workshop 13. ATLA,* 1996, 24, 81-106.

[22] Shah, VP; Flynn, GL; Yacobi, A; Maibach, HI; Bon, C; Fleischer, NM; Franz, TJ; Kaplan, SA; Kawamoto, J; Lesko, LJ; Marty, JP; Pershing, LK; Schaefer, H; Sequeira, JA; Shrivastava, SP; Wilkin, J; Williams, RL. AAPS/FDA Workshop Report: Bioequivalence of topical dermatological dosage forms – Methods of evaluation of bioequivalence. *Pharm. Res.,* 1998, 15, 167-171.

[23] Sauber, C; Schwarb, FP; Smith, EW. Tape-stripping technique. In: Bronaugh, RL; Maibach, HI, editors. *Percutaneous absorption: drugs – cosmetics – mechanisms – methodology.* Boca Raton, FL: Taylor & Francis Group; 2005, 399-410.

[24] European Commission - Scientific Committee on Consumer Non Food Products. Basic Criteria for the *in vitro* assessment of dermal absorption of cosmetic ingredients. SCCNFP/0750/03. Brussels, 2003.

[25] European Commission - Scientific Committee on Consumer Products. Opinion on Basic Criteria for the *in vitro* assessment of dermal absorption of cosmetic ingredients. SCCP/0970/06. Brussels, 2006.

[26] The European Cosmetic, Toiletry and Perfumery Association. Cosmetic ingredients: guidelines for percutaneous absorption/penetration. 2nd edition, August 1997.

[27] Organisation for Economic Co-operation and Development. Guidelines for testing of chemicals – Guideline 428: skin absorption: *In vitro* method, 2004.

[28] de Jager, M; Groenink, W; van der Spek, J; Janmaat, C; Gooris, G; Ponec, M; Bouwstra, J. Preparation and characterization of a stratum corneum substitute for *in vitro* percutaneous penetration studies. *Biochim. Biophys. Acta,* 2006, 1758, 636-644.

[29] Sartorelli, P; Andersen, HR; Angerer, J; Corish, J; Drexler, H; Göen, T; Griffin, P; Hotchkiss, SAM; Larese, F; Montomoli, L; Perkins, J; Schmelz, M; van de Sandt, J; Williams, F. Percutaneous penetration studies for risk assessment. *Environ. Toxicol. Pharmacol,* 2000, 8, 133-152.

[30] Wissing, SA; Müller, RH. Solid lipid nanoparticles as carrier for sunscreens: *in vitro* release and *in vivo* skin penetration. *J. Control. Release,* 2002, 81, 225-233.

[31] European Union: Commission Recommendation 2006/647/EC on the efficacy of sunscreen products and the claims made relating thereto [notified under document number C(2006) 4089].

[32] Iannuccelli, V; Sala, N; Tursilli, R; Coppi, G; Scalia, S. Influence of liposphere preparation on butyl-methoxydibenzoylmethane photostability. *Eur. J. Pharm. Biopharm.*, 2006, 63, 140-145.

[33] Walters, KA; Roberts, MS. Percutaneous absorption of sunscreens. In: Bronaugh, RL; Maibach, HI, editors. *Percutaneous absorption. Drugs – Cosmetics – Mechanisms – Methodology*. Boca Raton, FL: Taylor & Francis Group; 2005, 681-700.

[34] Iannuccelli, V; Coppi, G; Sergi, S; Mezzena, M; Scalia, S. *In vivo* and *in vitro* skin permeation of butyl methoxydibenzoylmethane from lipospheres. *Skin Pharmacol. Physiol.*, 2008, 21, 30-38.

[35] Jacobi, U; Weigmann, J; Ulrich, J; Sterry, W; Lademann, J. Estimation of the relative stratum corneum amount removed by tape stripping. *Skin. Res. Technol.*, 2005, 11, 91-96.

[36] Steinberg, DC. Regulations of sunscreens worldwide. In: Shaath, N. editor. *Sunscreens*. Boca Raton, FL: Taylor & Francis Group; 2005, 180-181.

[37] Bonda, CA. The photostability of organic sunscreen actives: a review. In: Shaath, N. editor. *Sunscreens*. Boca Raton, FL: Taylor & Francis Group; 2005, 342-343.

[38] Janjua, NR; Mogensen, B; Andersson, A; Petersen, JH; Henriksen, M; Skakkebæck, NE; Wulf, HC. Systemic absorption of the sunscreens benzophenone-3, octyl-methoxycinnamate, and 3-(4-methyl-benzylidene)camphor after whole-body topical application and reproductive hormone levels in humans. *J. Invest. Dermatol.*, 2004, 123, 57-61.

[39] Schauer, UMD; Völkel, W; Heusener, A; Colnot, T; Broschard, TH; von Landenberg, F; Dekant, W. Kinetics of 3-(4-methylbenzylidene)camphor in rats and humans after dermal application. *Toxicol. Appl. Pharmacol.*, 2006, 216, 339-346.

[40] Schlumpf, M; Schmid, P; Durrer, S; Conscience, M; Maerkel, K; Henseler, M; Gruetter, M; Herzog, I; Reolon, S; Ceccatelli, R; Faass, O; Stutz, E; Jarry, H; Wuttke, W; Lichtensteiger, W. Endocrine activity and developmental toxicity of cosmetic UV filters – An update. *Toxicology*, 2004, 205, 113-122.

[41] European Commission – Scientific Committee on Consumer Products. Opinion on methylbenzylidene camphor, SCCP/1042/0610, Brussels, 2006.

[42] Scalia, S; Mezzena, M; Iannuccelli, V. Influence of solid lipid microparticle carriers on skin penetration of the sunscreen agent, 4-methylbenzylidene camphor. *J. Pharm. Pharmacol.*, 2007, 59, 1621-1627.

[43] Müller, RH; Radtke, M; Wissing, SA. Solid lipid nanoparticles (SLN) and nanostructured lipid carriers (NLC) in cosmetic and dermatological preparations. *Adv. Drug Deliv. Rev.*, 2002, 54, S131-S155.

[44] Fartasch, M; Teal, J; Menon, GK. Mode of action of glycolic acid on human stratum corneum: ultrastructural and functional evaluation of the epidermal barrier. *Arch. Dermatol. Res.*, 1997, 289, 404-409.

[45] U.S. Food and Drug Administration: FDA Backgrounder. Alpha hydroxyacids in cosmetics. July 3, 1997.

[46] U.S. Food and Drug Administration: Center for Food Safety and Applied Nutrition – Office of Cosmetics and Colors. Guidance for Industry. Labeling for topically applied cosmetic products containing alpha hydroxyacids as ingredients. December 2, 2002.

[47] Jiang, M; Qureshi, SA. Assessment of *in vitro* percutaneous absorption of glycolic acid through human skin sections using a flow-through diffusion cell system. *J. Dermatol. Sci.*, 1998; 18, 181-188.

[48] Kraeling, MEK; Bronaugh, RL. *In vitro* percutaneous absorption of alpha hydroxy acids in human skin. *J. Soc. Cosm. Chem.*, 1997, 48, 187-197.

In: Skin Anatomy and Physiology Research Developments ISBN: 978-1-60741-469-8
Editor: Leon F. Bukowsky

Chapter 8

Skin Aging-The Effect of Menopause

Jean Calleja-Agius*

Department of Obstetrics and Gynaecology, Mater Dei Hospital, B'Kara, Malta,
12, 'Mon Nid', Gianni Faure Street, Tarxien, Malta TXN2421, USA

Abstract

Cutaneous ageing manifests itself as a progressive reduction in maximum function and reserve capacity of its constitutive tissues. The atrophy of collagen is a major factor in skin ageing. The menopause has been shown repeatedly to have a negative effect on the connective tissue of the skin. Such an effect is prevented and in some cases reversed with estrogen therapy. Large-scale clinical trials are necessary to help make informed recommendations regarding postmenopausal estrogen use and its role in prevention of skin ageing.

Keywords: Skin ageing; Collagen; Hormone Replacement Therapy.

Introduction

Cutaneous ageing manifests itself as a progressive reduction in maximum function and reserve capacity of its constitutive tissues. It is not a unique and uniform biological event. Factors aggravating the clinical aspects of ageing include the effects of past or present diseases, as well as diverse environmental influences and physiological variations (Table 1) (1;2). Collagen atrophy is a major factor in skin ageing. There are a number of functions of the skin which deteriorate with ageing (Table 2).

* Corresponding Author: Telephone number: (+356) 21693041, Fax number: (+356) 23331027, Email: jean@waldonet.net.mt

Table 1. The Seven Types of Cutaneous Ageing.

Ageing types	Determinant factor
Chronological	Passage of time
Genetic	Genetics (e.g. premature ageing syndromes, phototype, melanotype)
Photoageing	Ultraviolet and infrared irradiations
Behavioural	Diet, tobacco, alcohol abuse, drug addiction
Catabolic	Chronic intercurrent debilitating disease (e.g. infections, cancers)
Endocrine	Dysfunction or ageing of hormone systems (e.g. ovaries, testes, thyroid)
Gravitational	Gravitational force

Table 2. Functions of the Skin known to Decline with Ageing.

Epidermal turnover	Immune function
Wound healing	Vascular reactivity
Injury response	Sweat production
Barrier function	Sebum production
Sensory perception	Vitamin D production

A fairly consistent finding in work on the menopause and hormone replacement therapy (HRT) is the positive effect of estrogen on connective tissue and its turnover. The menopause has been shown repeatedly to have a negative effect on the connective tissue in the dermis of the skin. This is prevented and in some cases reversed with estrogen therapy. This effect probably also extends to the extracellular non-collagenous matrix in all these systems, i.e. skin, carotid and intervertebral discs. The common thread is that estrogen has profound effects on connective tissue turnover, no matter the site (3). This has implications not only in maintaining the structure and aesthetic appearance of tissue, but also the strength and stiffness of various tissues and the functioning of surrounding organs.

Skin Physiology

The skin is the largest organ in the body. It is the primary barrier against pathogen invasion and dehydration. There is a complex mosaic of a population of cells of diverse embryonic origin that, under normal conditions, co-exist side by side (Figure 1).

This organ is stratified into three layers-epidermis, dermis and subcutis. It is perforated by a variety of adjuncts to produce hair, sebum and sweat. The epidermis consists primarily of keratinocytes and melanocytes, and forms the thin outer layer. The dermis is the deeper layer, forming the main bulk of the skin. Its function is to provide a tough matrix to support the blood vessels, nerves and appendages that are embedded in it. The fibres present in the dermal connective tissue are predominantly collagen and elastin (4).

Eighty percent of the dry weight of adult skin consists of collagen. Collagen fibres are arranged parallel to the skin surface. This gives the skin a high tensile strength and prevents it from being torn by overstretching. In contrast, elastin constitutes about 5% of the dermis, and provides the skin with elasticity and resilience (5). Elastin fibres are arranged as a thinly distributed subepidermal network, and are also produced by fibroblasts. The dermal connective tissue also contains sensory receptors and the supportive glycosaminogylcans (GAGs) (6).

Skin quality deteriorates with age due to the synergistic effects of chronologic ageing, photoageing, hormonal deficiency and environmental factors. The ageing of the skin results from a decline in several metabolic activities. The dermis undergoes morphological, physical and chemical changes during ageing (4). Menopausal effects of the skin are thought to include atrophy; decreased collagen content, water content, and sebaceous secretions; loss of elasticity; and manifestations of hyperandrogenism. The cumulative effect of estrogen deficiency on the skin is thought to contribute to poor wound healing in older patients (7). In mice, oophorectomy alone was sufficient to accelerate skin ageing and increase sensitivity to ultraviolet radiation (8). This resulted in further deterioration of skin quality and increased wrinkling. This may account for the accelerated skin ageing seen in postmenopausal women.

Effects of Ageing on Structural Components of the Skin

Collagen

The predominant form of collagen found in adult human skin is Type I, followed by Type III (9). The genes for human collagen Type I are located on chromosomes 7 and 17 (10). Collagen is synthesised by fibroblasts from procollagen molecules by the action of neutral endoproteases. The fibrils of collagen undergo a series of post-translational modifications in order to enhance their stability and tensile strength. In young subjects, microscopic examination of collagen from the dermis of skin areas not exposed to the sun shows thin, wavy, uniform fibrillar units (11).

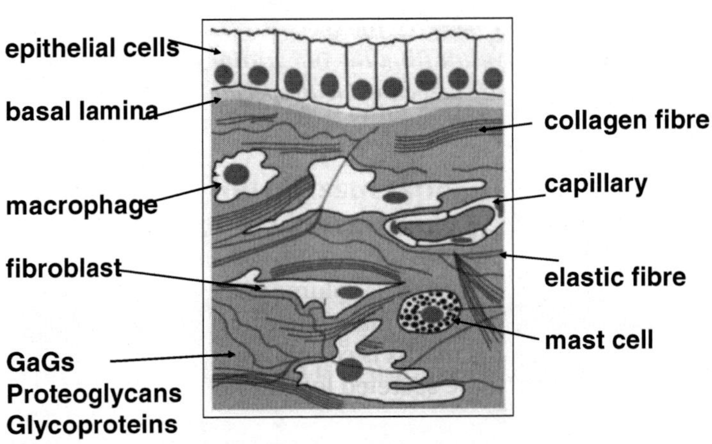

Figure 1. The structure of the skin.

The skin becomes thinner with age (12;13). In elderly subjects, the skin contains thickened, clumped basophilic collagenous material, indicating partial degradation of collagen (14). The atrophy of collagen is a major factor in skin ageing. Studies based on the amount of collagen in a specific area of the skin show a significant decline in the dermal quantity of collagen with ageing (15-17).

During ageing, there is a decrease in the enzymes concerned in post-translational processing of collagen. The amounts of hydroxyproline and glycosylated hydroxylysine in Type I collagen decrease with age (18;19). Collagen ageing results from progressive cross-linking between the collagen molecules (20). A larger proportion of the cross-links between collagen molecules become non-reducible, that is, the number of immature and reducible crosslinks decrease with age (21). The molar ratio of glycosylated hydroxylysine residues to unsubstituted hydroxylysine residues have been found to increase with ageing (22). There is a reduction in the number of fibroblasts that synthesize collagen and vessels that supply the skin. This leads to an increase in laxity, making wrinkles more evident (4).

The exact role of estrogen on collagen integrity is still unclear. Anabolic steroids have been shown to increase collagen synthesis in human dermal fibroblasts (23). In rats, estrogen has been shown to inhibit collagen degradation (24). However, estrogens have no stimulatory effect on procollagen synthesis in cultured human cells (25).

Studies show a strong correlation between skin collagen loss and estrogen deficiency due to menopause (26;27). As much as 30% of skin collagen (both Type I and III) is lost in the first five years after the menopause. Total collagen declines an average of 2.1% per postmenopausal year over a period of 15 years. The decrease in skin collagen content has been shown to correlate with age-related decreases in bone mineral density. This is consistent with the presence of Type I collagen in bone.

One study showed a closer correlation between collagen loss and chronologic age than between skin collagen loss and time since menopause. This finding may be explained by the fact that the study participants were between 40 and 55 years of age and had recently undergone surgical menopause, and consequently had not been estrogen deficient for a long time (28) **(Figure 2)** However, when more than one than one year elapsed since menopause, there is a more pronounced reduction in the skin collagen content.

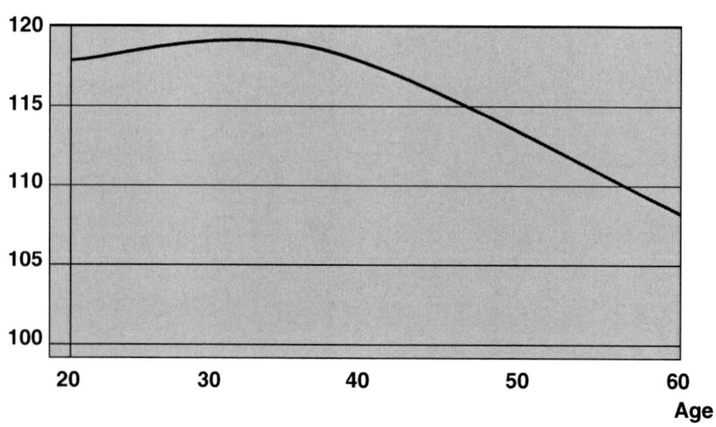

Figure 2. Changes in the collagen/protein ratio by age.

The decline in skin collagen content can be prevented in women receiving estrogen therapy (29). A beneficial effect of subcutaneous (13;26;30), topical (12;26;31;32) or oral (16;33) estrogen treatment has been demonstrated on the collagen content of skin. There was a variation in the extent of the estrogen-induced increase in collagen content, which depended upon the route of administration, dose and duration of hormone treatment. Moreover, there are differences in the methods employed to assess collagen levels, so results between studies are often not comparable (7).

It has been shown that the increase in collagen with estrogen is proportionate to baseline collagen levels (12;26). One study observed no change in collagen levels of postmenopausal women following one year of HRT (34). This can be explained by the fact that, given the short time since menopause, the amount and synthetic rate of collagen may have been optimal (35). It has been observed that there is a delay in the collagen decrease after the onset of menopause (15). Estrogen treatment may be prophylactic for women with high skin collagen levels and even therapeutic for women with low collagen content (12;26).

Elastin

Like collagen, elastin is a fibre-forming functional protein. Elastin fibres are closely linked and interwoven with the collagen fibrils so that they can recoil after transient stretching and are prevented from overstretching. Young women with premature menopause were observed to have accelerated degenerative changes in dermal elastic fibres (6). Histologic studies demonstrate that topical estrogen can increase the number and thickness of skin elastic fibres (36). Recent clinical trials demonstrated no observable improvement in elastin fibre content from baseline with systemic estrogen therapy (33;34;37). However, these studies either treated a small sample of women ($n \leq 21$) for 6 months (33;37), or involved very early postmenopausal women (34).

Water

Healthy skin needs substantial water content, which is determined by the cutaneous evaporation rate and epidermal hydration (7). Transepidermal water flux decreases with age (38). There are minor quantities of various glycosaminoglycans (including versican and heparan sulfate) in the dermis, which are closely associated with skin collagen. These glycosaminoglycans have a high water-binding capability, and are essential for the normal skin hydration. The total dermal glycosaminoglycan content decreases significantly with ageing (4). It has been postulated that collagen and glycosaminoglycans may interact to produce the age-related changes in the properties of collagen. It is possible that the state of hydration of the dermis, influenced by glycosaminoglycans, may be more important than the extent of collagen cross-linking (39).

Dry skin is one of the commonest dermatological conditions in older women (40). An epidemiological study showed that estrogen use was associated with a statistically significant decrease in the likelihood of senile dry skin (41). These positive effects may be related to estrogen-stimulated increases in mucopolysaccharides and hyaluronic acid levels in skin (42;43), which correlate to an increased dermal water content (44). There is also an increase in skin thickness, which subsequently elevates natural moisturizing factors (31).

Sebaceous Glands and Hair

It has been shown that sebaceous secretions decrease with age (45). Estrogen replacement alone has a sebum-suppressive action (46), but the addition of a progestin leads to significant increases in skin surface lipids (46;47). Overall, there is a 38% increase in sebum production in postmenopausal women taking hormone replacement therapy, when compared with controls (47).

Possible changes in postmenopausal women include an increase in facial hair; and a decrease in body and/or pubic hair. The onset of menopause can lead to a diffuse or an androgenic alopecia (48-50). Another type of hair loss, includes frontal fibrosing alopecia, which is a variant of lichen planopilaris. The latter has been associated with the postmenopausal phase, however the hair loss persists despite hormone treatment (51).

Effects of Ageing on Physical Characteristics of the Skin

Skin Thickness

There is an increase in skin thickness up to the age of 35 to 49, followed by an age-related thinning (7). For the initial 15 to 18 postmenopausal years, the decrease in skin thickness accelerates with as much as 1.13% annual decline (12;26). The thinning effect is due to decreases in collagen, water and glycosaminoglycans (7). There is a high incidence of thin skin in osteoporotic women (45;52). In fact, there is a strong correlation between skin thickness, collagen content and bone density in postmenopausal women (12;26;53). Most clinical trials have shown that postmenopausal women who take hormone replacement therapy have greater skin thickness when compared to non-users (16;37;47;54-56) (Figure 3).

Elasticity

Skin ageing, especially in the face, is associated with a progressive increase in extensibility and a reduction in skin elasticity (7). In postmenopausal women, skin elasticity decline 0.55% per year after menopause. Twelve months of hormone replacement therapy increased elasticity by 5.2% (57). Studies have shown that there hormone replacement therapy delays the process of deterioration in the extensibility of the skin, slowing the progress of cutaneous slackening that follows menopause(47;58).

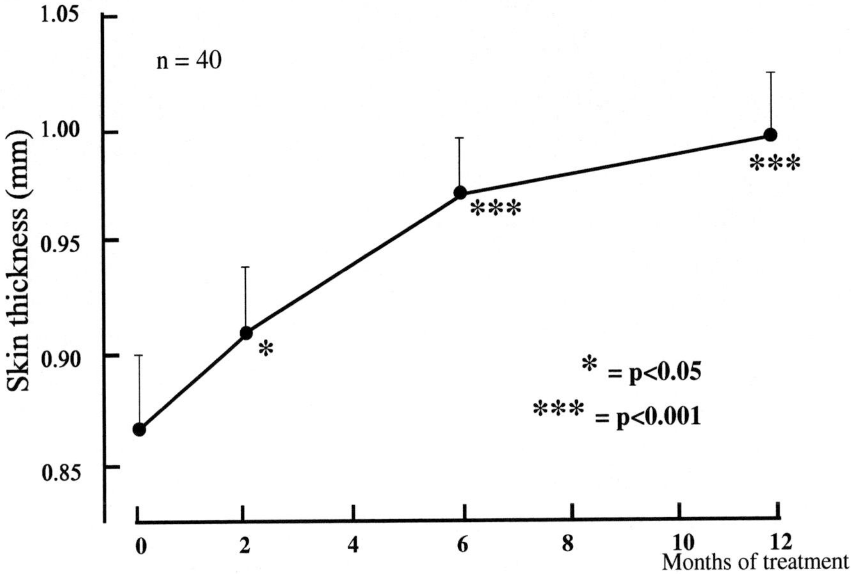

Figure 3. Skin thickness in women on 100mg estradiol implants (12;26).

Wrinkles

During the ageing process, there is a decrease in the collagen content and in the production of glycosaminoglycans in the connective tissue. There is also a higher intracellular concentration of protocollagen lysylhydroxyproline transferase, which is the enzyme responsible for collagen breakdown (59). The loss of connective tissue in cutaneous ageing results in increased distensibility and loss of tonicity, leading to a progressive deepening of facial creases and wrinkling (7). In untreated perimenopausal women, there is a rapid increase in skin extensibility, as detected in computerised measurements of skin deformability (60). The mechanical properties of the skin improve with estrogen (58;61;61). Facial wrinkling improved on estrogens (58) but worsened with smoking (60;62). However, few clinical studies have specifically examined hormone replacement therapy and facial wrinkling, due to technical challenges in quantitating a visual end point such as facial wrinkles (7).

Blood Flow

The dermis and epidermis are nourished by arterioles and capillaries, that pass upwards from the subcutaneous layer. The integrity in the structure and function of capillary blood vessels is important in healthy skin. There is a rich capillary network in the dermal papillae, which is responsible for the menopausal flush (63). Core temperature haemostasis is maintained with cutaneous circulation. Peripheral microcirculation at the level of the nail-fold capillaries decreases significantly with menopause (64). Six to twelve months of hormone replacement therapy was shown to increase capillary blood flow in the nail-fold by as much as 20-30% (64). The endothelium–dependent and –independent vascular reactivity in the cutaneous microcirculation improves substantially in postmenopausal women receiving estrogen (65).

Wound Healing

With increasing age, the skin becomes more fragile and susceptible to trauma, leading to more lacerations and bruising. Older women have been shown to heal less well, possibly due to low levels of transforming growth factor(TGF)-β (7). Venous ulcers and pressure sore are among the chronic wounds commonly suffered by the elderly. These cause significant suffering and cost, thus imposing a burden for patients and physicians alike (66). Cutaneous wound healing involves vascularization, granulation, collagen deposition and re-epithelialization (67). The effect of estrogen levels on the stages of wound healing is still unclear, because of contradictory findings in animal studies (7). Recent molecular and human studies appear promising. Estrogen has been shown to induce TGF-β secretion by dermal fibroblasts(68), and this can enhance the rate and quality of wound healing (31). Estriol iontophoresis has also been used for the treatment of atrophic acne scars (31).

Impact on Quality of Life

Quality of life is a subjective parameter. The World Health Organisation Criteria of Quality of Life (1991) define the following domains: physical, psychologic, level of independence, social relationships, environment and spirituality/personal beliefs (69). There are a number of standardized questionnaires which try to record all aspects of quality of life (70-72). Currently, the best methods available for determining quality of life include the Utian Quality of Life Index (73) and the Menopause Rating Scale I and II (74-76).

Bruises and wounds due to falls cause pain and discomfort. Dizzy spells and lack of sleep due to hot flushes lead to fatigue. Lack of libido and dyspareunia due to atrophic vaginitis can affect the sexual activity of postmenopausal women. Dry eyes and heavy sweating have a great impact on the patient's work capacity. There can be impairment in the process of thinking, memory and concentration due to sleep disturbances and depressive mood. Self-esteem can be badly affected due to urinary disorders and dry hair. In postmenopausal women, there is an increased risk of fractures, especially hip and vertebral, leading to decreased mobility and increased dependence on medical aids. The activities of daily living may be affected due more likelihood of forgetfulness, apathy and fatigue. Personal relationships may be impaired due to embarrassment with hot flushes. Marital relationships may become more stressful due to reduced libido and dyspareunia. Poor self-esteem and declining body image may also lead to poor performance at work and decreased work satisfaction. Dizzy spells, leading to fractures, can impair the physical safety and security of the environment. (Table 3)

The 'Skin-Ego' can have an adverse influence due to the change in the psychosexual role of the skin in the climacteric (77). Vessel dysregulation causes an increase in the vulnerability of the skin. The skin becomes drier and more acidic, especially due to the involution of sweat glands and sebaceous glands. There is a change in skin appearance and morphology, mainly due to wrinkling and change in hair distribution. Altered peripheral nerve function, especially in the genital area, lead to reduced libido and dyspareunia (78).

Table 3. Effects of Menopause on the Skin.

- Hot flushes; Altered hot/cold sensation
- Skin collagen changes:
  - tensile properties of the skin
  - wound healing
- Atrophic changes
  - Dry vulva
  - Dry eyes
  - Changes to Hair
  - Incontinence
  - Dyspareunia
  - Psychosexual role of the skin; effect on relationships
  - Transdermal role

Is Age Skin Deep? - The Impact on Intervertebral Discs and Carotid Arteries

The intervertebral discs are responsible for 20% of the spinal column height. Each disc is composed of high collagen content and glycosaminoglycans. They allow flexion and extension of the spine, and also act as "shock absorbers" of the spinal column. This may have an impact on osteoporotic compression fractures (79). In women under the age of 35 years, the intervertebral discs contain the more flexible collagen Types II, IV and IX, together with Type I collagen (80). There is a change in collagen type with the ageing process (81) and possibly with increasing years since menopause (82). The collagen Types I, III and VI predominate at the expense of collagen Types II, IV and IX. In the aged interverebral disc, there is also a significant decrease in glycosaminoglycans and elastin. These changes have significant effects on the shape and biomechanics of the intervertebral disc, which in turn may have an impact on vertebral body deformity and eventual fracture (79). A study confirmed that premenopausal women and hormone treated women had lumbar disc heights of 2.01 +/- 0.09cm and 2.15 +/- 0.08cm respectively, the latter results being significantly higher than the untreated postmenopausal group (height of three lumbar discs 1.82 +/- 0.06cm) and the osteoporotic fracture group (1.58 +/- 0.1cm) (p=<0.0001)(82).

The arteries, including the carotids, undergo postmenopausal connective tissue changes mimicking those in the skin and bone. The media is the layer containing the largest amount of collagen. HRT has a morphological effect on the carotid arteries in postmenopausal women. It has been suggested that HRT given to postmenopausal women differentially influences the layers of the carotid artery. Hormones seem to encourage thickening of the layers with the highest connective tissue component (externa and media) and to delay thickening of the atheromatous intima layer. Women with implants had thicker carotid artery wall measurements (0.84+/-0.26mm) than the other groups. The media (0.32 +/- 0.11mm) was significantly thicker in the implant group. This layer has a high connective tissue component including collagen Type I and III, and elastin fibers. The intima layer was thinner (0.25 +/- 0.09mm) in the oral HRT group compared with controls (0.29 +/- 0.1mm). The control group had a statistically significant higher intima-media ratio (1.17 +/-0.05), compared with both the oral HRT group (0.92 +/-0.04) and implant groups (0.94+/-0.03) (83).

Conclusion

The menopause has been shown repeatedly to have a negative effect on the connective tissue in the dermis of the skin. Such an effect is prevented and in some cases reversed with estrogen therapy. This is similar to what happens in bone matrix and the carotid artery media and intervertebral discs. The common thread is that estrogen has profound effects on connective tissue turnover, no matter the site. This has profound implications not only in maintaining the structure and aesthetic appearance of tissue, but also the strength and stiffness of various tissues and the functioning of neighbouring and surrounding organs.

References

[1] Pierard GE. EEMCO guidance to the in vivo assessment of tensile functional properties of the skin. Part 1: relevance to the structures and ageing of the skin and subcutaneous tissues. *Skin Pharmacol Appl Skin Physiol*, 1999, 12(6), 352-362.

[2] Calleja-Agius, J; Muscat-Baron, Y; Brincat, MP. Skin ageing. *Menopause Int*, 2007, 13(2), 60-64.

[3] Brincat, MP; Calleja-Agius, J; Baron, YM. The skin, carotid and intervertebral disc: making the connection! *Climacteric*, 2007, 10 Suppl 2, 83-87.

[4] Castelo-Branco, C. Skin collagen changes related to age, menopause and hormone replacement therapy. In: Brincat MP, editor. *Hormone Replacement Therapy and the Skin.*, UK: Parthenon Publishing, 2001.

[5] Uitto, J. Connective tissue biochemistry of the aging dermis. Age-related alterations in collagen and elastin. *Dermatol Clin.*, 1986, 4(3), 433-446.

[6] Bolognia, JL; Braverman, IM; Rousseau, ME; Sarrel, PM. Skin changes in menopause. *Maturitas*, 1989, 11(4), 295-304.

[7] Brincat, MP; Baron, YM; Galea, R. Estrogens and the skin. *Climacteric*, 2005, 8(2), 110-123.

[8] Tsukahara, K; Nakagawa, H; Moriwaki, S; Kakuo, S; Ohuchi, A; Takema, Y; et al. Ovariectomy is sufficient to accelerate spontaneous skin ageing and to stimulate ultraviolet irradiation-induced photoageing of murine skin. *Br J Dermatol*, 2004, 151(5), 984-994.

[9] Lovell, CR; Smolenski, KA; Duance, VC; Light, ND; Young, S; Dyson, M. Type I and III collagen content and fibre distribution in normal human skin during ageing. *Br J Dermatol.*, 1987, 117(4), 419-428.

[10] Kohn, RR; Schnider, SL. Collagen changes in aging skin. In: A. K. Balin, A. M. Kligman, (Eds.), *Aging and the Skin*. New York: Raven Press, 1989.

[11] Selmanowitz, VJ; Rizer, RL; Orentreich, N. Aging of the skin collagen. In: C. E. Finch, L. Hayflick, (Eds.), *Handbook of the biology of aging*. New York: Van Nostrand Reinhold, 1977.

[12] Brincat, M; Kabalan, S; Studd, JW; Moniz, CF; de Trafford, J; Montgomery, J. A study of the decrease of skin collagen content, skin thickness, and bone mass in the postmenopausal woman. *Obstet Gynecol.*, 1987, 70(6), 840-845.

[13] Brincat, M; Moniz, CJ; Studd, JW; Darby, A; Magos, A; Emburey, G; et al. Long-term effects of the menopause and sex hormones on skin thickness. *Br J Obstet Gynaecol*, 1985, 92(3), 256-259.

[14] Hall, DA. *The aging of connective tissue*. London: Academic Press, 1976.

[15] Brincat, M; Moniz, CF; Kabalan, S; Versi, E; O'Dowd, T; Magos, AL; et al. Decline in skin collagen content and metacarpal index after the menopause and its prevention with sex hormone replacement. *Br J Obstet Gynaecol*, 1987, 94(2), 126-129.

[16] Castelo-Branco, C; Duran, M; Gonzalez-Merlo, J. Skin collagen changes related to age and hormone replacement therapy. *Maturitas*, 1992, 15(2), 113-119.

[17] Shuster, S; Black, MM; McVitie, E. The influence of age and sex on skin thickness, skin collagen and density. *Br J Dermatol*, 1975, 93(6), 639-643.

[18] Barnes, MJ; Constable, BJ; Morton, LF; Royce, PM. Age-related variations in hydroxylation of lysine and proline in collagen. *Biochem J.*, 1974, 139(2), 461-468.

[19] Murai, A; Miyahara, T; Shiozawa, S. Age-related variations in glycosylation of hydroxylysine in human and rat skin collagens. *Biochim Biophys Acta*, 1975, 404(2), 345-348.

[20] Bailey, AJ; Robins, SP; Balian, G. Biological significance of the intermolecular crosslinks of collagen. *Nature*, 1974, 251(5471), 105-109.

[21] Hall, DA; Reed, FB; Nuki, G; Vince, JD. The relative effects of age and corticosteroid therapy on the collagen profiles of dermis from subjects with rheumatoid arthritis. *Age Ageing*, 1974, 3(1), 15-22.

[22] Schnider, SL; Kohn, RR. Effects of age and diabetes mellitus on the solubility and nonenzymatic glucosylation of human skin collagen. *J Clin Invest.*, 1981, 67(6), 1630-1635.

[23] Falanga, V; Greenberg, AS; Zhou, L; Ochoa, SM; Roberts, AB; Falabella, A; et al. Stimulation of collagen synthesis by the anabolic steroid stanozolol. *J Invest Dermatol*, 1998, 111(6), 1193-1197.

[24] Woessner, JF Jr. Total, latent and active collagenase during the course of post-partum involution of the rat uterus. Effect of oestradiol. *Biochem J.*, 1979, 180(1), 95-102.

[25] Mahonen, A; Jukkola, A; Risteli, L; Risteli, J; Maenpaa, PH. Type I procollagen synthesis is regulated by steroids and related hormones in human osteosarcoma cells. *J Cell Biochem.*, 1998, 68(2), 151-163.

[26] Brincat, M; Versi, E; Moniz, CF; Magos, A; de Trafford, J; Studd, JW. Skin collagen changes in postmenopausal women receiving different regimens of estrogen therapy. *Obstet Gynecol*, 1987, 70(1), 123-127.

[27] Affinito, P; Palomba, S; Sorrentino, C; Di Carlo, C; Bifulco, G; Arienzo, MP; et al. Effects of postmenopausal hypoestrogenism on skin collagen. *Maturitas*, 1999, 33(3), 239-247.

[28] Shah, MG; Maibach, HI. Estrogen and skin. An overview. *Am J Clin Dermatol*, 2001, 2(3), 143-150.

[29] Brincat, M; Moniz, CF; Studd, JW; Darby, AJ; Magos, A; Cooper, D. Sex hormones and skin collagen content in postmenopausal women. *Br Med J (Clin Res Ed)*, 1983, 287(6402), 1337-1338.

[30] Savvas, M; Bishop, J; Laurent, G; Watson, N; Studd, J. Type III collagen content in the skin of postmenopausal women receiving oestradiol and testosterone implants. *Br J Obstet Gynaecol*, 1993, 100(2), 154-156.

[31] Schmidt, JB; Binder, M; Demschik, G; Bieglmayer, C; Reiner, A. Treatment of skin aging with topical estrogens. *Int J Dermatol*, 1996, 35(9), 669-674.

[32] Varila, E; Rantala, I; Oikarinen, A; Risteli, J; Reunala, T; Oksanen, H; et al. The effect of topical oestradiol on skin collagen of postmenopausal women. *Br J Obstet Gynaecol*, 1995, 102(12), 985-989.

[33] Sauerbronn, AV; Fonseca, AM; Bagnoli, VR; Saldiva, PH; Pinotti, JA. The effects of systemic hormonal replacement therapy on the skin of postmenopausal women. *Int J Gynaecol Obstet*, 2000, 68(1), 35-41.

[34] Haapasaari, KM; Raudaskoski, T; Kallioinen, M; Suvanto-Luukkonen, E; Kauppila, A; Laara, E; et al. Systemic therapy with estrogen or estrogen with progestin has no effect on skin collagen in postmenopausal women. *Maturitas*, 1997, 27(2), 153-162.

[35] Oikarinen, A. Systemic estrogens have no conclusive beneficial effect on human skin connective tissue. *Acta Obstet Gynecol Scand.*, 2000, 79(4), 250-254.

[36] Punnonen, R; Vaajalahti, P; Teisala, K. Local oestriol treatment improves the structure of elastic fibers in the skin of postmenopausal women. *Ann Chir Gynaecol Suppl.*, 1987, 202, 39-41.

[37] Kalogirou, D; Aroni, K; Kalogirou, O; Antoniou, G; Botsis, D; Kontoravdis, A. Histological changes induced by tibolone and estrogen/glucocorticoid on aging skin. Int *J Fertil Womens Med.*, 2000, 45(4), 273-278.

[38] Wilhelm, KP; Cua, AB; Maibach, HI. Skin aging. Effect on transepidermal water loss, stratum corneum hydration, skin surface pH, and casual sebum content. *Arch Dermatol*, 1991, 127(12), 1806-1809.

[39] Elden, HR. *Advances of biology of the skin*. In: W. Montagna, J. P. Bentley, & R. L. Dobson (Eds.), The dermis. New York: Appleton Century Crofts, 1970.

[40] Beauregard, S; Gilchrest, BA. A survey of skin problems and skin care regimens in the elderly. *Arch Dermatol*, 1987, 123(12), 1638-1643.

[41] Dunn, LB; Damesyn, M; Moore, AA; Reuben, DB; Greendale, GA. Does estrogen prevent skin aging? Results from the First National Health and Nutrition Examination Survey (NHANES I). *Arch Dermatol*, 1997, 133(3), 339-342.

[42] Sobel, H; Cohen, RA. Effect of estradion on hyaluronic acid in the skin of aging mice. *Steroids*, 1970, 16(1), 1-3.
[43] Uzuka, M; Nakajima, K; Ohta, S; Mori, Y. The mechanism of estrogen-induced increase in hyaluronic acid biosynthesis, with special reference to estrogen receptor in the mouse skin. *Biochim Biophys Acta*, 1980, 627(2), 199-206.
[44] Grosman, N; Hvidberg, E; Schou, J. The effect of oestrogenic treatment on the acid mucopolysaccharide pattern in skin of mice. *Acta Pharmacol Toxicol (Copenh)*, 1971, 30(5), 458-464.
[45] Jacobsen, E; Billings, JK; Frantz, RA; Kinney, CK; Stewart, ME; Downing, DT. Age-related changes in sebaceous wax ester secretion rates in men and women. *J Invest Dermatol*, 1985, 85(5), 483-485.
[46] Sator, PG; Schmidt, JB; Sator, MO; Huber, JC; Honigsmann, H. The influence of hormone replacement therapy on skin ageing: a pilot study. *Maturitas*, 2001, 39(1), 43-55.
[47] Callens, A; Vaillant, L; Lecomte, P; Berson, M; Gall, Y; Lorette, G. Does hormonal skin aging exist? A study of the influence of different hormone therapy regimens on the skin of postmenopausal women using non-invasive measurement techniques. *Dermatology*, 1996, 193(4), 289-294.
[48] Rebora, A. Pathogenesis of androgenetic alopecia. *J Am Acad Dermatol*, 2004, 50(5), 777-779.
[49] Hoffmann, R; Niiyama, S; Huth, A; Kissling, S; Happle, R. 17alpha-estradiol induces aromatase activity in intact human anagen hair follicles ex vivo. *Exp Dermatol*, 2002, 11(4), 376-380.
[50] Wallace, ML; Smoller, BR. Estrogen and progesterone receptors in androgenic alopecia versus alopecia areata. *Am J Dermatopathol*, 1998, 20(2), 160-163.
[51] Kossard, S; Lee, MS; Wilkinson, B. Postmenopausal frontal fibrosing alopecia: a frontal variant of lichen planopilaris. *J Am Acad Dermatol*, 1997, 36(1), 59-66.
[52] Black, MM; Shuster, S; Bottoms, E. Osteoporosis, skin collagen, and androgen. *Br Med J.*, 1970, 4(5738), 773-774.
[53] Baron, YM; Brincat, M; Galea, R. Increased reduction in bone density and skin thickness in postmenopausal women on long-term corticosteroid therapy. A suggested role for estrogen add back therapy. *Adv Exp Med Biol.*, 1999, 455, 429-436.
[54] Pierard-Franchimont, C; Letawe, C; Goffin, V; Pierard, GE. Skin water-holding capacity and transdermal estrogen therapy for menopause: a pilot study. *Maturitas*, 1995, 22(2), 151-154.
[55] Baron, YM; Brincat, M; Galea, R. Increased reduction in bone density and skin thickness in postmenopausal women on long-term corticosteroid therapy. A suggested role for estrogen add back therapy. *Adv Exp Med Biol.*, 1999, 455, 429-436.
[56] Maheux, R; Naud, F; Rioux, M; Grenier, R; Lemay, A; Guy, J; et al. A randomized, double-blind, placebo-controlled study on the effect of conjugated estrogens on skin thickness. *Am J Obstet Gynecol.*, 1994, 170(2), 642-649.
[57] Sumino, H; Ichikawa, S; Abe, M; Endo, Y; Ishikawa, O; Kurabayashi, M. Effects of aging, menopause, and hormone replacement therapy on forearm skin elasticity in women. *J Am Geriatr Soc.*, 2004, 52(6), 945-949.

[58] Pierard, GE; Letawe, C; Dowlati, A; Pierard-Franchimont, C. Effect of hormone replacement therapy for menopause on the mechanical properties of skin. *J Am Geriatr Soc.*, 1995, 43(6), 662-665.

[59] Anttinen, H; Orava, S; Ryhanen, L; Kivirikko, KI. Assay of protocollagen lysyl hydroxylase activity in the skin of human subjects and changes in the activity with age. *Clin Chim Acta*, 1973, 47(2), 289-294.

[60] Henry, F; Pierard-Franchimont, C; Cauwenbergh, G; Pierard, GE. Age-related changes in facial skin contours and rheology. *J Am Geriatr Soc.*, 1997, 45(2), 220-222.

[61] Kafantari, H; Kounadi, E; Fatouros, M; Milonakis, M; Tzaphlidou, M. Structural alterations in rat skin and bone collagen fibrils induced by ovariectomy. *Bone*, 2000, 26(4), 349-353.

[62] Castelo-Branco, C; Figueras, F; Martinez de Osaba, MJ; Vanrell, JA. Facial wrinkling in postmenopausal women. Effects of smoking status and hormone replacement therapy. *Maturitas*, 1998, 29(1), 75-86.

[63] Brincat, MP; Baron, YM; Galea, R. Skin and connective tissues. In: J. Studd, & C. Lauritzen, (Eds.), *Current Management of the Menopause*. London: Taylor & Francis, 2001.

[64] Haenggi, W; Linder, HR; Birkhaeuser, MH; Schneider, H. Microscopic findings of the nail-fold capillaries--dependence on menopausal status and hormone replacement therapy. *Maturitas*, 1995, 22(1), 37-46.

[65] Arora, S; Veves, A; Caballaro, AE; Smakowski, P; LoGerfo, FW. Estrogen improves endothelial function. *J Vasc Surg.*, 1998, 27(6), 1141-1146.

[66] Ashcroft, GS; Greenwell-Wild, T; Horan, MA; Wahl, SM; Ferguson, MW. Topical estrogen accelerates cutaneous wound healing in aged humans associated with an altered inflammatory response. *Am J Pathol.*, 1999, 155(4), 1137-1146.

[67] Calvin, M. Oestrogens and wound healing. *Maturitas*, 2000, 34(3), 195-210.

[68] Ashcroft, GS; Dodsworth, J; van Boxtel, E; Tarnuzzer, RW; Horan, MA; Schultz, GS; et al. Estrogen accelerates cutaneous wound healing associated with an increase in TGF-beta1 levels. *Nat Med.*, 1997, 3(11), 1209-1215.

[69] Lauritzen, C. Benefits, Risks and Costs of Estrogen and Hormone Replacement Therapies. In: C. Lauritzen, & J. Studd, (Eds.), *Current Management of the Menopause*. UK: Taylor & Francis, 2005.

[70] Kaplan, RM; Andersen, JP; Ganiats, T. The quality of well-being scale: rationale for a single quality of life index. In: S. Walker, & M. Roser, (Eds.), *Quality of Life Assessment*: Key issues in the 1990s. Dordrecht: Kluwer Academic Press, 1993.

[71] Hunt, SM; McKenna, SP; McEwen, J; Williams, J; Papp, E. The Nottingham Health Profile: subjective health status and medical consultations. *Soc Sci Med [A]*, 1981, 15(3 Pt 1), 221-229.

[72] McHorney, CA; Ware, JE Jr; Raczek, AE. The MOS 36-Item Short-Form Health Survey (SF-36): II. Psychometric and clinical tests of validity in measuring physical and mental health constructs. *Med Care*, 1993, 31(3), 247-263.

[73] Utian, WH; Yanata, JW; Kingsberg, SA; Patrick, LD. Determinants of quantification of quality of life after the menopause: the Utian Menopause Quality of Life score. In: T. Aso, editor. *The menopause at the millenium*. NY: Parthenon Publishing, 2000.

[74] Schneider, H. Quality of life assessed by menopause rating scales. In: H. Schneider, editor. *Menopause. The State of the Art*. London: Parthenon, 2003.

[75] Schneider H, Behre HM. Contemporary evaluation of climacteric complaints, its impacts on quality of life. In: Schneider H, editor. Hormone Replacement Therapy and Quality of Life. London: Parthenon, 2003.

[76] Schneider, HP; Heinemann, LA; Rosemeier, HP; Potthoff, P; Behre, HM. The Menopause Rating Scale (MRS): comparison with Kupperman index and quality-of-life scale SF-36. *Climacteric*, 2000, 3(1), 50-58.

[77] Graziottin, A. Psychosexual role of the skin in the climacteric. In: Brincat MP, editor. *Hormone Replacement Therapy and the Skin*. Lancaster: Parthenon, 2001.

[78] Graziottin, A. *Libido: the biologic scenario*. Maturitas 2000, 34 Suppl 1, S9-16.

[79] Brincat, MP; Baron, YM; Galea, R. Connective tissue changes in the menopause and with HRT. In: R. A. Lobo, editor. *Treatment of the postmenopausal woman: basic and clinical aspects*, 2007.

[80] Nerlich, AG; Schleicher, ED; Boos, N. 1997 Volvo Award winner in basic science studies. Immunohistologic markers for age-related changes of human lumbar intervertebral discs. *Spine*, 1997, 22(24), 2781-2795.

[81] Boos, N; Weissbach, S; Rohrbach, H; Weiler, C; Spratt, KF; Nerlich, AG. Classification of age-related changes in lumbar intervertebral discs: 2002 Volvo Award in basic science. *Spine*, 2002, 27(23), 2631-2644.

[82] Baron, YM; Brincat, MP; Galea, R; Calleja, N. Intervertebral disc height in treated and untreated overweight post-menopausal women. *Hum Reprod.*, 2005, 20(12), 3566-3570.

[83] Baron, YM; Galea, R; Brincat, M. Carotid artery wall changes in estrogen-treated and -untreated postmenopausal women. *Obstet Gynecol.*, 1998, 91(6), 982-986.

In: Skin Anatomy and Physiology Research Developments
Editor: Leon F. Bukowsky
ISBN: 978-1-60741-469-8

Chapter 9

Distributed Parameter Estimation of Dermal Absorption of Chemicals using a Physiologically Inspired Boundary Conditions

L. Simon *

Otto H. York Department of Chemical, Biological and Pharmaceutical Engineering
New Jersey Institute of Technology, University Heights, Newark, NJ 07102, USA

Abstract

A spatial-temporal framework representing dermal absorption of chemicals is important for toxicological risk assessment. Failure to adequately estimate the amount of chemicals entering the body through the skin may compromise the ability of physiologically-based pharmacokinetic (PBPK) models to predict concentration-time profiles in individual tissue compartments. This contribution considers the conventional PBPK model equations as a boundary condition to a diffusive mass transport problem. The partial differential equation (PDE), representing the uptake of dibromomethane (500 to 10000 ppm) in the skin, is discretized into ordinary differential equations (ODEs) by orthogonal collocation techniques. The resulting system is solved in the Mathematica® environment to evaluate the fate of dibromomethane in the liver, fat, rapidly and slowly perfused compartments and to monitor its evolution in the different layers of the skin. This approach, which uses published physicochemical properties, predicts laboratory data very well. Cumulative amounts of dibromomethane into and out of the skin are also computed and compared to those obtained by applying a perfect sink boundary condition at the skin-capillary interface. Discrepancies between the two model predictions become more pronounced with increased exposure time. The steady-state dibromomethane concentration and the time to reach equilibrium values increased with the exposure level and stratum corneum depth. The proposed methodology may help to explore and

* Corresponding author. Tel.: 973-596-5263; fax: 973-596-8436; e-mail: laurent.simon@njit.edu

elucidate potential links among exposure-time, concentration, skin depth and the onset of skin irritation.

1. Introduction

Physiologically based pharmacokinetic (PBPK) models have been applied, successfully, to assess risk posed by toxic chemicals and to elucidate their biological mechanisms as they are transported to specific organs and tissues. In the PBPK modeling framework, the body is divided into several physiological compartments, such as the liver and lung. Material balance equations are written to represent chemical uptake in the various tissues. The transport phenomena, occuring in each organ, are complex and involve convection and diffusion contributions that are rigorously described using partial differential equations (PDEs). Assumptions (e.g., homogeneous compartments, perfusion- or diffusion-limited processes) are usually made to address certain aspects of the problem and to limit the scope of modeling. The well-mixed compartment approach, often adopted by researchers in the field, leads to stiff ordinary differential equations (ODEs) that are solved using softwares such as acslXtreme® (AEgis Technology Group) and Berkeley Madonna™ (Macey & Oster). Since a comprehensive database of biochemical, physiological and physicochemical parameters are compiled for a large number of compounds [1], model developers can easily compare their predictions with experimental concentration data. The findings of such investigations are instrumental in promoting a better understanding of the dominant mechanisms that control the absorption and distribution of toxic agents throughout the body. Nestorov (2003) offered a comprehensive review of PBPK structures that describes model development methodologies, implementations, limitations and research orientation [2].

PBPK models, developed to predict biological tissue distribution of chemicals, are often applied to describe percutaneous absorption. Such approaches allow researchers to assess dermal absorption from soil contamination by Volatile Organic Compounds (VOCs), such as perchloroethylene (PCE) [3]. The mathematical framework also facilitated the simulation of worst-case scenarios for dermal exposures to methyl chloroform found in contaminated soil [4]. In those examples, ordinary differential equations were written to explain chemical concentration changes in subcutaneous tissues. Although the skin offers a complex heterogenous medium, the simplified representations have been successful in explaining laboratory data collected from rats and humans. Work on drug release from transdermal systems shows that PDE-based models are more suitable to describe the transport of medicaments via this route. The skin is composed of the epidermis (stratum corneum and viable epidermis), the dermis and the subcutaneous fat region. The stratum corneum, consisting of dead cells, constitutes the main resistance to drug permeation [5]. The nature of the epidermis (i.e., aqueous and lipid regions) has a profound impact on drug diffusivity [6]. However, only a few examples in the literature use PDEs because of the relative simplicity of PBPK models, the physiologically meaningful nature of the parameters [7], and the large database of information for animal species and humans,

The "well-stirred" homogeneous skin model has been critical in the generation of model parameters that can be determined experimentally [8]. As in distributed-parameter systems, the accumulation of penetrants in homogeneous skin models is governed by Fick's laws of diffusion as they traverse the dermal layers and blood flow rate. However, in the common PBPK framework, mass transfer resistance is mainly due to a very thin-layer representation of the stratum corneum. An implication of this analogy, unsubstantiated by experimental work with volatile organic compounds, is that chemicals do not accumulate in the skin's main barrier [9]. A drawback of this approach is that risk assessment, based on such analysis, only provides temporal concentration data. Poet and McDougal (2002) noted that accurate information, concerning both the absorption and penetration of chemicals into and through the layers of the skin, is indispensable for reliably predicting local and systemic toxicity [10]. In studies addressing jet prollant-8 (JP-8) irritation potential, researchers reasoned that the ability to ascertain the JP-8 concentration, that induces dermal irritation, is important and may result in the development of therapeutic intervention strategies to help individuals exposed to jet fuel [11]. Elucidating the mechanism of skin irritation in a spatial-temporal context is a critical step to fully comprehend the toxicity and irritation potency of chemicals. A firm understanding of the concentration and location of chemicals in the skin layers and how they relate to biological responses may promote perspectives not found in the well-stirred compartment model. In addition, the ability to predict the time it takes a compound, in each skin layer, to reach a steady-state concentration, is paramount to efforts toward a comprehensive risk assessment of dermal exposure to toxic compounds. Similar investigations were undertaken to estimate brain equilibrium half-life (i.e., time to reach 50% of its plateau level after single intravenous bolus dose) based on PBPK models [12].

2. Pbpk Modeling of Dermal Chemical Absorption

Physiologically-based pharmacokinetic skin models were initially proposed in an effort to standardize and simplify parameter estimation through laboratory experiments and enable the extrapolation of results across species [8]. Dermal absorption is modeled using skin permeation values in lieu of Fick's second law of diffusive transport adopted in drug-delivery research. Chinery and Gleason (1993) employed different skin permeability coefficients to construct a PBPK model for dermal absorption of chloroform from exposure to an aqueous medium [13]. Guidance on how PBPK models can be used to study toxicity after dermal exposure can be found in the work of Anderson and Keller [14].

The steady-state permeation flux can be calculated using Fick's first law of diffusion:

$$J_{ss} = \frac{DK}{l}\Delta C = P\Delta C \qquad (1)$$

where D is the diffusion coefficient of the penetrant, l is the thickness of the membrane, K is the membrane/donor partition coefficient, ΔC is the difference between the concentration in the vehicle and the concentration in the sink (i.e., receiver chamber), P is the permeability coefficient. The dermal uptake and assessment of potential toxicity of chemical agents are based on the P value, the applied concentration and the surface area and time of exposure. An average flux is usually calculated in animal studies [15]:

$$J_{ave} = \frac{M}{A \times t} \tag{2}$$

In this formulation, M is the total mass of chemical absorbed, t is the time and A is the exposed area. It is customary to express the permeability coefficient as:

$$P = \frac{J_{ave}}{C_{sfc}} \tag{3}$$

where C_{sfc} is the vehicle concentration. Combining Eqs. (2) and (3) gives:

$$M = PAC_{sfc}t \tag{4}$$

Methodologies are proposed to relax the assumption of steady-state conditions embedded in Eq. (4) and to account for the fact that, in a PBPK model, mass balance equations have to include chemicals entering the skin from the arterial blood and exiting via the venous blood [15].

2.1. Homogeneous One Compartment Skin Model (1-CSM)

A single homogeneous compartment is developed to represent the skin [8]:

$$V_{sk}\frac{dC_{sk}}{dt} = P_{sk}A_{sk}\left(C_{sfc} - \frac{C_{sk}}{R_{sk/sfc}}\right) + Q_{sk}\left(C_a - \frac{C_{sk}}{R_{sk/b}}\right) \tag{5}$$

Equation (5), based on mass conservation, describes the accumulation of permeant. The lumped-parameter approach treats the skin as a process unit in which concentration changes due to a) the blood flow to the skin (Q_{sk}), the skin permeability and area (P_{sk}, A_{sk}, respectively), b) concentrations in the arterial blood and in the skin (C_a and C_{sk}, respectively), and c) the skin to surface and skin to blood partition coefficients ($R_{sk/sfc}$ and $R_{sk/b}$). Compound accumulation in the skin is the result of material transported by the blood flow and mass transfer from the surface. The model assumes an infinitely thin resistance layer and tends to underestimate the amount of chemical initially absorbed into the skin [16].

2.2. Homogeneous Two-Compartment Skin Model (2-CSM)

Booktout et al. (1996) wrote a two-subcompartment model made up of the stratum corneum (I) and a lumped region (II) composed of the viable epidermis, dermis and subcutaneous fat. Blood only flows in the latter region (II). In this approach, the stratum corneum and subcompartment II are described by:

$$V_{sc}\frac{dC_{sc}}{dt} = P_{sc}A_{sc}\left(C_{sfc} - \frac{C_{sc}}{R_{sc/sfc}}\right) + P_{cd}A_{cd}\left(C_{cd} - \frac{C_{sc}}{R_{sc/cd}}\right) \tag{6}$$

and

$$V_{cd}\frac{dC_{cd}}{dt} = P_{cd}A_{cd}\left(C_{cd} - \frac{C_{sc}}{R_{sc/cd}}\right) + Q_{cd}\left(C_{a} - \frac{C_{cd}}{R_{cd/b}}\right), \tag{7}$$

respectively. Volumes of regions I and II are V_{sc} and V_{cd}; C_{sc} and C_{cd} are the concentration in regions I and II; P_{sc} and P_{cd} are the drug permeability in sections I and II; A_{sc} and A_{cd} are the surface areas of I and II; $R_{sc/sfc}$, $R_{sc/cd}$ and $R_{cd/b}$ are the blood partition coefficients at the following interfaces: stratum corneum to surface, stratum corneum to compartment II, and region II to blood, respectively; Q_{cd} is the blood flow rate to region II. The mass transfer resistance of the stratum corneum is at a thin interfacial layer between the exposure medium and the stratum corneum [9]. An additional mass transport resistance is due to a similarly thin layer, situated between the stratum corneum and the viable skin. Although the model defined by Eqs. (6) and (7) may lead to more accurate predictions than the one-compartment construct, the dermal resistances, represented by two infinitesimally thin layers, underestimate the chemical accumulation in the stratum corneum [9]. In addition, since not all of the new parameters are measurable, regression techniques are usually applied to estimate the permeability constants and partition coefficients [8]. However, the 2-CSM does not allow the monitoring of compounds at different depths of the skin layers. A three subcompartment skin model, derived from the homogeneous representation, was also described in [8]. It should be noted that one of the main attractions of PBPK models is the presence of meaningful and measurable parameters in the mathematical description of permeant uptake through the body. Consequently, the results of increasingly complex models have to be interpreted and extrapolated with caution. In section 2.4, Fickian diffusion and orthogonal collocation methods are used to estimate the dermal absorption at different skin layers.

2.3. Homogeneous Three-Compartment Skin Model (3-CSM)

The 2-CSM was expanded to a three sub-compartment skin model [8]:

$$V_{sc}\frac{dC_{sc}}{dt}=P_{sc}A_{sc}\left(C_{sfc}-\frac{C_{sc}}{R_{sc/sfc}}\right)+P_{ve}A_{ve}\left(C_{ve}-\frac{C_{sc}}{R_{sc/ve}}\right) \tag{8}$$

$$V_{ve}\frac{dC_{ve}}{dt}=P_{ve}A_{ve}\left(\frac{C_{sc}}{R_{sc/ve}}-C_{ve}\right)+P_{cd}A_{cd}\left(C_{cd}-\frac{C_{ve}}{R_{ve/cd}}\right) \tag{9a}$$

and

$$V_{cd}\frac{dC_{cd}}{dt}=P_{cd}A_{cd}\left(\frac{C_{ve}}{R_{ve/cd}}-C_{cd}\right)+Q_{cd}\left(C_{a}-\frac{C_{cd}}{R_{cd/b}}\right). \tag{9}$$

Equations (8), (9a) and (9) are written for the stratum corneum (*sc*), viable epidermis (*ve*), and composite dermal compartment (*cd*), respectively. The latter compartment is composed of the dermis and subcutaneous fat. These equations were written by Bookout et al. (1996) and are repeated here for completeness. Definitions of the quantities are provided in the Nomenclature section. It is worth noticing that blood only flows through the composite dermal. Experiments show that the three sub-compartment model results in more accurate blood concentration estimations of dibromomethane [8]. The disadvantage of this procedure is that some of the new parameters would have to be estimated or optimized.

2.4. Membrane Skin Model (MSM)

Equations (5)-(9) are useful in addressing the resistance offered by the skin layers and the contribution of skin physiology in influencing the distribution of a chemical through tissues. The skin tissues include i) the stratum corneum, the outermost epidermal layer, that has a thickness ranging from 10 to 40 μm and is composed of dead cells containing keratin; ii) the viable skin made of the viable epidermis (50-100 μm) and the dermis (500-3000 μm) [9]. The stratum corneum offers the most significant mass transfer resistance for most compounds [17]. Describing chemical absorption through the skin using the structures outlined above assumes that the major resistance to the transport of molecules simply occurs at some interfaces. The spatial variation of drugs in the layers is not captured by these models. To maintain the PBPK modeling framework and to represent the physiology of the skin, Roy et al. (1996) proposed a distributed parameter (DP-PBPK) representation of dermal absorption where the resistance is distributed all throughout the stratum corneum [9]. The accumulation of mass in the viable skin is a function of the mass flux at the stratum corneum/viable skin interface. The equations used can be summarized as:

$$\frac{\partial C_{sc}}{\partial t} = \frac{\partial}{\partial x}\left(D_{sc} \frac{\partial C_{sc}}{\partial x} \right) \tag{10}$$

$$C_{sc}\ \ 0,t\ = C_{sfc} R_{sc/sfc} \tag{11}$$

$$C_{sc}\ \ h,t\ = \frac{C_{vs}}{R_{vs/sc}} \tag{12}$$

$$C_{sc}\ \ x,0\ = 0 \tag{13}$$

$$V_{vs} \frac{dC_{vs}}{dt} = J\ \ h,t\ \ A_{vs} + Q_{sk}\left(C_a - \frac{C_{vs}}{R_{vs/b}} \right) \tag{14}$$

Equation (10) is Fick's second law applied to the stratum corneum. The diffusion coefficient in the stratum corneum, D_{sc}, is not a function of time or the drug concentration. The donor cell concentration, C_0, does not change significantly during the course of exposure. As a result, the concentration on the surface of the stratum corneum, $C_{sc}\ \ 0,t$, remains constant (Eq. (11)). Equation (12) is a local equilibrium partition condition at the stratum corneum/viable skin interface. The skin is initially free of drug (Eq. (13)). The mass accumulation in the viable skin is represented by Eq. (14) and $J\ \ h,t$ is the transient flux at the stratum corneum/viable skin interface. Roy et al. (1996) proposed a numerical scheme based on a central difference formula to convert Eqs. (10)-(14) into a set of ODEs. An orthogonal collocation methodology, that provides increased accuracy, is implemented in this contribution.

3. Orthogonal Collocation Techniques

The method of orthogonal collocation consists of writing the concentration of chemicals in the stratum corneum as a finite series:

$$C_{sc}(\zeta,t) \approx a(t) + \zeta b(t) + \zeta(1-\zeta)\sum_{i=1}^{N} a_i(t) P_{i-1}(\zeta) \qquad (15)$$

after scaling the thickness of the layer to 1. In this formulation, $\{P_i(\zeta)\}$ represents a set of polynomials such that $P_n(\zeta)$ is orthogonal to $P_m(\zeta)$ when $m \neq n$, over some interval. The locations of the collocation points (ζ) are given by the roots of $P_n(\zeta)$. System nonlinearities and the level of model accuracy required by the user influence the selection of the number of internal collocation points (N). A system of ODEs is generated by substituting Eq. (15) in the original partial differential equation.

A dimensionless version of Eqs. (10)-(13) is first written and solved by the orthogonal collocation method and by the built-in solver, *NDSolve* in Mathematica®. According to this method, the normalized concentration of the dissolved chemical (C_{1sc}) in the stratum corneum is expressed by linear combinations of Jacobi polynomials, $P_i\ \zeta_j$, as the basis functions. A weight function $W\ \zeta$ was written to satisfy the orthogonality condition:

$$\langle P_m\ \zeta\ , P_n\ \zeta\ \rangle_W = \int_0^1 W\ \zeta\ \times P_m\ \zeta\ \times P_n\ \zeta\ d\zeta = 0 \qquad (16)$$

where $\langle f_1, f_2 \rangle_W$ stands for the inner product of functions f_1 and f_2 with respect to $W\ \zeta$. The internal collocation points, ζ_j, were chosen as the positive roots of the equation:

$$P_N\ \zeta\ = 0 \qquad (17)$$

Equation (15) is rewritten as:

$$C_{1sc}\ \zeta_j, \tau\ = \sum_{i=1}^{N+2} d_i\ \tau\ \zeta_j^{(i-1)} \qquad (19)$$

The first derivative of Eq. (19) with respect to ζ is:

$$\frac{\partial}{\partial \zeta} C_{1sc}\ \zeta_j, \tau\ = \sum_{i=1}^{N+2} d_i\ \tau\ (i-1)\zeta_j^{i-2} \qquad (18)$$

The vector-matrix forms of Eq. (19) and (18) are:

$$\mathbf{c} = \mathbf{Z}\mathbf{d} \tag{19}$$

and

$$\frac{\partial \mathbf{c}}{\partial \zeta} = \mathbf{Q}\mathbf{d} \tag{20}$$

where $\mathbf{c} = C_{1sc}(\zeta_j, \tau)$ and $\mathbf{d} = d_i(\tau)$ represent vectors; $\mathbf{Z} = \zeta_j^{i-1}$, $\mathbf{Q} = (i-1)\zeta_j^{i-2}$ are matrices. The solution of $\mathbf{d}$ in Eq. (19) is substituted in eq. (20) to yield:

$$\frac{\partial \mathbf{c}}{\partial \zeta} = \mathbf{Q}\mathbf{Z}^{-1}\mathbf{c} = \mathbf{A}\mathbf{c} \tag{21}$$

With these results, the normalized PDE problem is reduced to a system of ODEs in $C_{1sc}(\zeta_j, \tau)$ from which a set of $dC_{sc}(x_j, t)/dt$ can be easily obtained after converting the transformed variables back to their original scale. All the boundary conditions are incorporated in the ODEs, which are now written in terms of C_{vs}. Because C_{vs} is connected to other tissue compartments, such as liver and brain, the whole-body PBPK representation can be effectively formulated as a biologically-inspired boundary condition to a diffusive mass transport problem. Although no numerical benefit is gained from this perspective, the new paradigm has the advantage of placing the skin at the center of the analysis. In this framework, the design of novel and more complex transdermal drug-delivery devices can be fully investigated. The difficulty with this approach is that it involves a mixed system of ODEs and PDEs, which are not easily solved by software packages. However, this method makes it easy to visually represent the spatial-temporal evolution of toxic chemicals in the skin following dermal exposure and to explore potential links among exposure-time, concentration, skin depth and the onset of skin irritation.

A more detailed description of orthogonal collocation techniques is offered in [18] and [19]. Implementations of the method and advances can be found in [20-22]. The solution strategy significantly reduced the number of spatial nodes used in finite difference-based methods and required less computational resources to achieve similar performance [18]. The methodology is carried out using in-house codes written in Mathematica®.

4. Tissue Compartments in the Body

The PBPK model used in this work is similar to the one described by Bookout et al. [8]. The transport equations apply to solutes with large permeability across the capillary wall.

Except for the lung, absorption of the compound into the various tissues is only limited by the blood perfusion rate (i.e., perfusion-limited PBPK). Material balances around the tissues yield (Fig. 1):

$$V_r \frac{dC_r}{dt} = Q_r \left(C_a - \frac{C_r}{R_{r/b}} \right) \tag{22}$$

$$V_l \frac{dC_l}{dt} = Q_l \left(C_a - \frac{C_l}{R_{l/b}} \right) - \frac{k_f C_l V_l}{R_{l/b}} - \frac{V_{max} C_l}{K.R_{l/b} + C_l} \tag{23}$$

$$V_s \frac{dC_s}{dt} = Q_s \left(C_a - \frac{C_s}{R_{s/b}} \right) \tag{24}$$

$$V_f \frac{dC_f}{dt} = Q_f \left(C_a - \frac{C_f}{R_{f/b}} \right) \tag{25}$$

$$C_a = \frac{Q_c C_v}{\left(\frac{Q_a}{R_{b/air}} + Q_c \right)} \tag{26}$$

$$C_v = \frac{1}{Q_c} \left(\frac{Q_p C_p}{R_{p/b}} + \frac{Q_r C_r}{R_{r/b}} + \frac{Q_l C_l}{R_{l/b}} + \frac{Q_s C_s}{R_{s/b}} + \frac{Q_f C_f}{R_{f/b}} \right) \tag{27}$$

Equations (22)-(27) are solved along with models 1-CSM, 2-CSM, 3-CSM, or MSM. The subscript "*p*" stands for "*sk*", "*cd*" or "*vs*". The composite dermal compartment "*cd*" is represented by Eq. (7) (2-CSM) or Eq. (9) (3-CSM); "sk" and "*vs*" are used for models 1-CSM and MSM, respectively. Subscript "*a*" represents arterial, "*v*", venous and "*c*" stands for cardiac blood. Equations (22)-(25) are the mass-balance equations around the rapidly perfused tissue ("*r*"), liver ("*l*"), slowly perfused tissue ("*s*") and fat tissue ("*f*"). By assuming that the amount of chemical in the lung does not change with time, and that concentration in the surrounding air is negligible, Eq. (26) is written [23]. Equation (27) is employed to show the solute behavior in the large venous compartment; a steady-state assumption is made [23].

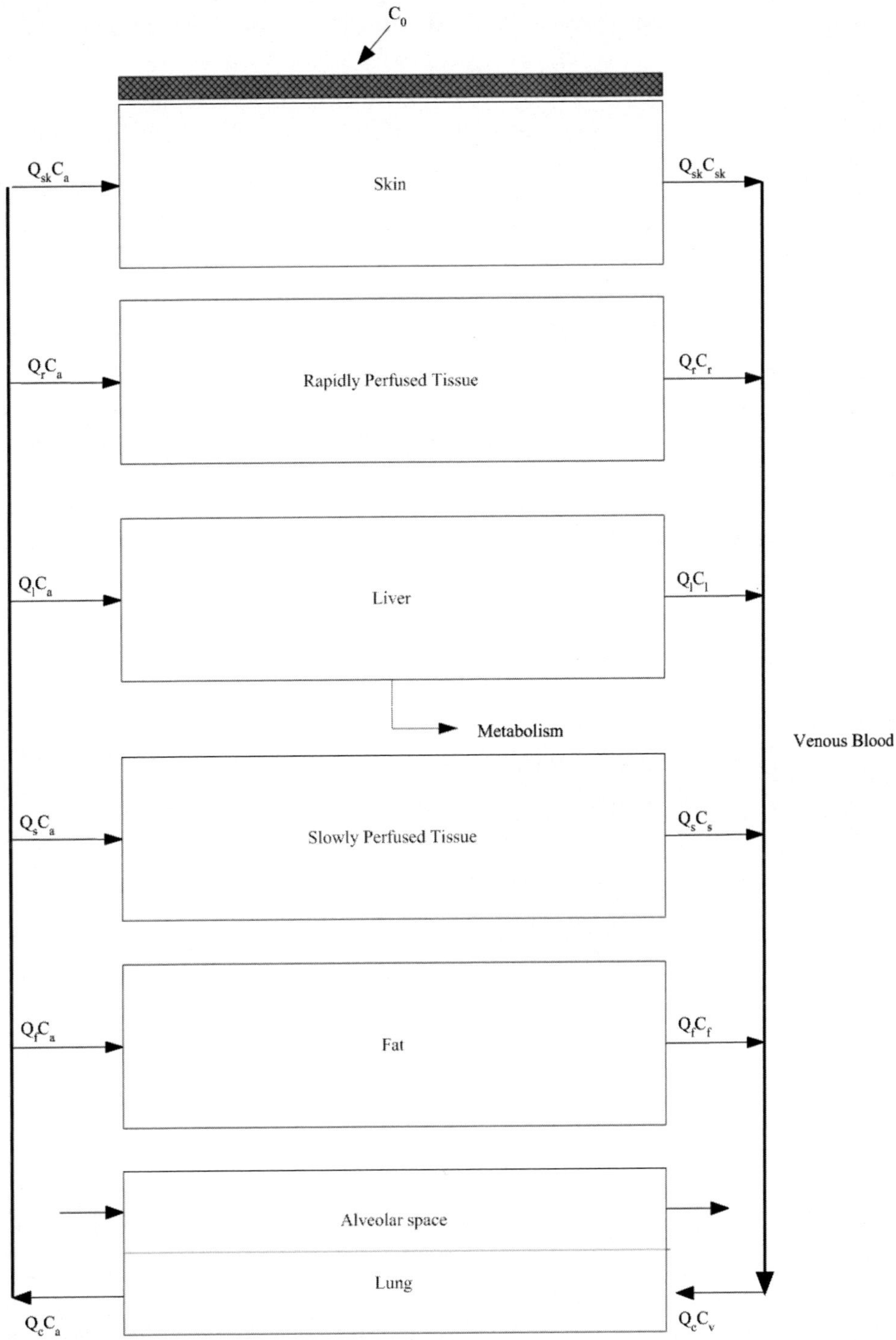

Figure 1. PBPK schematic representing the different tissues.

5. Numerical Results

The lumped-parameter models were solved using Mathematica®, which offers an integrated environment for statistical analysis, visualization and solutions for stiff and non-stiff ordinary equations. Physiologically-based pharmacokinetic modeling studies, such as the one conducted by Loizou et al. [24], are essential for a better understanding of the dermal absorption of solvent liquids and vapors. In that study, *m*-Xylene (50 ppm) was absorbed in humans by the inhalation and dermal routes. The compartments were liver, fat, skin and richly- and poorly-perfused tissues. Numerical simulations facilitated the estimation of dermal concentration exposure necessary to produce the same body burden from inhalation of 50 ppm *m*-Xylene [24].

In this contribution, the study was based on the work by Bookout et al. (1996). Because results of 1-CSM, 2-CSM, 3-CSM approaches are already shown in [8], only the 1-CSM is reproduced here for illustration. Second, the membrane skin model was solved for the absorption of dibromomethane by using orthogonal collocation techniques. The spatial-temporal concentration profiles at different skin depths were plotted. Third, values for the cumulative amounts of the chemical into and out of the skin were computed and compared to those obtained by applying a "perfect sink" boundary condition at the skin-capillary interface. Fourth, the time it would take distinct skin layers to become saturated with dibromomethane was investigated.

5.1. Well-stirred Single Compartment Model

The model parameters were found in [8]. Dibromomethane vapor concentrations varied from 500 to 10,000 ppm. As expected, the amount of chemical in the venous blood increased with the time and level of dibromomethane exposure (Fig. 2). The profiles are identical to those generated in [8]. The model validity was tested, in the original work, by comparing experimental data with simulated values. A good agreement was achieved. One of the advantages of this effort is that other exposure scenarios can be tested, as well, and the findings extrapolated across various species. The mathematical framework can be used to estimate dermal exposure concentration.

5.2. Diffusive Transport Model

The 1-CSM did not provide information about chemical concentration in the skin layers. Orthogonal collocation techniques were applied using a total of 8 internal collocation points. A higher number did not increase model accuracy. The various tissues were assumed free of the drug at the beginning of the experiment. Estimation of the stratum corneum diffusion coefficient is based on the steady-state permeability of the stratum corneum from the environmental medium ($K_{sc/sfc}$), the effective thickness of the stratum corneum (h) and the equilibrium partition coefficient between the stratum corneum and the environmental medium ($R_{sc/sfc}$) [25]:

$$D_{sc} = \frac{K_{sc/sfc}h}{R_{sc/sfc}} \quad (28)$$

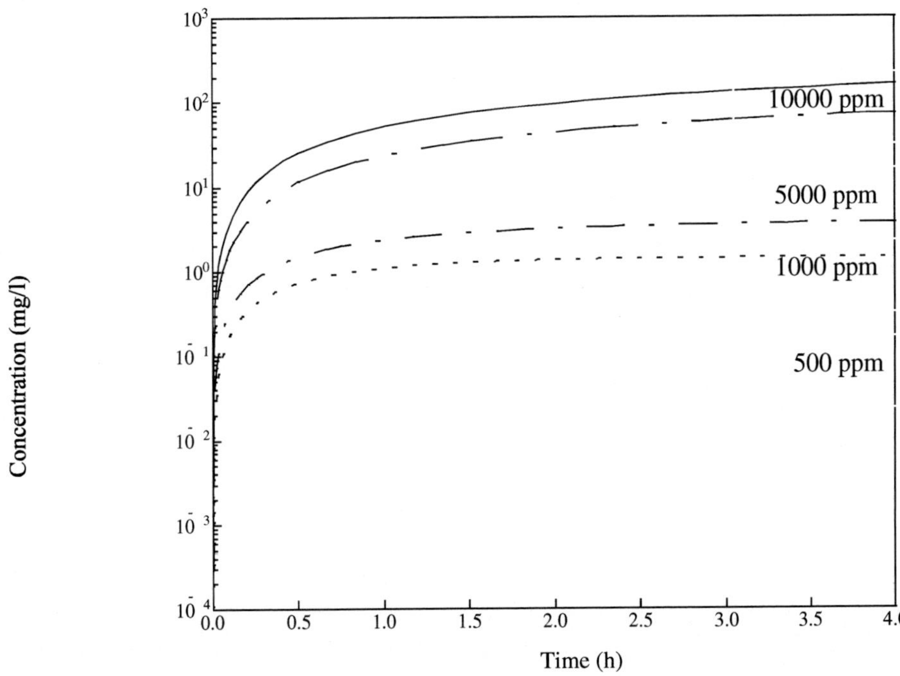

Figure 2. Venous blood concentration of dibromomethane using a well-stirred single compartment model. The exposure level varied from 500 to 10000 ppm.

The value for $R_{sk/b}$ was used in place of $R_{vs/b}$ in this example. This approximation should not introduce significant error in the calculation based on reported values of skin/air and viable epidermis-dermis-subcutaneous fat/air partition coefficients (266.0 and 259.3, respectively) [8]. The overall skin permeability ($K_{sk/sfc}$) was employed in Eq. (28) as an estimation of $K_{sc/sfc}$. Simulation results (Fig. 3) show that the diffusive transport model predicts well the chemical concentration in venous blood when compared to experimental data in [8]. In addition, Fig. 3 agrees with the trend shown in Fig. 2. The detailed description makes it possible to monitor the evolution of chemicals in the different skin layers. Such a feature was tested with the same conditions as in the single compartment model (i.e., 500 to

10000 ppm). The results are shown in Figs. 4 to 7. Steady-state dibromomethane concentration increased with the stratum corneum depth and exposure level.

Investigators outline other benefits associated with the distributed parameter model. Roy et al. (1996) reported that the end-exposure dose estimated by such methodologies is more consistent with the prediction of EPA-recommended Cleek and Bunge method for short-term exposure [25]. More recently, studies, using chloroform as a test compound, show that the homogeneous skin model predicts a very rapid initial uptake, as indicated by the quick appearance of chloroform in exhaled breath once the exposure begins [26]. The initial lag, supported by experimental data, was not observed.

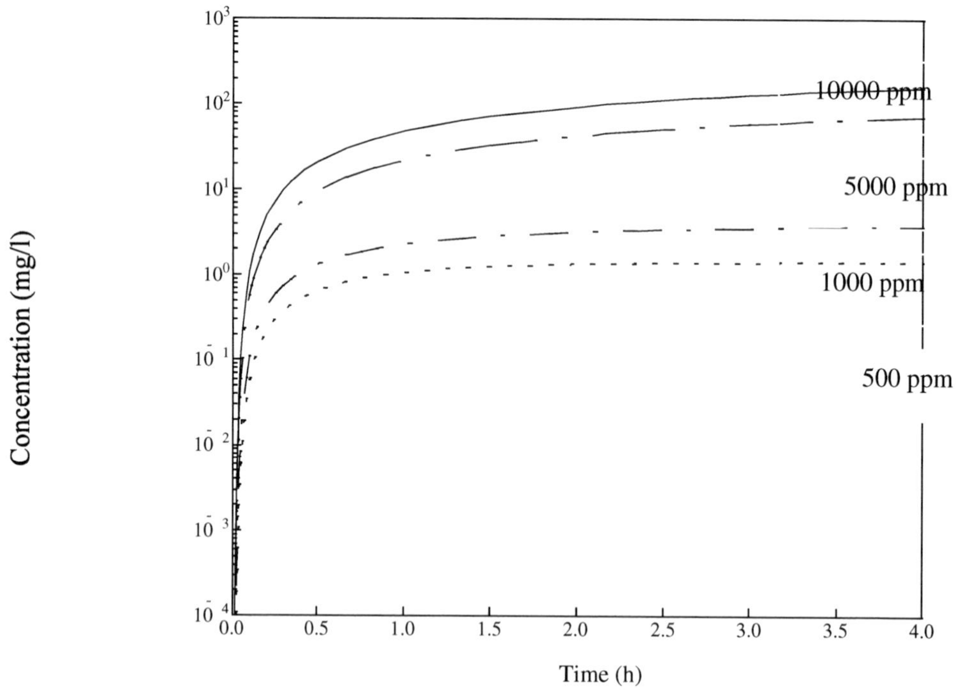

Figure 3. Venous blood concentration of dibromomethane using a membrane model of the skin. The exposure level varied from 500 to 10,000 ppm.

A membrane model, implemented using a finite-difference scheme, exhibited a better fit to actual data [26] than the homogenous representation. Similar to findings made by Roy et al. (1996), a lag-time was apparent in the exhaled breath concentration profile [9]. In studies conducted by Norman et. al. (2008), a lower cumulative uptake was also reported when the well-stirred skin approach was used [26]. PBPK model prediction capability improved, significantly, when the skin was represented by a membrane where diffusive transport took place. With fewer nodes than finite difference formula, the orthogonal collocation method gives a more accurate estimation of fluxes and concentrations. This feature may help increase the popularity of Fickian diffusion equation in aqueous dermal exposure. In addition, the reduced number of nodes, necessary to achieve acceptable model accuracy, makes the procedure easily transportable to other software packages.

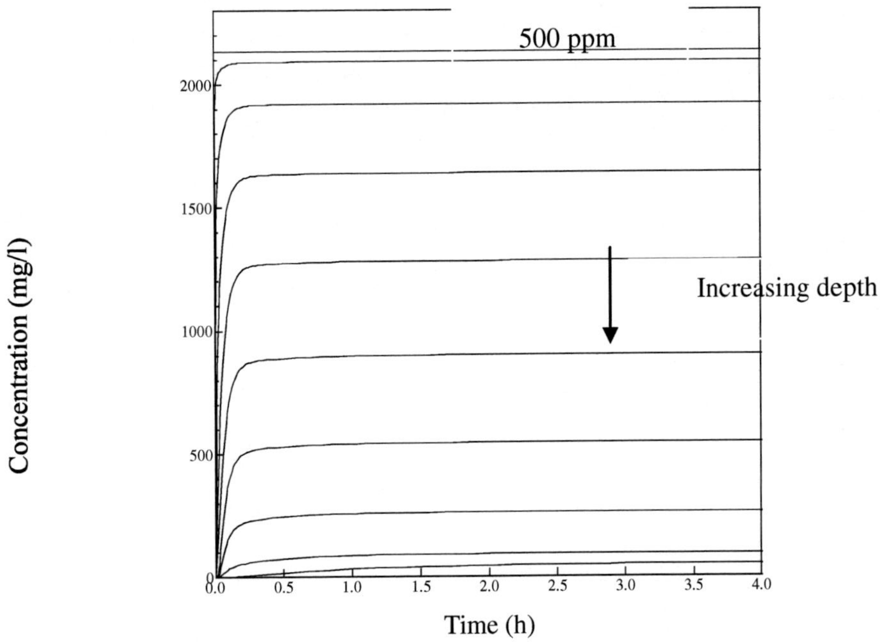

Figure 4. Dibromomethane concentration in the stratum corneum. The depths (dm), based on the internal collocation points, are 0, 2.055×10-6, 1.052×10-5, 2.455×10-5, 4.226×10-5 6.124×10-5, 7.895×10-5, 9.298×10-5, 1.014×10-4, 1.035×10-4. An exposure level of 500 was used.

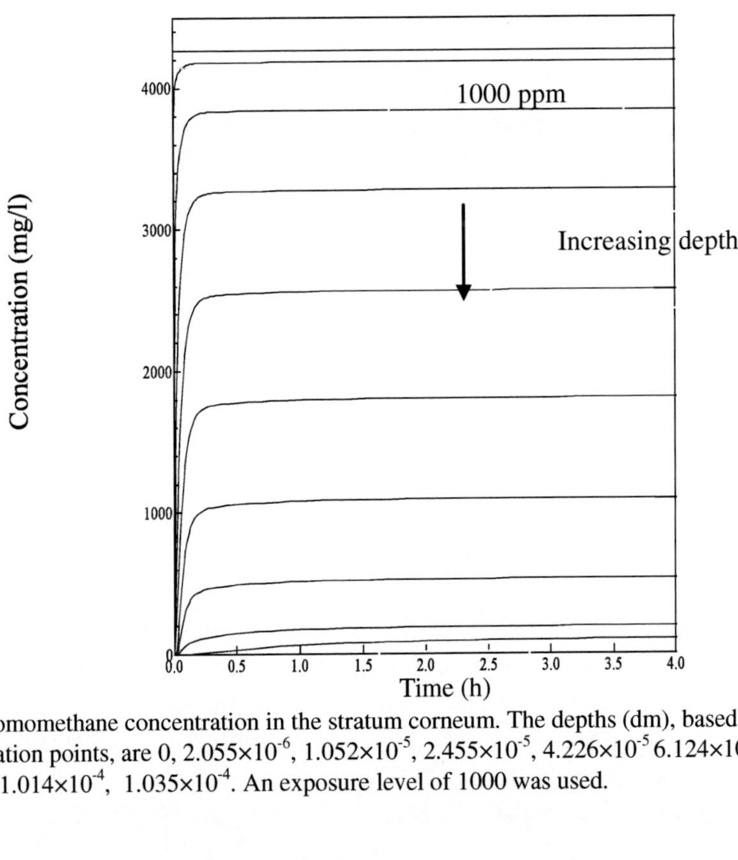

Figure 5. Dibromomethane concentration in the stratum corneum. The depths (dm), based on the internal collocation points, are 0, 2.055×10^{-6}, 1.052×10^{-5}, 2.455×10^{-5}, 4.226×10^{-5} 6.124×10^{-5}, 7.895×10^{-5}, 9.298×10^{-5}, 1.014×10^{-4}, 1.035×10^{-4}. An exposure level of 1000 was used.

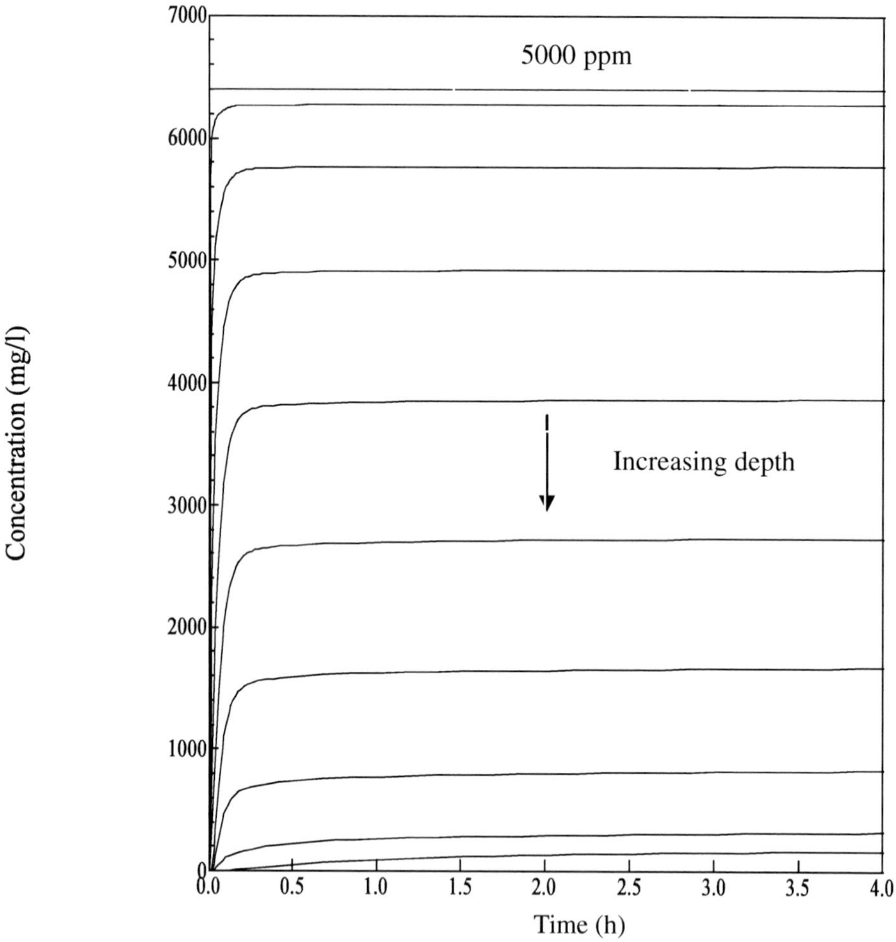

Figure 6. Dibromomethane concentration in the stratum corneum. The depths (dm), based on the internal collocation points, are 0, 2.055×10^{-6}, 1.052×10^{-5}, 2.455×10^{-5}, 4.226×10^{-5} 6.124×10^{-5}, 7.895×10^{-5}, 9.298×10^{-5}, 1.014×10^{-4}, 1.035×10^{-4}. An exposure level of 5000 was used.

5.3. Amount of Chemical Released Through the Skin

The incorporation of a non-homogeneous skin model into the whole body PBPK structure can alternatively be represented as a Fickian diffusion transport problem. One of the boundary conditions is set by the remaining ODEs. It would be enlightening to compare the widely used "perfect sink" condition, assumed in the modeling of controlled-release systems, to the physiologically-based boundary condition. Amounts of chemical from the environment into the stratum corneum (M_{sc}) and from the stratum corneum into the viable skin (M_{vs}), or a receiver, are chosen to guide the analysis since the difference (M_{sc}-M_{vs}) represents chemical accumulation in the stratum corneum. In the long run, the "perfect sink" assumption overestimates the total dose absorbed in both layers as a result of the infinitely fast clearance, which creates a higher driving force (Fig. 8). The exposure level was fixed at 500 ppm for this simulation.

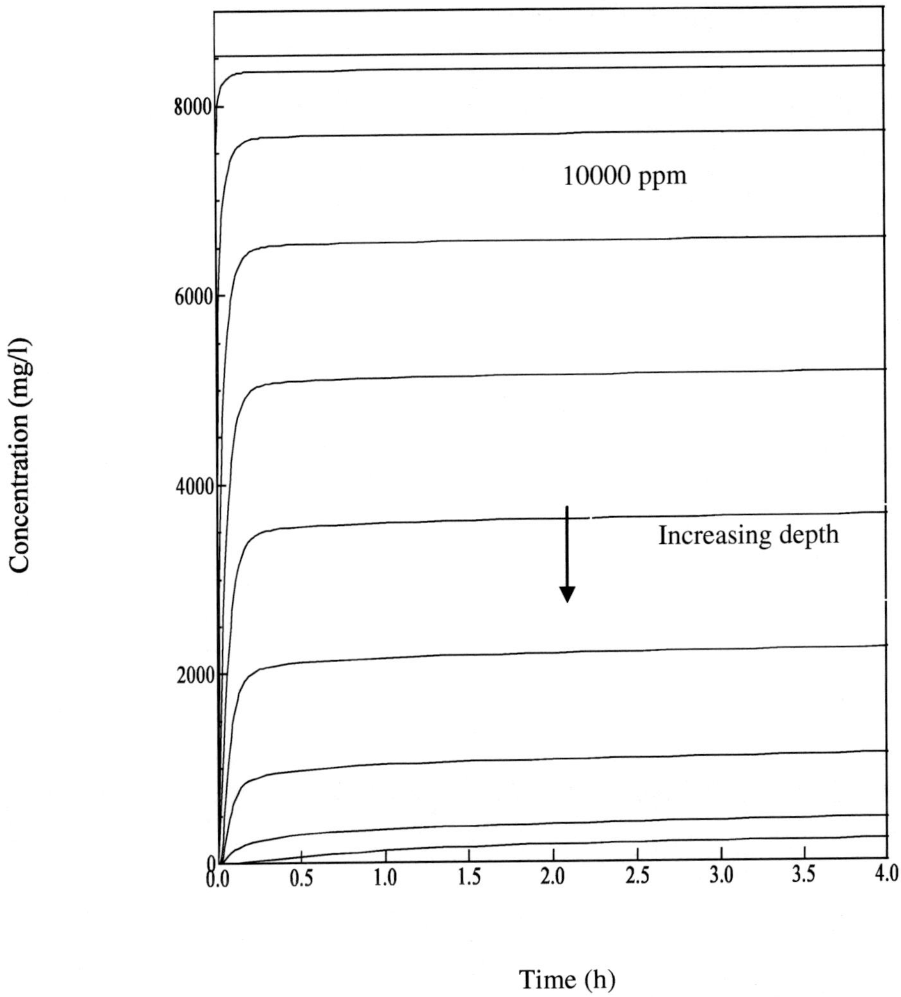

Figure 7. Dibromomethane concentration in the stratum corneum. The depths (dm), based on the internal collocation points, are 0, 2.055×10^{-6}, 1.052×10^{-5}, 2.455×10^{-5}, 4.226×10^{-5} 6.124×10^{-5}, 7.895×10^{-5}, 9.298×10^{-5}, 1.014×10^{-4}, 1.035×10^{-4}. An exposure level of 10,000 was used.

5.4. Time Required to Reach Equilibrium Concentrations

The speed at which the skin becomes saturated after coming in contact with a chemical agent is a question of utmost importance for toxicological assessment. It is well known that thermal relaxation time varies with the distance along a uniformly insulated bar when one end is brought to a new temperature [27]. In designing novel patches for drug release, the time to reach a constant delivery rate is also critical [28]. For the above mentioned systems, it was possible to estimate a time constant directly from the closed-form solution in the Laplace or time domain. Such options are not available for the present distributed-parameter model due to the nonlinear Michaelis-Menten equation for the liver. To address the problem, a response time defined by how long it takes to reach 98% of the steady-state value is chosen in agreement with process control theory. The exposure concentration of dibromomethane was allowed to vary from 500 to 1000 ppm for the illustration. The routine "FindRoot"' in Mathematica® was invoked to estimate the time elapsed (t) when $C_{sc}\ x_i,t\ = 0.98C_{sc,ss}\ x_i,t_{\text{large}}$. In this formulation, x_i represents the stratum corneum depth of interest (i.e., scaled collocation point); the subscript "*ss*" implies a steady-state value and t_{large} is set at 100 hours. The result of the investigation is shown in Fig. 9. The response time increases with the depth and exposure level.

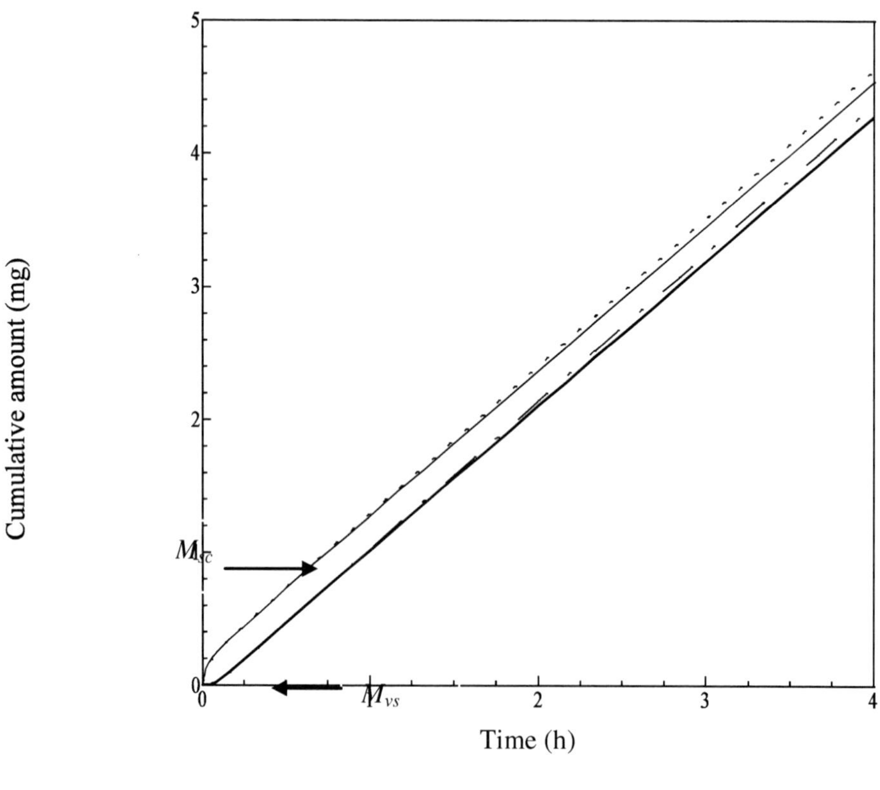

Figure 8. Amount of dibromomethane from the environment into the stratum corneum (M_{sc}) and from the stratum corneum into the viable skin (M_{vs}). The "perfect sink" assumption (--- and ____ _ ____) was compared to the physiologically based boundary condition (____ and ____)

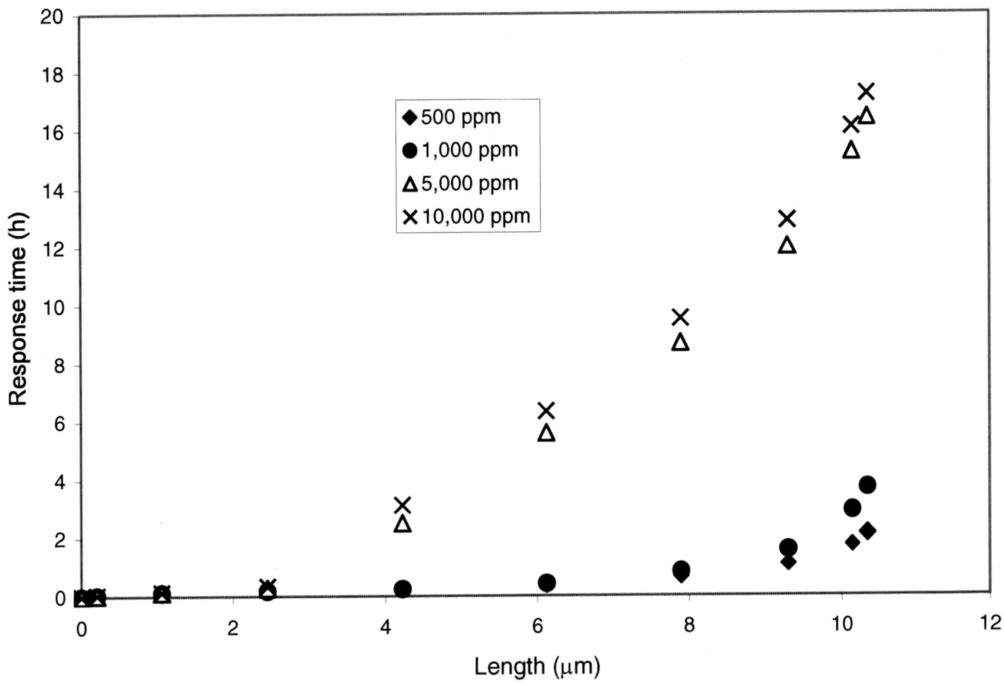

Figure 9. Response time for stratum corneum layers to become saturated with dibromomethane following exposure.

6. Conclusion

Fick's second law was used to analyze diffusive chemical transport through the skin. The boundary condition corresponded to a physiologically-based pharmacokinetic model. Orthogonal collocation procedures were implemented to discretize the partial differential equation in a Mathematica® environment and the results compared to a 1-compartment homogeneous skin model. The diffusive transport model predicted venous blood dibromomethane concentrations very well when compared to experimental data and results from the well-stirred 1-compartment model. This framework facilitated the monitoring of the chemical concentration at various stratum corneum depths. A rise in the exposure level was accompanied by an increase in the equilibrium dibromomethane concentration as the chemical penetrates deeper layers of the tissue. The relaxation time toward saturation in this region was an increasing function of depth and dibromomethane concentration in the environment. Compared to the "perfect sink" assumption, the cumulative amount of chemicals absorbed in the stratum corneum and the viable skin was less when the PBPK boundary condition was invoked.

Nomenclature

J permeation flux (mg/h)
D diffusion coefficient (dm^2/h)
K membrane/donor partition coefficient
l membrane thickness (dm)
P permeability coefficient (dm/h)
C concentration (mg/l)
M total mass of chemical absorbed (mg)
t time (h)
A exposed area (dm^2)
V volume (l)
R partition coefficient
Q blood flow (l/h)
x space variable (dm)
h stratum corneum thickness (dm)
a coefficient in Eq. (15)
b coefficient in Eq. (15)
P Jacobi polynomial
d coefficient in Eq. **Error! Reference source not found.**
W weight function

Subscripts

ss steady state
ave average
sfc vehicle
sk skin
a arterial
b blood
sc stratum corneum
cd composite dermal (2-CSM and 3-CSM)
ve viable epidermis
vs viable skin
i series index in Eq. (15)
1sc scaled value in the stratum corneum
r rapidly perfused tissue
l liver
s slowly perfused tissue
f fat tissue
ss steady state

Greek letters

ζ scaled space variable

References

[1] Meulenberg, C. J. W. & Vijverberg, H. P. M. (2003). Empirical relations predicting human and rat tissue: Air partition coefficients of volatile organic compounds. *Toxicol. Appl. Pharmacol.,* 165, 206-216.

[2] Nestorov, I. (2003). Whole body pharmacokinetic models. *Clin. Pharmacokinet.,* 42, 883-908.

[3] Poet, T. S., Weitz, K. K., Gies, R. A., Edwards, J. A., Thrall, K. D., Corley, R. A., Tanojo, H., Hui, X., Maibach, H. I. & Wester, R. C. (2002). PBPK modeling of the percutaneous absorption of perchloroethylene from a soil matrix in rats and humans. *Toxicol. Sci.,* 67, 17-31.

[4] Poet, T. S., Thrall, K. D., Corley, R. A., Hui, X., Edwards, J. A., Weitz, K. K., Maibach, H. I. & Wester, R. C. (2000). Utility of real time breath analysis and physiologically based pharmacokinetic modeling to determine the percutaneous absorption of methyl chloroform in rats and humans. *Toxicol. Sci.,* 54, 42-51.

[5] Blank, I. H. (1965). Cutaneous barriers. *J. Invest. Dermatol.,* 45, 249–256.

[6] Goyal, A., Mandapuram, S., Michniak, B. & Simon, L. (2007). Application of orthogonal collocation and regression techniques for recovering parameters of a two-pathway transdermal drug-delivery model. *Comput. Chem. Eng.,* 31, 107-120.

[7] Spcar, R. (1997). Large simulation models: calibration, uniqueness and goodness of fit. *Environ. Modell. Softw.,* 12, 219-228.

[8] Bookout, R. L. J., McDaniel, C. R., Quinn, D. W. & McDougal, J. N. (1996). Multilayered dermal subcompartments for modeling chemical absorption. *SAR QSAR Environ Res,* 5, 133-50.

[9] Roy, A., Weisel, C., Lioy, P. & Georgopoulos, P. (1996). A distributed parameter physiologically-based pharmacokinetic model for dermal and inhalation exposure to volatile organic compounds. *Risk Analysis,* 16, 147-160.

[10] Poet, T. S. & McDougal, J. N. (2002). Skin absorption and human risk assessment. *Chem. Biol. Interact.,* 140, 19-34.

[11] Pinheiro, J. & Bates, D. (2000). *Mixed-effects models in S and S-Plus.* New York: Springer.

[12] Liu, X., Smith, B. J., Chen, C., Callegari, E., Becker, S. L., Chen, X., Cianfrogna, J., Doran, A. C., Doran, S. D., Gibbs, J. P., Hosea, N., Liu, J., Nelson, F. R., Szewc, M. A. & Van Deusen, J. (2005). Use of a physiologically based pharmacokinetic model to study the time to reach brain equilibrium: an experimental analysis of the role of blood-brain barrier permeability, plasma protein binding, and brain tissue binding. *J. Pharmacol. Exp. Ther.,* 313, 1254-1262.

[13] Chinery, R. L. & Gleason, A. K. (1993). A compartmental model for the prediction of breath concentration and absorbed dose of chloroform after exposure while showering. *Risk Anal.,* 13, 51–63.

[14] Andersen, M. E. & Keller, W. C. (1984). Toxicokinetic principles in relation to percutaneous absorption and cutaneous toxicity. In V. A. Drill & P. Lazar (Ed.), *Cutaneous Toxicity* (pp. 9-27). New York:Raven Press.

[15] Jepson, G. W. & McDougal, J. N. (1997). Physiologically based modeling of nonsteady state dermal absorption of halogenated methanes from an aqueous solution. *Toxicol. Appl. Pharmacol.,* 144, 315-324.

[16] McKone, T. E. (1993). Linking a PBPK model for chloroform with measured breath concentrations in showers: implications for dermal exposure models. *J. Exp. Anls. & Env. Epi.,* 3, 339-365.

[17] Kalia, Y. & Guy, R. (2001). Modeling transdermal drug release. *Adv. Drug Del. Rev.,* 48, 159–172.

[18] Finlayson, B. A. (1981). *Nonlinear Analysis in Chemical Engineering.* New York: McGraw-Hill.

[19] Srivastava, R. K. & Joseph, B. (1985). Reduced-order models for separation columns — V. Selection of collocation points. *Comput. Chem. Eng.,* 9, 601–613.

[20] Adrover, A., Continillo, G., Crescitelli, S., Giona, M. & Russo, L. (2000). Wavelet-like collocation method for finite-dimensional reduction of distributed systems. *Comp. and Chem. Eng.,* 24, 2687-2703.

[21] Cruz, P., Mendes, A. & Magalhaes, F. D. (2002). Wavelet-based adaptive grid method for the resolution of nonlinear PDEs. *AIChE J.,* 48, 774-785.

[22] Simon, L. (2005). Observing biomass concentration in a fixed-bed bioreactor. *Chem. Eng. Comm.,* 192, 272–285.

[23] Albanese, R. A., Banks, H. T., Evans, M. V. & Potter, L. K. (2002). Physiologically based pharmacokinetic models for the transport of trichloroethylene in adipose tissue. *Bull Math Biol,* 64, 97-131.

[24] Loizou, G., Jones, K., Akrill, P., Dyne, D. & Cocker, J. (1999). Estimation of the dermal absorption of m-xylene vapor in humans using breath sampling and physiologically based pharmacokinetic analysis. *Toxicol. Sci.,* 48, 170-179.

[25] Cleek, R. L. & Bunge, A. L. (1993). A new method for estimating dermal absorption from chemical exposure. 1. General approach. *Pharm Res,* 10, 497-506.

[26] Norman, A. M., Kissel, J. C., Shirai, J. H., Smith, J. A., Stumbaugh, K. L. & Bunge, A. L. (2008). Effect of PBPK model structure on interpretation of in vivo human aqueous dermal exposure trials. *Toxicol Sci,* 104, 210-7.

[27] Collins, R. (1980). The choice of an effective time constant for diffusive processes in finite systems. *J. Phys. D: Appl. Phys.,* 13, 1935-1947.

[28] Simon, L. (2007). Analysis of heat-aided membrane-controlled drug release from a process control perspective. *Int. J. Heat Mass Transfer,* 50, 2425-2433.

In: Skin Anatomy and Physiology Research Developments
Editor: Leon F. Bukowsky
ISBN: 978-1-60741-469-8

Chapter 10

Advances in Ablative Laser Treatment for Cutaneous Facial Rejuvenation

Mario A. Trelles*
Instituto Médico Vilafortuny/Fundación
Antoni Gimbernat E-43850 Cambrils (Tarragona), Spain

Introduction

Conventional ablative laser resurfacing is still considered the gold standard in the treatment of the sequelae associated with severe facial aging. However, because the post-treatment effects require long recovery periods and patients cannot return to their normal activities during this down time, a technique called fractional laser resurfacing has been proposed as an alternative. Fractional laser resurfacing techniques can offer good results when fighting skin deterioration such as textural changes, tissue laxness and pigmentation occurring with aging while maintaining well-controlled side effects normally associated with laser photothermal action.

With fractional resurfacing, laser radiation does not produce thermal damage to the whole of the cutaneous surface. In this case, therapeutic damage is induced to a small volume of tissue as a result of thousands of microscopic thermal columns. As only partial ablation occurs, the typical, slow wound healing stage of conventional ablative laser resurfacing is shortened and tissue recovery and reepitheliazation occurs quickly due to the active migration of keratinocytes from the neighboring non-treated tissue. In addition, the procedure can be carried out with topical anesthesia, producing only mild discomfort and the side effects, mainly edema and erythema, are milder in intensity and have a much shorter duration than those that occur in conventional ablative laser resurfacing.

Regardless of the laser wavelength, in fractional resurfacing the main objective of treatment is to produce small areas of photothermal microlesions in the target tissue separated

* Corresponding Author: E-mail: imv@laser-spain.com

by areas of untreated skin which help in the healing process, allowing rapid skin recovery. When laser energy is delivered, there is a thermal effect following interaction. Depending on the laser wave length, effects are first located in the epidermis or in the dermis. Treatment produces cause residual thermal damage (RTD) in adjacent tissue. The RTD is recognized as kick-starting the body's own wound healing process, resulting in neocollagenesis, neoelastinogenesis and neovascularization, all of which are essential in obtaining better structured, younger-looking skin.

In brief, the purpose of fractional resurfacing is to obtain the best possible result in the treated area with well controlled damage and side effects. These aims are achieved due to the fact that the degree of RTD in tissue occurs only in determined points, isolated among the untreated areas with no RTD. The extent of each of these controlled therapeutic lesions depends on the dose used, the pulse width and the number of laser passes over the target area or, in other words, the number of laser pulses per treatment area, known as pulse density.

The system of "fractionating" the laser beam will often vary according to the manufacturer. Ablative and non-ablative lasers, when designed for treatment in fractional mode, can do so by splitting the main beam using a dividing lens. When laser energy is pulsed on the skin with these fractionated beams the technique is known as stamping or stacking (Figure 1). On the other hand, in the scanner, or sweeping, technique, the laser beam partially covers the surface of the skin with programs of different computer-guided designs.

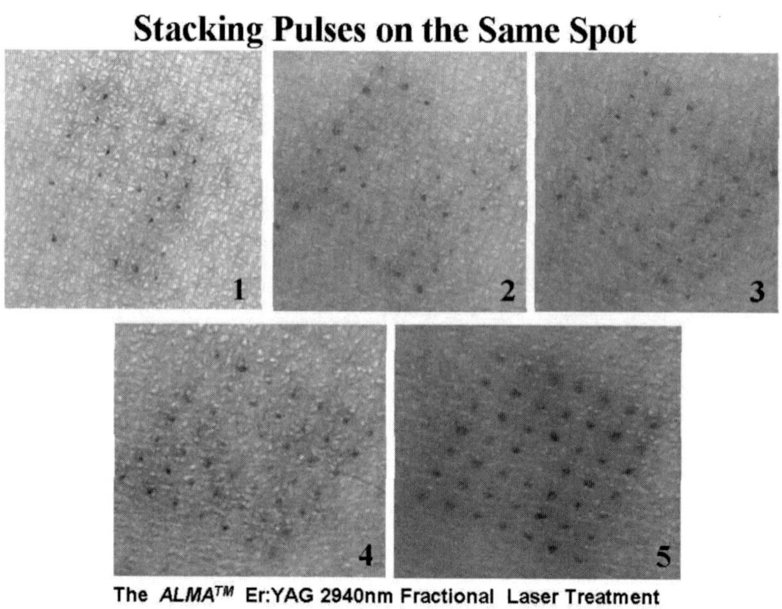

Figure 1. Skin surface microphotography showing effects of the Er:YAG laser (Alma Lasers®) in ablative fractional mode. Left (1): Note the small perfectly aligned ablations produced by the microbeams, obtained as a result of the lens splitter. The same image is repeated in 2,3,4 and 5, representing the number of pulses on the same spot, done without moving the laser hand-piece in the "stacking" mode. Effects on the skin are seen to increase with multiple pulses. Microbeams are separated 50 μm from each other forming a square grid of 11 mm x 11 mm, with a total of 49 beams. If the hand piece is slightly moved, rotating it on its vertical axis, greater impact point density of micro-beams per surface unit of the skin will be achieved.

In ablative fractional resurfacing, the most typical lasers are the CO_2 and Er:YAG lasers which enable precise elimination of tissue starting with the epidermis. This is due to the characteristics of their wavelengths, both of which are well absorbed by water, although absorption is better with the Er:YAG. The Er:YAG laser wavelength is absorbed by water 10 times more than that of a CO_2 laser, and hence the therapeutic lesion created by this laser can be efficiently limited to the superficial layers of the epidermis (Figure 2).

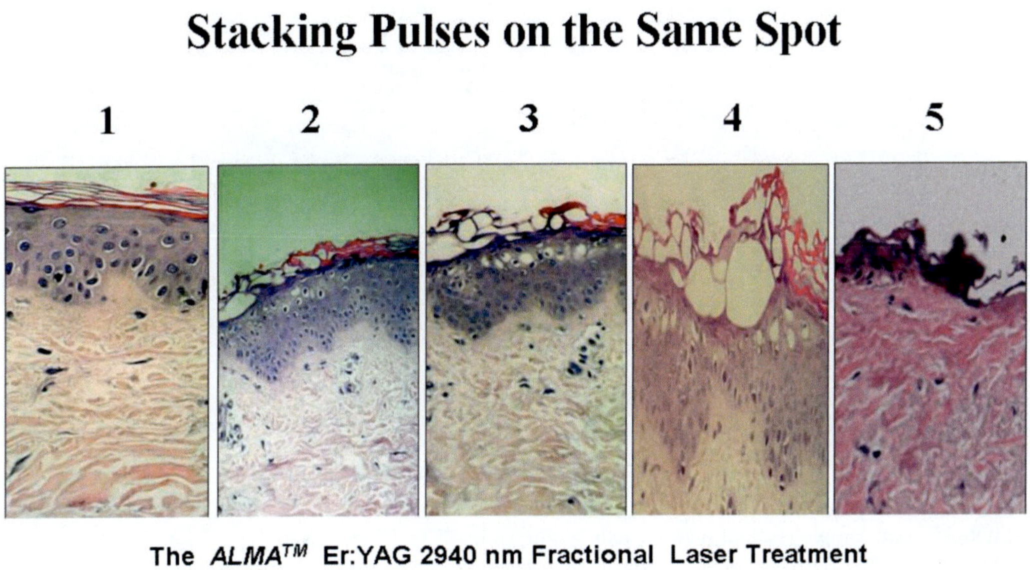

Figure 2. Skin samples (Hematoxylin /Eosin x 250). Histologies correspond to effects produced by one of the various microbeams. Several Er:YAG fractional Pixel™ pulses have been delivered in stacking mode. Images are correlated with number of laser pulses of Figure 1. Note that as the number of pulses on the same spot increases, the epidermis is progressively "erased" until it is fully eliminated. Pulses enter the dermis leaving some thermal deposit as seen in (5) right (1200 mJ, 200 ms pulse).

A single ablative fractional treatment session with the Er:YAG laser, set at low fluences, does not achieve excellent results. Usually several treatment sessions are recommended in order to obtain rejuvenation effects on the skin. But, if a single session is carried out using high fluence settings, tissue requires a longer recovery period and can potentially induce more side effects (such as erythema) in the post-operative period. The same applies when using the CO_2 laser in a single session, but this laser produces greater RTD on the skin than the Er:YAG, with a potential for increased side effects (Figure 3).

When carrying out a fractional laser treatment, the wavelength of the different systems defines where the energy acts: either on the skin surface or deep in the dermis. Two modes are possible in the fractional approach for skin rejuvenation, depending on the photothermal reaction between the laser wavelength and parameters and the target tissue: (a) the ablative mode, in which thermal action includes elimination of epidermis with a minimal amount of RTD in the dermis and (b) the non-ablative mode, in which the aim is to achieve zones of coagulation in the dermis with absence of or minimal damage to the epidermis.

Alma™ Pixel™ CO_2 laser high fluence effects on the skin produced by a single pass during fractional resurfacing

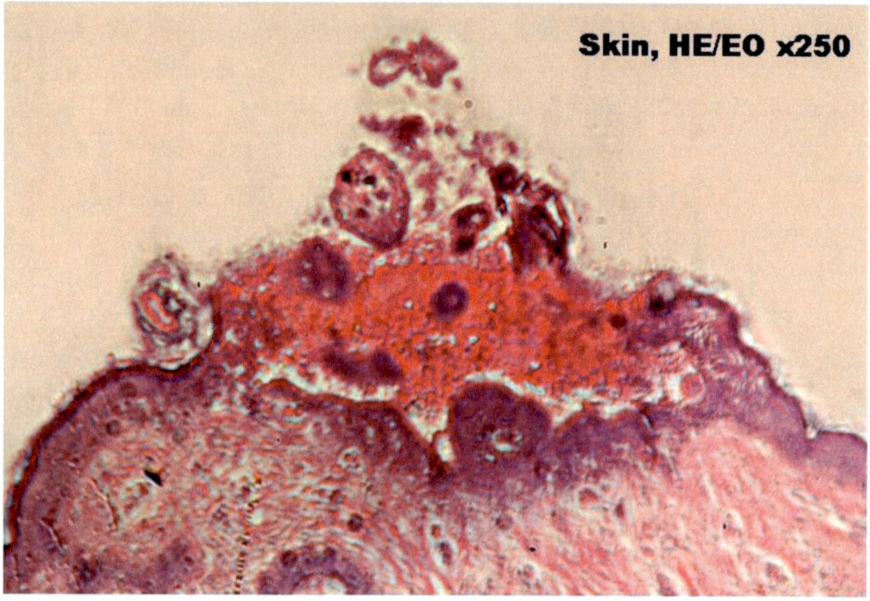

Programmation in superpulsed mode

Figure 3. Skin sample (Hematoxylin /Eosin x 400) of one CO_2 laser pass in Pixel® fractional mode (Alma Lasers®) carried out with a high fluence. The energy delivered by the laser is in superpulsed mode, i.e., several peaks of high energy are shot during the period that the laser action lasts. Laser pulse frequency was 300 Hz with a time period of 200 ms. The total of the epidermis is seen eliminated, with noticeable but very well delimited RTD.

Ablative and Nonablative Fractional Lasers

Ablative Systems

The pixel™ mode in the Er:YAG laser and in the CO_2 laser

The Pixel™ System (Alma Lasers™, Israel) can be used by both the Er:YAG and CO_2 lasers. In both systems, the hand-piece is equipped with a splitter, a lens which divides the laser beam into several microbeams.

The rapid ablation of the epidermis produced by the Er:YAG laser, due to its very high absorption in water, causes minimal secondary thermal damage in the neighboring skin. When using the fractional mode, the Er:YAG laser properties enable the safe treatment of patients with sensitive or dark skins as well as defects, such as lines and wrinkles, especially those which are not of an advanced degree (Figure 4).

Depending on whether a lesser or a greater effect is required in the tissue, the treatment setting must be adapted, in order to obtain tissue elimination with or without RTD.

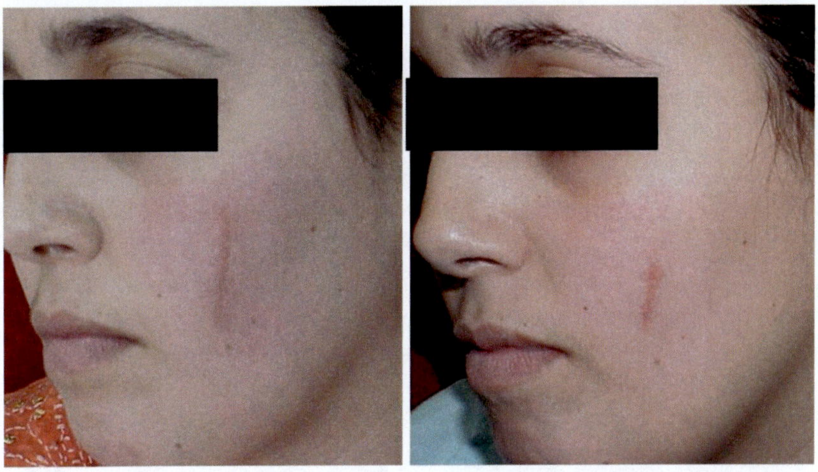

Figure 4. Female, phototype IV, presenting a scar on the left cheek. Tissue is depressed and atrophic. The Er:YAG fractional laser in Píxel mode mode was used for treatment (Alma Lasers®). Notice improvement achieved after three sessions of treatment (1000 mJ, 150 ms pulse). Fractional resurfacing with Er:YAG laser of scar tissue is very effective with the advantage of rapid skin condition recovery.

If signs of skin aging are of a lower degree, low fluences should be used and conversely, higher ones should be selected if lesions are more evident. Likewise, one single or several treatment sessions may be required in accordance with the particular conditions of each case (Figure 5).

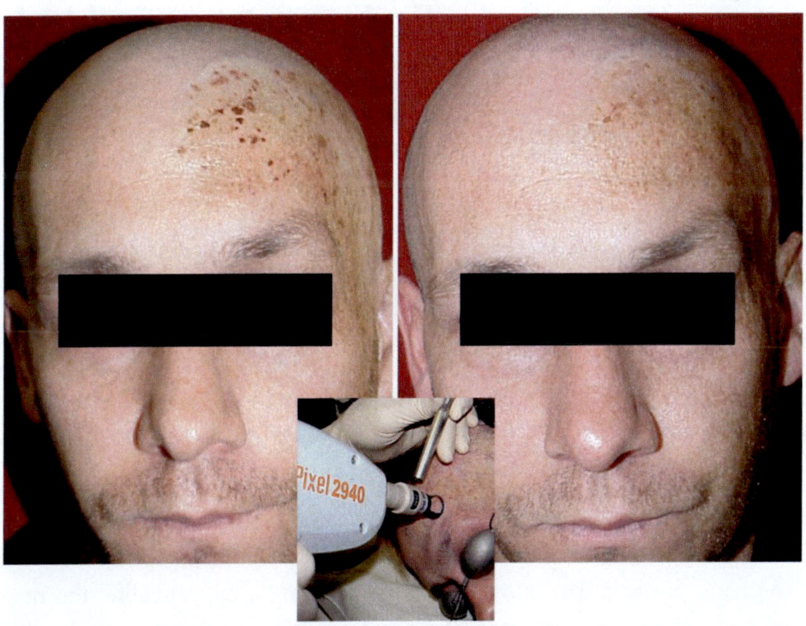

Figure 5. Male, phototype III, presenting residual scarring and reactive pigmentation on the head due to accidental burning. The Er:YAG laser in Pixel® mode was used for fractional resurfacing. Observe effects achieved two months after four treatments (800 mJ, 100 ms pulse). Treatment sessions were every 15 days and proved highly efficacious in order to progressively "peel" the skin achieving pigment elimination and enhanced skin texture.

With the Er:YAG laser, settings for low fluence emission, ranging between 800 and 900 mJ/cm^2, carried out with a few passes, will achieve the mild, controlled elimination of just a few layers of epidermal cells.

The Er:YAG laser beam, set to emit at low fluences, acts efficaciously as a highly superficial peel. Pulse duration (the longer the pulse, the greater the energy as is the case of the Alma Lasers™ Er:YAG laser), facilitates achieving treatments at a variety of depths in the skin by eliminating the tissue to the required depths. Several passes over the skin with this laser at low fluences give rise to an ablation effect with some RTD. This effect is seen to increase when higher fluences in the order of 1400 mJ/cm^2 are used. Subsequently a stimulation of neocollagenesis and elastinogenesis, is observed producing tissue tightening, thereby achieving skin rejuvenation.

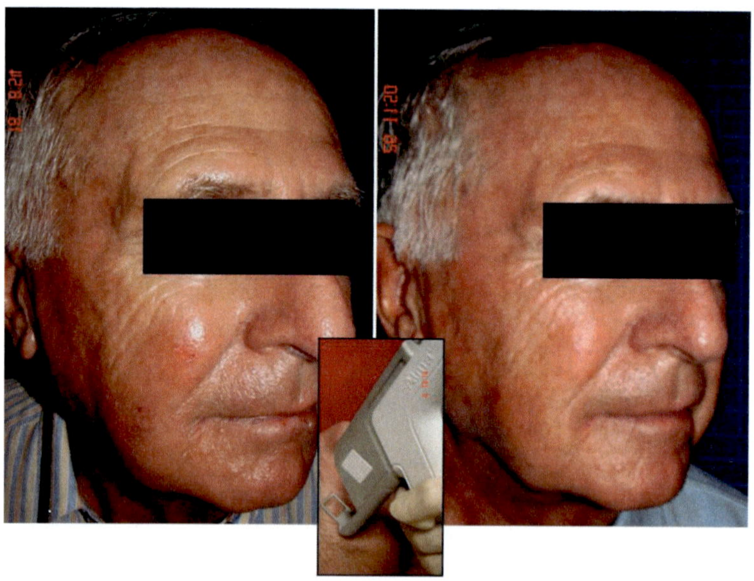

Figure 6. The graph represents several pulses of the Er:YAG laser in Pixel fractional mode (Alma Lasers®) carried out on the same point of impact, by keeping the hand piece static during pulses. The successive pulses "drill" the skin and repetition enables the laser energy to penetrate deeper into tissue. As the time between pulses is relatively short, energy builds up and the thermal effect propagates. Increased formation of RTD and heat propagation is produced in relation to programmed fluence, pulse width, pulse repetition rate and delay time. The different passes carried out in this fashion leave residual heat in tissue, which will positively influence the formation of new collagen during the tissue recovery stage.

Treatments are carried out by resting the end of the hand piece on the skin and firing the laser. The micro-beams impact the skin surface, visibly "marking" the skin as if it was being stamped. The hand piece is then moved to a neighboring area, repeating the maneuver until the whole of the treatment is completed. If a greater number of "marks" on the skin is desired, (or a greater number of pulses per area), the hand piece is rotated on its axis filling the treatment surface with more laser pulses. This degree of treatment effect can also be accomplished by repeatedly passing the laser hand-piece over the cutaneous surface while firing the laser. However, if more than one pulse is delivered on the same spot, laser energy will "perforate" the skin more deeply with each extra pulse. In this mode, known as stacking of laser pulses, RTD will accumulate progressively in the tissue (Figure 6).

The energy setting in Pixel ™ mode of the Er:YAG by Alma™, uses variable pulse duration, which is correlative with the fluences. Since this laser emits at a pre-set power, the duration of each pulse, which is controlled by the software installed in the system console, will depend on the fluence selected.

The CO_2 laser beam is also absorbed very well by water, but about one-tenth less than that of the Er:YAG laser. This means that CO_2 laser energy can penetrate deeper than the corresponding amount of Er:YAG energy, but can still be well-controlled by its absorption in water, which constitutes a major part of the skin. Fractional treatment using the CO_2 laser manages to rejuvenate the skin significantly. With this laser, the decision as to the treatment program must be taken on the basis of selecting the power, duration of laser shot, and the frequency with which the shots act on the skin. The therapeutic action of the CO_2 laser is more evident from the point of view of residual thermal damage (RTD) if a relatively long shot time is selected. Also, if laser shots are delivered at high frequency, skin elimination is accompanied by heat propagation to the tissue adjacent to the target. This RTD is greater than that associated with the Er:YAG laser and hence it gives rise to a greater stimulus in the dermis, which results in the active formation of new collagen (Figure 7).

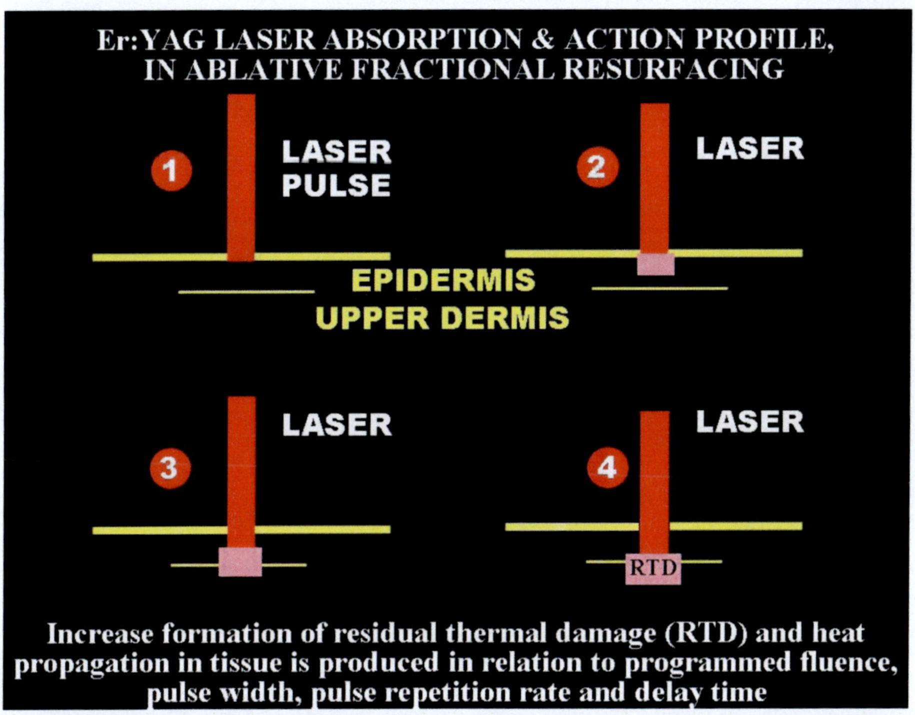

Figure 7. Male, phototype II, presenting extensiveskin photodamage and keratosis. Skin also has signs of elastosis. Pictures are of before and three weeks after a single session of full face treatment with the CO_2 laser in Pixel™ mode (Alma Lasers®) at high fluence, two passes. The improved condition of the skin achieved is obvious, with less keratotic tissue.

With high power settings, short shots and relatively long pauses between shots, residual damage is minor and thermal propagation can be better controlled. This approach makes skin recovery faster.

The Scanner Mode of the PULSED CO_2 Laser

One pulsed CO_2 system which can serve as an example of an ablative resurfacing system is the Activa™ FX CO_2 laser (Lumenis™, Israel). It offers two modes of scanning pulses: the sequential mode or the non-sequential, quasi-random mode. This system delivers pulses to the skin which are of a predetermined width (time) and spot size. Because the system can be set automatically, the power and frequency of the pulse can be adapted according to user's needs. Moreover, its sophisticated computer program allows the pulses to be delivered to the skin in several different designs, sizes and densities, that is to say, with a variable number of pulses per unit of area over the selected pattern shape.

In the sequential fractional mode, one shot follows the next, with greater or lesser density, i.e., nearer to or further from the other in the treatment area, until the surface of the selected design is completed. Then, the hand piece must be moved and the laser fired again, and so on until treatment is complete (Figure 8).

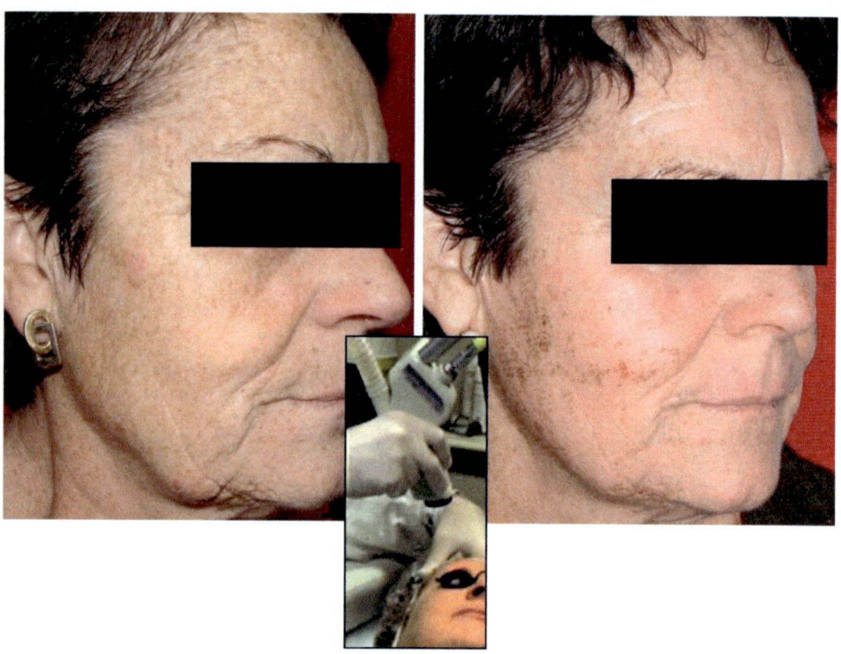

Figure 8. The Activa Ultrapulse™ CO_2 laser (Lumenis®) incorporates several lenses in the handpiece that permit maintaining focalization of the beam without contacting the skin surface. This technology is known as collimated laser beam, which facilitates treatment obtaining a homogenous image of energy distribution. Picture shows before and after of a female, phototype III, suffering from aging skin. A single session has been carried out with 100 mJ, 100 Hz and density 5. Skin looks much better only a week after treatment but there is still some residual scabbing but only mild erythema.

In the non-sequential, quasi-random mode, a pulse does not follow its neighbor, i.e. pulses are not located one beside the other but the pulses "jump" to a distant point within the treatment design area in order to avoid irradiating a spot immediately beside another. Pulses continue to be fired in the quasi-random mode until the area of the design is completed, according to the pulse density programmed. This sequence of pulses aims to help avoid thermal build-up in the treatment area.

The treatment technique using this laser system for ablative fractional resurfacing is identical in both modes (sequential and non-sequential), but the fact that the tissue accumulates less residual heat in the non-sequential mode makes skin recovery quicker, decreasing the setbacks or side effects such as prolonged edema and erythema and possible secondary hyperpigmentation (Figure 9).

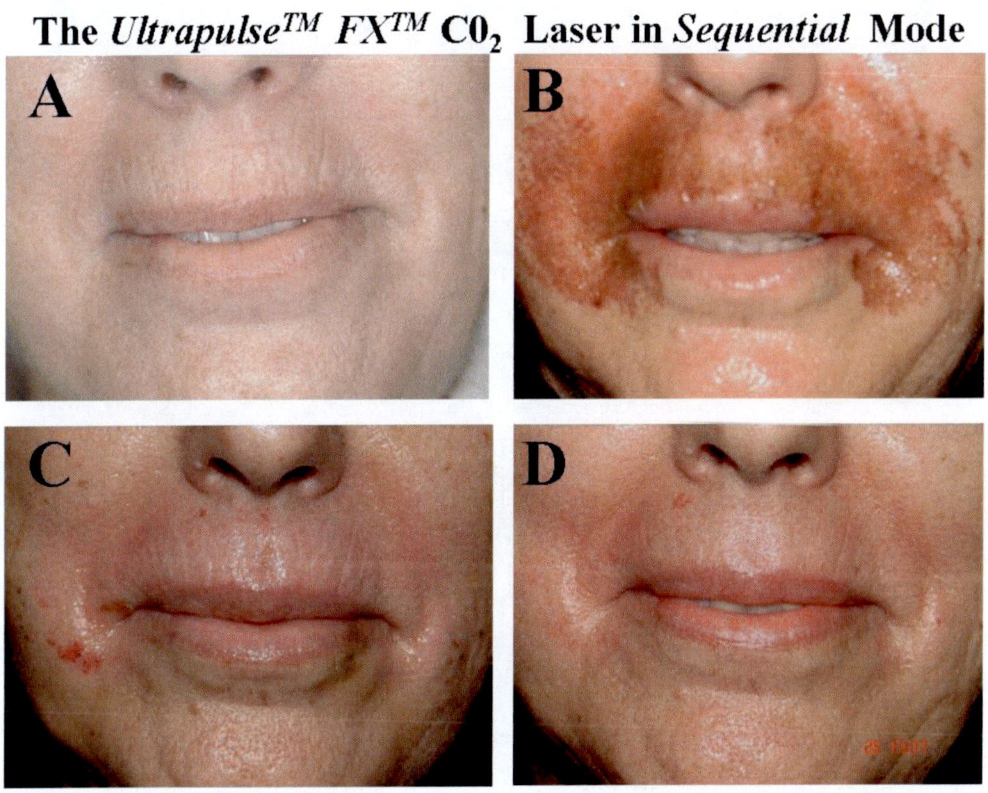

Figure 9. Sequence of treatment of upper lip wrinkles in a female, phototype II. Only one ablative fractional resurfacing treatment session with the CO_2 **Ultrapulse Active™ laser** (Lumenis®) in sequential fractional mode, 125 mJ/100 Hz and density 5 has been practiced. Pictures present the "before" condition (A), 48 hours after treatment (B), seven days after treatment (C) and 12 days after treatment (D). Notice the rapid recovery with improvement in wrinkle aspect Some erythema is present that can be easily covered with make-up.

If the pulsed CO_2 laser is to be used for fractional resurfacing, the practitioner must bear in mind the correlation that exists between pulse width which is fixed (in microseconds), the emission power, pulse frequency and pulse density in the area designed for treatment. The decision as to the selection of the different programs must be in accordance with the skin condition, the size of the area for treatment and the desired treatment effects.

Note that a program using high frequency pulses per area in the selected design will produce greater elimination of the tissue leaving evident thermal damage. This treatment should be used in order to achieve more evident results (Figure 10).

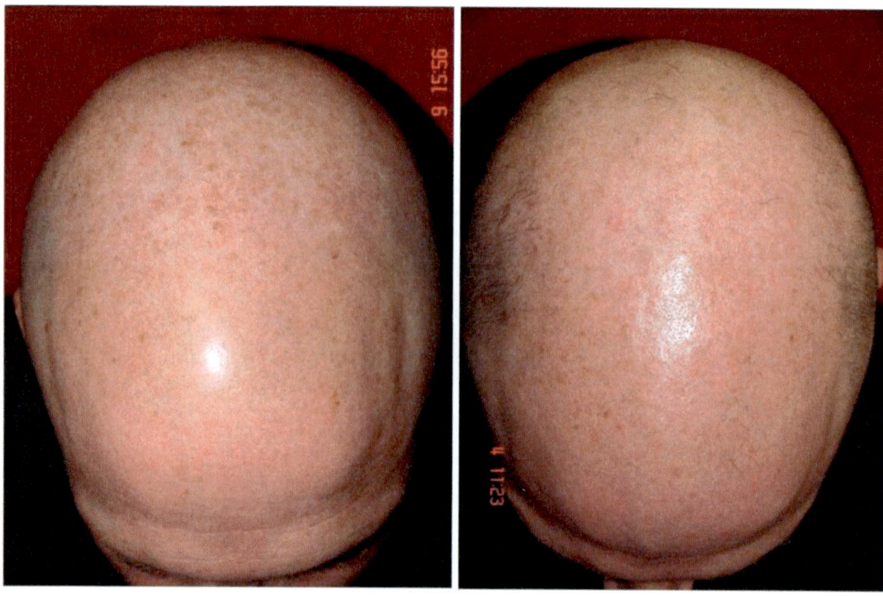

Figure 10. Male, phototype II, often exposed to sun radiation (sailor), presenting lentigo, keratosis and signs of elastosis. Pictures show before and 10 days after treatment with the CO_2 **Ultrapulse Active™** laser (Lumenis®) using 125 mJ/100 Hz density 6 in a single session. Excellent results have been achieved and patient was highly satisfied.

Nonablative Systems

Among the range of available techniques used for the treatment of aged skin, ablative laser resurfacing has always been presented as a high risk treatment, and non-ablative techniques, on the other hand, have been presented as involving less risk but only achieving very limited clinical improvement.

Currently used non-ablative fractional lasers emit in the spectrum of wavelengths between 1300 and 1600 nm, and pass through the epidermis to reach the dermis where they induce precise zones of thermal micro-coagulation following absorption. Columnar zones of coagulation can be observed in histological images of approximately 50 μm in diameter with a range of between 50 and 150 μm in depth.

Non-ablative fractional lasers offer a number of beam designs delivered for treatment with a variety of wavelengths, and induce thermal damage in the dermis. Just as for ablative fractional lasers, pulses can be delivered to the skin **in three different modes: a 'stamping'** mode (using a beam splitter), the randomly delivered pulses, or in scanned mode. All of these fractional non-ablative treatment modes seek to take the energy to the interior of the skin, respecting the integrity of the epidermis.

The first contribution in fractional photothermolysis to treat a small fractions of the skin with laser light was the 1540 nm Er:glass laser-based Fraxel® system by Reliant Technologies, (CA, USA). The partial action exerted in the dermis by the fractionated delivery of this laser energy was designed to create a unique reaction to stimulate the healing of the wound triggered by the islets of healthy tissue that are not treated by the laser. The smaller the size of the lesion in the dermis, the shorter the time taken by the skin to repair itself.

Fraxel ™ Mode

Each area treated using this fractional technology typically comprises thousands of individualized microthermal zones, produced by a 1540 nm laser, accompanied by normal peripheral tissue whose task is to repair the affected areas.

Upon termination of irradiation of the surface in question, the patient experiences a slight burning sensation, similar to that of overexposure to the sun. The discomfort lasts for a few hours and then the skin adopts a light red tone for five to seven days, which is to be interpreted as a normal sign of healing. Tumefaction is normally minimal and generally disappears in two to three days.

One advantage of this approach is that make-up may be applied a few days after treatment since, at average intensity, the skin reepithelizes within 24 hours. A kind of tan appears a few days after treatment and remains for between three and 14 days, when flaking begins, which is similar to that which takes place with a mild burn, but without any pain.

Fractional skin rejuvenation using the laser in the Fraxel® mode leaves the skin's stratum corneum intact. Treatment covers between 12% and 20% of the area of the skin selected, allowing the intact tissue to help rapid recovery and healing. Its effects, which may also act on the deep dermis, stimulate neocollagenesis thus remodeling the deep layers.

Depending on the nature and degree of cutaneous aging, three to five treatments are needed at intervals of approximately seven days, and visible improvement is usually noticed six months after the treatment.

Mosaic ™ Mode

This treatment mode is a characteristic of the 1550 nm Mosaic™ laser (Lutronic, Inc., Seoul, Korea). This system offers an advanced solution in the practice of non-ablative fractional resurfacing since it achieves tangible improvements of the skin in patients of all photo-types.

The Mosaic™ laser operates by irradiating multiple forms at random, in which the laser beam is aimed at the dermis in the form of microscopic beams of energy. Absorption of the laser energy produces deep, thermal micro-wounds which are narrow and cylindrical in shape.

The significance of action present in tissue is represented by columns of coagulated tissue microscopically visible beneath the epidermis. The depth of penetration in the dermis is very much correlated with the energy used for treatment. Delineation of the necrotic area from healthy tissue is very well achieved.

The hand-piece of this laser controls and processes the information of the selected program, with the pulses of laser energy being delivered randomly in what the manufacturers refer to as controlled chaos technology (CCT). Despite the fact that pulse distribution is random on tissue, its action uniformly covers the area of treated skin. This mode of fractional treatment differs from the typical "painting" mode of other fractional lasers.

The CCT irradiation mode increases the application of conventional non-ablative modes since at a velocity of up to 700 spots per second, it can achieve a treatment of a highly natural, uniform aspect.

The range of technological ability offered by this Lutronic™ system is interesting since in addition to the "chaos" mode, it also offers a standard fractional irradiation mode in "stamp" form. During treatment, it is possible to switch between the two, enabling the performance of precise treatments according to the conditions of the tissue and the dimensions of the area being treated (Figure 11)

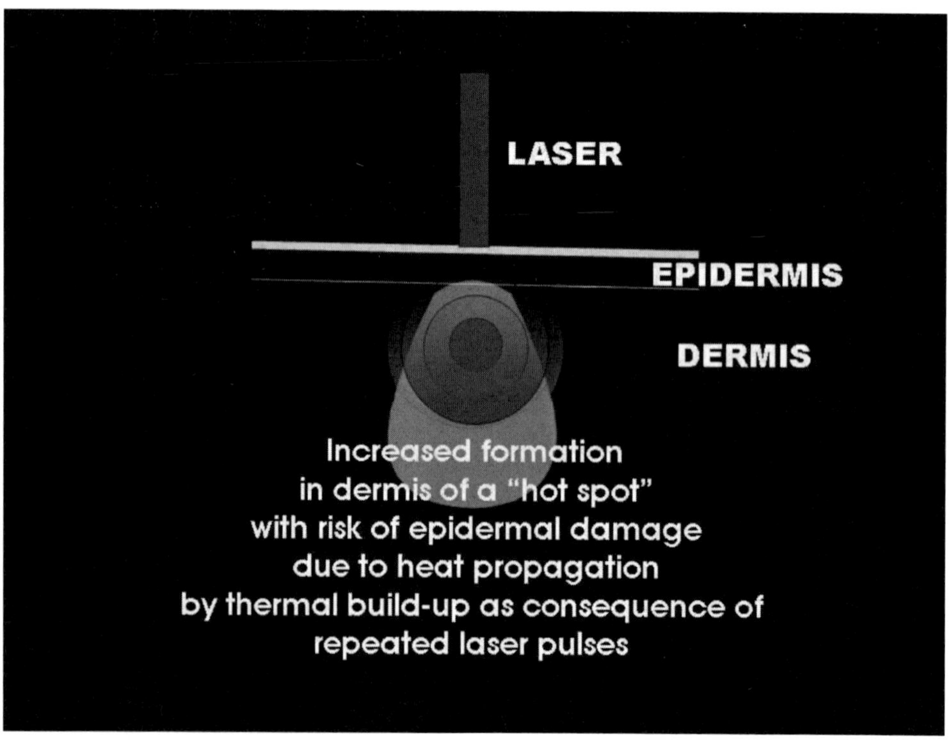

Figure 11. Full face non-ablative fractional resurfacing with a pulsed 1550 nm laser (Mosaic™, Lutronic®, South Korea). The patient, a female, phototype IV, received three treatment sessions, one every other week. Pictures show before and one month after last session. Observe the improved quality of skin showing a tightening effect. Some color of the pigmented lesions was eliminated due to a mild epidermal "peel" observed a few days after each (of three) treatment sessions.

In "chaos" mode, treatment is done at high speed. It is a *dynamic* mode which continuously supplies fractionated laser beam pulses, rapidly covering large surface areas. On **the other hand, "stamp" mode eradication is advisable for** the treatment of small lesions or scars, since *statically* between 50 and 500 spots/cm^2 are distributed instantaneously, with a tolerable pain profile.

Discussion

In general, fractional resurfacing is presented as a technique that can be carried out without the need for anesthesia. In practice, and especially if repeated laser passes are performed at high energy settings or when the interval between pulses is short, some pain is inevitable and is difficult to tolerate. In fact, thermal build-up in the treated area leads to the patient experiencing pain.

A direct relationship exists between pain intensity and the different laser passes during treatment. In addition, the frequency of laser pulses and energy density deposited in the skin are important. Particularly in these circumstances, a topical anesthetic is recommended and should be applied two hours before surgery, removing any residue before proceeding with treatment. Following fractional resurfacing, patients are recommended to use a non-fluorinated topical corticoid in combination with an antibiotic (such as gentamicin) preferably in the form of an ointment.

There is no need to cover the treated area with occlusive dressings. Ointments should be applied three times a day in small amounts (using them as a moisturizing cream), and should continue until the fine crusting that forms in the treated areas falls off spontaneously.

In our experience, there is no need for oral medication, although it is prudent to recommend topical anti-herpetic creams, especially if treatment is done on the lips, and to combat any possible discomfort Paracetamol 500 mg is indicated to be taken every four hours.

Pain and discomfort, such as stinging, burning and smarting, are usually more apparent than with conventional resurfacing practice. The fact that the superficial *nociceptive* receptors are not totally eliminated during fractional resurfacing, especially the ablative type, would be the cause of the pain and discomfort felt by patients. Certainly the nerve endings in the islets of untreated tissue **"warn" the neighboring lesion, converting that information into pain.**

In general, with both ablative and non-ablative fractional lasers, if multiple passes are carried out, progressive heat build-up takes place in the tissue. If ablative fractional resurfacing is performed, the absorption of the laser energy in the epidermis produces partial or total elimination. However, if fractional treatment is delivered with non-ablative lasers, energy absorption is carried out within the dermis producing a coagulation effect therein. If low energy levels are set when using the non-ablative fractional laser technique, collagen formation can be activated in the different treatment sessions, tightening and rejuvenating the skin. Depending on the energy setting for treatment and the number of sessions, the improvement in the cutaneous aspect will range from very slight to very clear from the aspect of lines and wrinkles, but several treatment sessions will always be required (Figure 12).

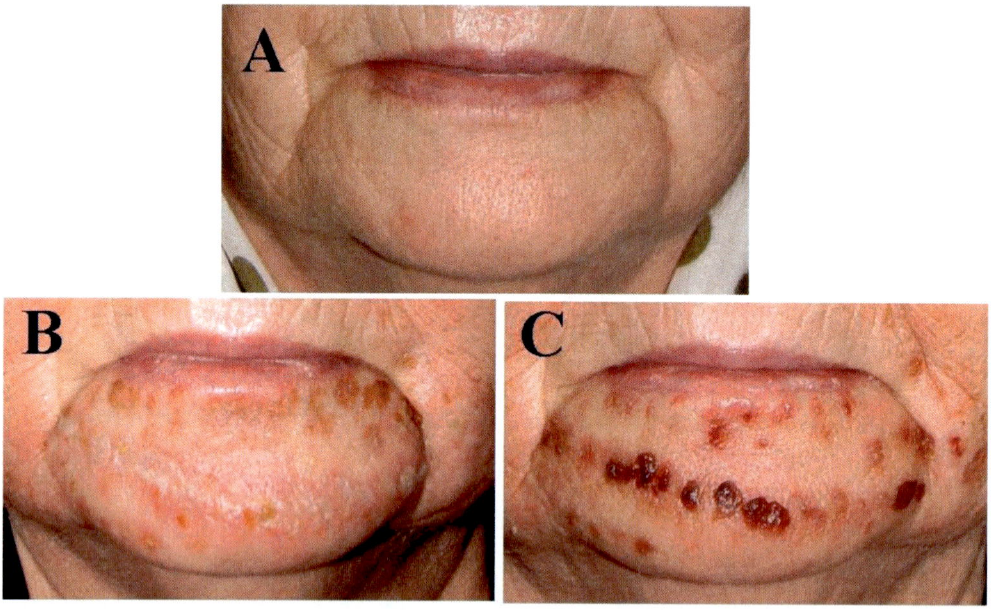

Figure 12. The graph represents several laser pulses with a non-ablative laser 1540 nm at 20 mJ. The multiple micro beams **can deliver high energies in each of the multiple micro beams after the "main"** beam of the laser is divided by the splitter lens. Although, due to the wave length, energy is addressed for absorption in the dermis, repeated laser pulses will build up thermal effects and propagation of heat to neighboring tissue also damaging the epidermis with detachment.

Note, however, that if high levels of energy are set or several laser passes are done over the same area in the same session in treatment using the non-ablative fractional laser mode, the epidermis will detach as a consequence of thermal propagation from inside the dermis, which is where the energy of non-ablative lasers is first absorbed.

Lasers that act in the ablative fractional mode, such as the Er:YAG or the CO_2, are absorbed by the water in the target tissue and hence their action takes place first in the epidermis, improving the external characteristics of the skin, with immediate changes in aspect. These lasers offer a good means to improve skin presenting superficial pigmentation. If the aim is to improve lines and wrinkles, the action of the laser should reach the dermis and produce residual thermal damage, irritating the skin, kick-starting the wound healing process and activating collagen formation. These results can be obtained in a single session, or, more generally, in several treatment sessions if low energy settings are used, especially if more prolonged post-operative side effects are to be avoided.

Performing just one treatment session and not several as is usually recommended in fractional resurfacing has its advantages, but usually involves more side effects and slower skin recovery. Thus, each case must be evaluated and patients, having been presented with the relevant explanations, must decide whether they prefer a program involving several sessions or just one. In any case, patients must assiduously comply with their post-operative skin care instructions, and they must be prepared to wait for around two to three weeks before obtaining enhanced healthier, more youthful looking skin, which will then continue to improve as the remodeling phase of wound healing proceeds. Good patient education and management of patient expectations will ensure patient compliance with all instructions.

In our experience, regardless of whether we use ablative or non-ablative fractional resurfacing, patients report greater compliance when just one treatment session is carried out. Our impression is that no significantly different final results are seen between a single session using higher energy settings, in comparison with 2 or 3 treatment sessions with more conservative energy levels.

In the case of both ablative and non-ablative fractional lasers, the longer the pulse width, the higher the fluence. This achieves the required effects at a greater depth in the dermis, which are necessary in order to get the desired results in the treatment of wrinkles and scars (Figure 13).

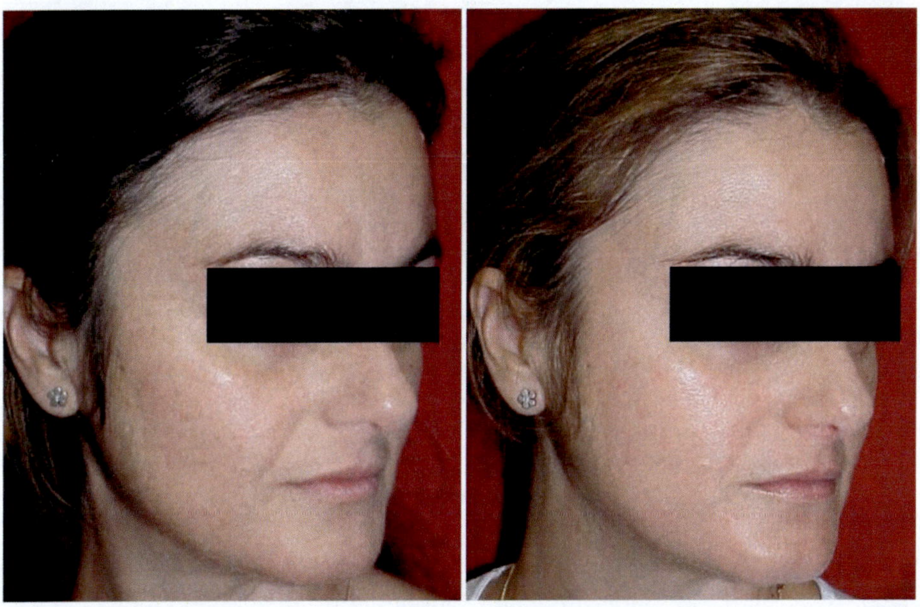

Figure 13. Female, phototype III, before and 7 days after treatment of the chin area with 1540 nm non-ablative fractional mode laser. Single laser pulse, high energy was used producing coagulation of the dermis and secondary epidermis lesion, well visible. Negative reaction is seen because of the excessive fluence. Laser pulse delivered was of 20 mJ in each micro-beam fractionated by the lens splitter. In order for the beam to deliver such energy, an excessive pulse width of the laser was necessary leading to possible over dosage regarding pulse time and undesired effects.

In principle, non-ablative fractional treatment is more suitable in order to improve facial lines and wrinkles, for cutaneous remodeling and in the treatment of residual acne scarring. In the case of non-ablative treatments using high fluences, thermal diffusion starts at the point of energy absorption in the dermis and is conducted in all directions including backwards towards the epidermis, even blistering and marking the skin. The epithelium can detach using non-ablative lasers and hence, at the skin surface, when effects are moderate they can translate into a mild lightening of the superficial pigmentation present in the skin (Figure 14).

The decision to carry out several fractional passes on the skin with the non-ablative laser approach must take treatment objectives into account. Based on histological studies, we know that the greater the depth of action, the greater the volume of tissue treated and, obviously, the more efficacious the cutaneous remodeling achieved. Non-ablative fractional mode permits treatment of skin types I to V with relatively high fluences and with several laser passes and a low risk of adverse reactions.

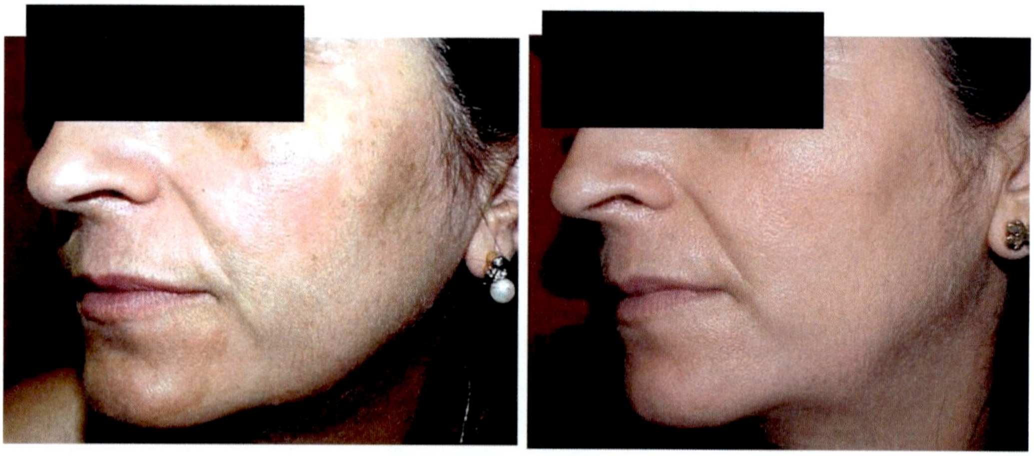

Figure 14. Non-ablative fractional treatment using 1540 nm Er:Glass laser (**Matisse™ Quanta Systems,** Milan italy) in a young female, phototype III, Energy used was of 10 mJ and two passes were carried out. This treatment manages to build up a thermal effect in the dermis quite efficiently preserving the epidermis. A nice skin **"lifting effect" is observed with a healthier aspect of tissue** one month after a single treatment. Rejuvenation effect is more remarked in middle-aged patients when non-ablative fractional laser treatments are used.

Post-operative pain in non-ablative treatments is better tolerated than when treatment is given with ablative lasers; however, pain is closely related to high fluences. When treating using the different fractional modes, significant side effects are not usually observed. Nevertheless, in order to obtain substantial results with non-ablative fractional resurfacing, more treatment sessions are required than with the ablative mode. The application of cold air over the skin surface alleviates the pain and discomfort that occur during treatment. Its use is especially advisable if topical anesthetics prove insufficient and the patients indicate that they are experiencing excessive pain.

The indices of the responses of the skin following treatment depend on age, sex and skin phototype. The maxim that the fewer the signs of cutaneous aging, the better the results, is valid; therefore, it is of utmost importance to select patients correctly and to match the best type of treatment for them on an individual basis.

As already mentioned, educating the patient regarding the treatment technique and how to proceed with post-treatment skin care is extremely important in order to control patient expectations and to ensure that they accept the reality of the possible results. If the aim is to treat degree II and III wrinkles, the patient must be told that at greater treatment intensity, which is necessary in order to achieve the best results, greater recovery time will be needed.

Conclusion

Fractional laser skin rejuvenation in both the ablative and non-ablative modes is without any doubt a valid and elegant approach to reversing the signs of cutaneous aging due to both chronological (intrinsic) and photoaging (extrinsic) factors. It offers advantages over the gold standard of full-face ablative laser resurfacing, particularly regarding the prolonged downtime and potential for adverse side effects associated with that approach. Each fractional mode has its own advantages. It is most important that the clinician is thoroughly conversant with the photobiological principles inherent in the delivery of the chosen wavelength, and the laser-tissue interactions embodied in each wavelength coupled with the importance of the other parameters selected. Good laser surgeons must make science work for them to achieve the optimum effect in their patients on a truly individual basis, which goes hand in hand with establishing and maintaining an excellent physician-patient rapport.

References

Alster, TS; Tanzi, EL; Lazarus, M. The use of fractional laser photothermolysis for the treatment of atrophic scars. *Dermatol Surg.*, 2007, 33, 295-9.

Behroozan, Ds; Goldberg, LH; Dai, T et al. Fractional photothermolysis for the treatment of surgical scars, a case report. *J Cosmet laer Ther.*, 2006, 8, 35-8.

Bitter, PH. Noninvasive rejuvenation of photoaged skin using serial full-face intense pulsed light treatments. *Dermatol Surg.*, 2000, 26, 835-843.

Buis, J; Mazer, JM. Le relissage fractionné par laser Fraxel® , un traitement complementaire possible pour la chirurgie du rajeunissement facial. *Ann Chir Plat Esthet.*, 2007, (in press).

Camacho, FM. Remodelamineto cutáneo, perspectiva histórica. *Piel*, 2005, 20, 504-17.

Chan, H. Effective and safe use of lasers, light sources and radiofrequency devices in the clinical management of Asian patients with selected dermatoses. *Laser Surg Med.*, 2005, 31, 1243-4.

Dawson, E; Willey, A; Lee, K. Adverse events associated with nonablative cutaneous laser, radiofrequency, and light-based devices. *Semin Cutan Med Surg.*, 2007, 26, 1521.

Fisher, GH; Geronemus, Rg. Short-term side effects of fractional photothermolysis. *Dermatol Surg.*, 2005, 31, 1245-9.

Fitzpatrick, RE; Goldman, MP. Resurfacing of photodamage of the neck using the Ultrapulse CO_2 laser. *Lasers Surg Med.*, 1997, 21-33.

Geronemus, RG. Fractional photothermolysis, current and future applications. *Lasers Surg Med.*, 2006, 38, 169-76.

Glaich, As; Rahman, Z; Goldberg, LH; Friedman, PM. Fractional resurfacing for the treatment of hypopigmented scars, a pilot study. *Dermatol Surg.*, 2007, 33, 289-94.

Gold, MH. Fractional technology, a review and clinical approaches. *J Drugs Dermatol.* 2007, Aug, 6(8), 849-52.

Goldberg, DJ. Nonablative subsurface remodeling, clinical and histological evaluation of a 1320 nm Nd,YAG laser. *J Cutan Las Ther.*, 1999, 1, 153-157.

Goldberg, DJ. Full-face nonablative dermal remodeling with a 1320 nm Nd,YAG laser. *Dermatol Surg.*, 2000, 26, 915-918.

Hantash, BM; Bedi, VP; Sudireddy, V; et al. Laser-induced transepidermal elimination of dermal content by fractional photothermolysis. *J Biomed* opt., 206, 11, 041115.

Hantash, BM; Bedi, VP; Chan, KF; Zachary, CB. Ex vivo histological characterization of a novel ablative fractional resurfacing device. *Lasers Surg Med.*, 2007, 39, 87-95.

Hantash, BM; Mahmood, MB. Fractional photothermolysis, A novel aesthetic laser surgery modality. *Dermatol Surg Med.*, 2007, 33, 525-34.

Hasegawa, T; Matsukura, T; Mizuno, Y. et al. Clinical trial of a laser device called fractional photothermolysis system for acne scars. *J Dermatol*, 2006, 33, 623-7.

Laubach, H; Chan, HH; Rius, F; Anderson, RR. Effects of skin temperature on lesions size in fractional photothermolysis. *Lasers Surg Med.*, 2007, 39, 14-8.

Lee, MW. Combination visible and infrared lasers for skin rejuvenation. *Semin Cutan Med Surg.,* 2002, 21, 288-300.

Lee, MW. Combination 532-nm and 1064-nm lasers for noninvasive rejuvenation and toning. *Arch Dermatol*, 2003, 139, 1265-1276.

Manstein, D; Herron, GS; Sink, RK; et al. Fractional photothermolysis, a new concept for cutaneous remodelling using microscopic patters of thermal injury. *Lasers Surg Med.*, 2004, 34, 426-38.

Marra, De, Yip, D; Fincher, EF; Moy, RL. Systemic toxicity from topically applied lidocaine in conjunction with fractional photothermolysis. *Arch Dermatol*, 2006, 142, 1024-6.

McDaniel, DH; Ash, K; Lord, J; Newman, J. The erbium,YAG laser, a review and preliminary report on resurfacing of the face, neck and hands. *Aesthet Plast Surg.*, 1997, 17, 157-64.

Menaker, GM; Wrone, DA; Williams, RM; Moy, Rl. Treatment of facial Rhytides with a nonablative laser, a clinical and histological study. *Dermatol Surg.*, 1999, 25, 440-444.

Miller, LD. The erbium laser gains a role in cosmetic surgery. *BiophotonInt*, 1997, (May/June), 38-42.

Narurkar, VA. Skin rejuvenation with microthermal fractional photothermolysis. *Dermatol Ther.*, 2007, 20, S10-S13.

Pozner, JN; Glanz, S; Goldberg, DJ; Fractional erbium resurfacing, histologic and early clinical experience. *Lasers in Surgery and Medicine*, 2007, 39, S19, 73.

Rokhsar, C; Fitzpatrick, RE. The treatment of melasma with fractional photothermolysis. *Dermatol Surg.*, 2005, 31, 1645-50.

Tannous, ZA; Astner, S. Utilizing fractional photothermolysis in the treatment of therapy-resistant melasma. *J. Cosmet Laser Ther.*, 2005, 7, 39-43.

Tanzi, EL; Williams, CM; Alster, TS. Treatment of facial rhytides with a nonablative 1,450-nm Diode laser, A controlled and histologic study. *Dermatol Surg.*, 2003, 29, 124-128.

Trelles, MA. Red light-emitting diode (LED) therapy assisted healing improves results of facial skin fractional resurfacing. *16th European Academy of Dermatology and Venereology Congress*, 2007, May.

Trelles, MA. Laser ablative resurfacing for photorejuvenation based on more than a decade's experience and 1200 patients, personal observations. *J Cosmetic Dermatology*, 2004, 2-13.

Trelles, MA; Allones, I; Luna, R. Facial rejuvenation with a nonablative 1320 nm Nd,YAG laser, a preliminary clinical and histological evaluation. *Dermatol Surg*, 2001, 27, 111-116.

Trelles, MA; Allones, I; Luna, R. One-pass resurfacing with a combined-mode erbium,YAG/CO_2 laser system, a study in 102 patients. *Brit J Derm.*, 2002, 146, 473-480.

Trelles, MA; Allones, I; Velez, M. Nonablative facial skin photorejuvenation with an intense pulsed light system and adjunctive epidermal care. *Lasers in Medical Science*, 2003, 18, 104-111.

Trelles, MA; García-Solana, L; Calderhead, RG. Skin Resurfacing Improved with a New Dual Wavelength Er,YAG / CO_2 Laser System, A Comparative Study. *J Clin Laser Med Surg.*, 1999, 17, 99-104.

Trelles, MA; Levy, JL; Pardo, L; Kontoes, V; Soria, C. Complication du relissage laser CO_2, une revue de 728 patients. *J. Med Esth et Chir Derm.*, 9/2000, Vol XXVII, 107, 169-74.

Trelles, MA; Mordon, S; Benítez, V; Levy, JL. Er,YAG Laser resurfacing using Combined Ablation and Coagulation Modes. *Dermatol Surg.*, 2001, 27, 727-734.

Trelles, MA; Soria, C; Pardo-Mateu, L; Chamorro, JJ; Makaron, T; Buezo, O. renovación anatómica y estética de los labios, con ayuda del láser. *Cir. Plas. Iberolatinoam*, 1998, 24, 1, 63-71.

Weiss, Ra; Weiss, MA. Devices for nonabaltive photorejuvenation. In, Goldman MP, ed. *Cutaneous and Cosmetic Laser Surgery*. Philadelphia, Mosby Elseier Ed, 2006, 249-62.

Wanner, M; Tanzi, EL; Alster, TS. Fractional photothermologysis, treatment of facial and nonfacial cutaneous photodamage with a 1550 nm erbium-doped fiber laser. *Dermatol Surg.*, 2007, 33, 23-8.

In: Skin Anatomy and Physiology Research Developments ISBN: 978-1-60741-469-8
Editor: Leon F. Bukowsky

Chapter 11

Study of Temperature Distribution within Heated Skin Tissue Using the Boundary Element Method

E. Y. K. Ng*, F. Xu[1], T. J. Lu[2], A. L. Y. Cheng and E. H. Ooi
School of Mechanical & Aerospace Engineering,
Nanyang Technological University, Singapore
[1]Engineering Department, Cambridge University, Cambridge, UK
[2]MOE Key Laboratory of Strength and Vibration, School of Aerospace,
Xi'an Jiaotong University, P.R. China

Abstract

With the advancement in computer technology, numerical simulation has been a useful tool in assisting the medical field in areas such as skin burns. Successful modeling of the skin can aid doctors in estimating the amount of the damaged skin to be removed to prevent development of poison due to harmful agents that enters the body. This chapter presents a two-dimensional human skin model developed to obtain temperatures within the skin due to heating under thermal steady state conditions. Simulations are carried out using the boundary element method (BEM) and the results are verified against the solutions obtained using the finite element method (FEM). The BEM proved to be a good alternative to using FEM. Advantages of BEM include improved accuracy, less required computer memory and more efficient computation. A parametric study is conducted using six factors: dermis thermal conductivity, subcutaneous fat thermal conductivity, blood perfusion rate, temperature of heating disk, heat transfer coefficient and ambient temperature. Results show that varying the temperature of the heating disk greatly affects the temperature within the affected tissue dominantly as compared to the other five factors.

---

* Author of correspondence: Adjunct NUH Scientist, Office of Biomedical Research, National University Hospital of Singapore. Email: mykng@ntu.edu.sg

Keywords: boundary element, skin burn, simulation, temperature, bioheat transfer

1. Introduction

Skin burn is heavily researched as it causes a tremendous amount of physical stress and trauma in burn victims. In 2006, the number of fire causalities in Singapore was 94, comprising 91 injured persons and 3 fatalities [1]. In Singapore General Hospital Burns Centre, a mean of 200 patients are admitted annually. Generally, burns are caused by many types of interaction with high temperature sources such as exposure to hot fire, contact with a hot solid or liquid, breathing in of hot vapor or electrical dissipation [2].

In the past, when computer technology was less advanced and widely available, very few experiments were conducted on humans and testing was mostly done on pigs. As Information Technology (IT) becomes more advanced, these methods were considered unnecessary and less favored. Accurately predicting the temperature within the skin tissue with the use of computer program codes could efficiently predict the seriousness of different burns accurately.

A serious wound generally requires a longer time for the removal of dead skins before it can heal on its own. If the dead skins are not removed it may produce further injury and cause additional systemic complications such as developing poisons in the body due to harmful agents entering the blood stream from the wounds. Thus, the computer program codes are potentially useful as surgical assistance to doctors; providing information needed to determine the amount of dead skins to be removed during surgery.

In this chapter, the Pennes bioheat equation, a simple yet useful model, is used for determining the steady state temperature distribution in the tissue involved [3]. It is the starting point of scientific modeling work in bioheat transfer. Although various improved and alternative models have emerged, the Pennes model is still widely in use due to its simplicity.

The numerical method used here is the boundary element method (BEM). The BEM is different compared to the more popular finite element method (FEM) and finite difference method (FDM) in that it only requires the boundaries of the solution domain to be discretized. This is unlike the FEM and FDM, which requires a full domain discretization [4]. Depending on the complexity of the geometry, this feature can result in important time saving in the creation and modification of the. This leads to less required computer memory and a more efficient computation.

The pioneers of skin burn injury, Henriques and Moritz [5], showed that a burn injury of standard threshold severity can be produced by progressively decreasing temperatures as the thermal insult period is logarithmically increased. From then on, many investigators have discussed burn injuries for different situations. Diller and Hayes [6] produced a finite element model of burn injuries in skin that contained the blood perfusion term. Torvi and Dale [7] presented a finite element model of skin for a flash fire exposure and discussed the sensitivity of burn predictions to variations in thermal physical properties. Ng and Chua [8], using the finite element method, presented a mesh-independent model to predict skin burn injuries. They also compared one- and two-dimensional programs for predicting skin burns, showing that the temperature distributions predicted by both programs were comparable [9].

2. Model of the Human Skin

A two-dimensional model of the human skin based on the work by Ng and Chua [8], such as the model shown in Figure 1, is considered here. In reality, the human skin consists of three layers, namely the epidermis, dermis and subcutaneous fat layer. For simplicity, since the epidermis layer is relatively thinner, it is modeled together with the dermis layer as one homogeneous region. A heating disk of 363K (90°C) is applied on the surface of the skin and is assumed to be in perfect thermal contact (i.e. zero thermal resistance) with the dermis. Blood perfusion is considered to be present inside the dermal layer only to aid in the parametric study. Homogeneous and isotropic thermal properties are assumed in each layer of skin tissue. Heat is assumed to be conducted inside the skin model.

Boundary conditions used are illustrated in Figure 1 and may be summarized as follows:

1. At both sides of the skin, they are assumed to be under adiabatic condition, thus $\frac{\partial T}{\partial n} = 0$.
2. At the location where the dermis is exposed to the heating disk, the temperature is 363K (90°C).
3. At the locations where dermis is exposed to ambient air, it undergoes natural convective heat transfer giving $-k_1 \frac{\partial T}{\partial n} = h(T - T_{amb})$, where k_1 is the thermal conductivity of the dermis, T is the tissue temperature, h is the convective heat transfer coefficient and T_{amb} refers to the ambient temperature.
4. The bottom of the skin is assumed to be at body's core temperature of 310K (37°C).

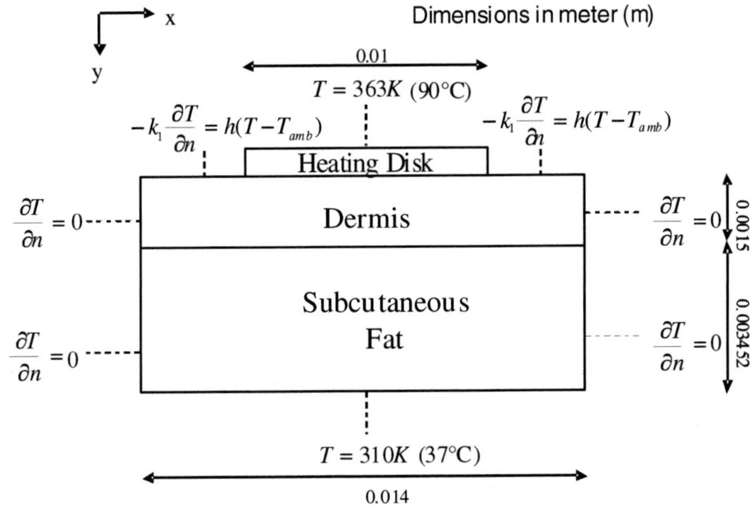

Figure 1. Model of the skin and its boundary conditions

The length of the heating disk and skin are 0.01m (1cm) and 0.014m (1.4cm) respectively. The thickness of dermis layer is 0.0015m (1.5mm) and the subcutaneous fat layer is 0.03452m (3.452mm). Values of various parameters used in describing the heat flow and the boundary conditions of the model are listed in Table 1. These values are similar to those chosen Torvi and Dale [7] and Ng and Chua [8].

Table 1. Important parameter values used for the skin model

Parameter	Symbol	Value (unit)
Thermal conductivity of Dermis	k_1	0.37 W/mK
Thermal conductivity of Subcutaneous Fats	k_2	0.16 W/mK
Convective Heat Transfer coefficient	h	7.0 W/m^2K
Length of Disk (in *x*-direction)	L_D	0.01m (1cm)
Total length of skin (in *x*-direction)	L_S	0.014m (1.4cm)
Temperature of arterial blood	T_a	310K (37°C)
Temperature of ambient air	T_{amb}	298K (25°C)
Temperature of heating disk	T_{disk}	363K (90°C)
Density of blood	ρ_b	1100 kg/m^3
Specific heat of blood	c_b	3300J/kgK
Blood perfusion rate	ω_b	2.4 x $10^{-2} m^3/(sm^3)$

3. The Boundary Element Method

As mentioned earlier, the equation governing the flow of heat inside the skin model is given by the steady-state Pennes bioheat equation, which comes in the form of

$$\nabla \cdot \left(k\nabla T(x,y)\right) + S(x,y) = 0 \qquad (1)$$

where k is thermal conductivity, T is temperature and $S(x,y)$ can be expressed as

$$S(x,y) = \omega_b \rho_b c_b (T_b - T) + Q_m \qquad (2)$$

where ρ_b, c_b and ω_b are the density, specific heat and blood perfusion rate respectively and Q_m is the metabolic heat generated by the skin. In this study, Q_m is taken to be zero since the heat generated from the metabolism of the human skin is very much smaller than the heat from the heating disk.

To carry out the BEM, the integral representation of (1) has to be derived, which is given by

$$\gamma(\xi,\eta)T(\xi,\eta) = \int_{\Gamma} T(x,y)\frac{\partial}{\partial n} w(x,y;\xi,\eta)d\Gamma - \int_{\Gamma} w(x,y;\xi,\eta)\frac{\partial}{\partial n} T(x,y)d\Gamma \\ - \int_{\Omega} S(x,y)\nabla^2 w(x,y;\xi,\eta)d\Omega \tag{3}$$

where $\gamma(\xi,\eta) = 0.5$ if the point (ξ,η) lies in the smooth path of Γ, $\gamma(\xi,\eta) = 1$ if (ξ,η) lies in the interior of the domain, Ω and $w(x,y;\xi,\eta)$ is the fundamental solution of the two-dimensional Laplace equation given by

$$w(x,y) = \frac{1}{2\pi}\ln\sqrt{(x-\xi)^2 - (y-\eta)^2} \tag{4}$$

To deal with the domain integral in (3), the dual reciprocity boundary element method (DRBEM) approximation is used such that

$$S(x,y) = \sum_{j=1}^{N+L} \beta_j f_j \tag{5}$$

where N is the total number of boundary nodes, L is the total number of interior collocation nodes, β_j is a set of unknown coefficients to be determined, and f_j is a set of interpolation function which comes in form of

$$f = 1 + r(x,y;\xi,\eta)^2 + r(x,y;\xi,\eta)^3 \tag{6}$$

Replacing (5) into (3), we obtain

$$\gamma(\xi,\eta)T(\xi,\eta) = \int_{\Gamma} T(x,y)\frac{\partial}{\partial n} w(x,y;\xi,\eta)d\Gamma - \int_{\Gamma} w(x,y;\xi,\eta)\frac{\partial}{\partial n} T(x,y)d\Gamma \\ - \sum_{j=1}^{N+L} \beta_j \int_{\Omega} f_j \nabla^2 w(x,y;\xi,\eta)d\Omega \tag{7}$$

Using Green's second identity on the domain integral, (7) becomes:

$$\gamma(\xi,\eta)T(\xi,\eta) = \int_\Gamma T(x,y)\frac{\partial}{\partial n}w(x,y;\xi,\eta)d\Gamma - \int_\Gamma w(x,y;\xi,\eta)\frac{\partial}{\partial n}T(x,y)d\Gamma$$
$$-\sum_{j=1}^{N+L}\beta_j\left\{\int_\Gamma \chi(x,y)\frac{\partial}{\partial n}w(x,y;\xi,\eta)d\Gamma - \int_\Gamma w(x,y;\xi,\eta)\frac{\partial}{\partial n}\chi(x,y)d\Gamma\right\} \quad (8)$$

where c is the particular solution defined by

$$\chi(x,y) = \frac{1}{4}r^2(x,y;\xi,\eta) + \frac{1}{16}r^4(x,y;\xi,\eta) + \frac{1}{25}r^5(x,y;\xi,\eta) \quad (9)$$

The coefficients β_j from (8) can be determined from equation (5). In matrix notation, we get

$$\{\beta\} = [\mathbf{F}]^{-1}\{\chi(x,y)\} \quad (10)$$

where $\mathbf{F}$ is the matrix generated from the collocation of the interpolation function.

Substituting the expression in (2) and the approximation in (10) into (8), we get

$$\gamma(\xi,\eta)T(\xi,\eta) = \int_\Gamma T(x,y)\frac{\partial}{\partial n}w(x,y;\xi,\eta)d\Gamma - \int_\Gamma w(x,y;\xi,\eta)\frac{\partial}{\partial n}T(x,y)d\Gamma$$
$$+\rho_b c_b \omega_b \sum_{j=1}^{N+L} W_j(\xi,\eta)(T - T_b) \quad (11)$$

where $W_j(\xi,\eta)$ is given by $[\mathbf{F}]^{-1}\Lambda$ and Λ is given by

$$\Lambda(x,y;\xi,\eta) = \chi(x,y)\frac{\partial}{\partial n}w(x,y;\xi,\eta)d\Gamma - \int_\Gamma w(x,y;\xi,\eta)\frac{\partial}{\partial n}\chi(x,y)d\Gamma \quad (12)$$

Using (11) and the boundary conditions specified earlier and following the discretization of the boundaries, a system of linear algebraic equation can be set up to determine the respective unknowns on the boundaries as well as at the interior collocation nodes. Interface between the dermal layer and the subcutaneous fat layer are treated using the continuity principle.

Domain 1, i.e., the dermal layer, consists of six different boundaries. Boundary 1: interface between domains 1 and 2, boundaries 2 and 6 with heat flux known and temperature unknown, boundaries 3 and 5 where temperature is unknown and boundary 4 where temperature is known and heat flux is unknown. Domain 2 consists of 4 boundaries. Boundary 1 is the interface between domain 1 and 2, boundaries 7 and 9 where heat flux is known and temperature is unknown and boundary 8 where temperature is known and heat flux is unknown. These are illustrated in Figure 2.

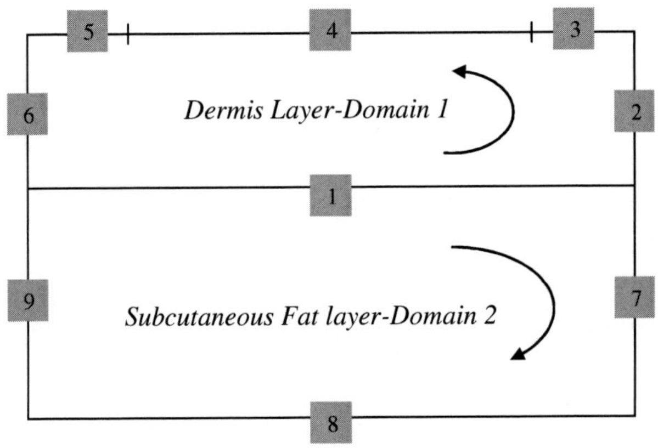

Figure 2. Domains and boundaries of the BEM skin model

4. Numerical Results

4.1 Validation

The BEM code is verified against the results obtained using COMSOL Multiphysics 3.2 (a partial differential equation calculator that utilizes the FEM) at 10 randomly and spatially well-spread chosen points. This is presented in Table 2. A convergence test is conducted with 100 interior points (L=100), 20 boundary nodes on domain 1 and 15 boundary nodes on domain 2. This is further illustrated in Figure 3.

4.2 Sensitivity analysis

A sensitivity analysis is carried out and observation is made at various depths of the skin model at x = 0.007m (middle of heating disk). Nine points along are selected along x = 0.007m such as illustrated in Figure 4. The parameters to be varied are dermis thermal conductivity, subcutaneous thermal conductivity, blood perfusion rate, ambient temperature, disk temperature and heat transfer coefficient. The reference baseline values are obtained so as to compare with FEM results [12]. To study the effect of dermis thermal conductivity, the baseline value of 0.37W/mK is reduced and increased by 50%. The same goes for the fat thermal conductivity of 0.16W/mK and heat transfer coefficient of 12500W/m^{2}K as baseline values. For the blood perfusion rate, the study is conducted using full blood perfusion

($0.024 m^3 s^{-1} m^{-3}$), half blood perfusion and no blood perfusion. For the study of ambient temperature effects, 298K (25°C) was taken as the baseline value. Values of 313K (40°C) and 291K (18°C) are used to simulate the skin under hot and cold ambient conditions respectively. The temperature of disk is also varied, with 363K (90°C) as baseline value and 333K (30°C) and 393K (120°C) as the cooler and hotter disk temperatures respectively. The various values of different parameters used are summarized in Table 3. In carrying out the sensitivity analysis of each parameter, the other parameters are maintained at their baseline values.

Table 2. Comparison of temperatures from Matlab BEM code and COMSOL Multiphysics 3.2

x	y	Temperature (K)	
		BEM	FEM
0.0023	0.0016	328.3597	328.7782
0.0023	0.0030	320.2389	320.5722
0.0023	0.0044	312.9140	313.0065
0.0070	0.0004	354.6507	355.9682
0.0070	0.0016	344.1421	344.6841
0.0070	0.0030	329.2715	329.2685
0.0070	0.0044	315.3514	315.3537
0.0117	0.0016	328.3597	328.7775
0.0117	0.0030	320.2389	320.5721
0.0117	0.0044	312.9140	313.0065

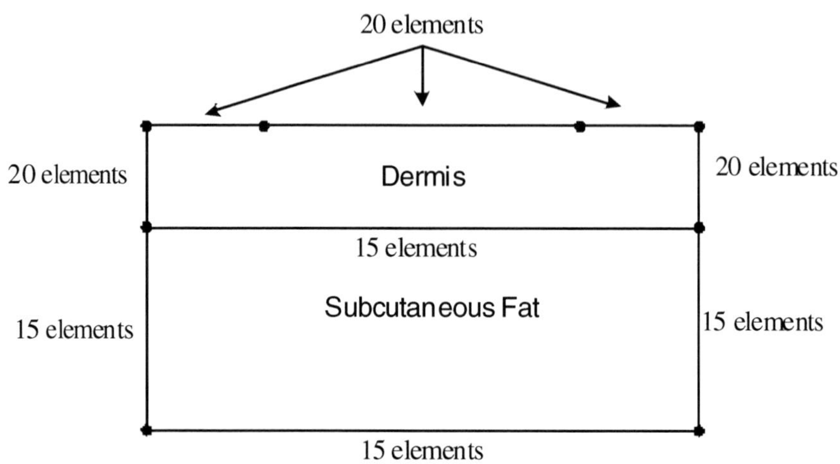

Figure 3. Numbers of elements used for each side and its discretized form

The effect of different values of dermis thermal conductivity is shown in Figure 5. It can be seen that a larger dermis thermal conductivity causes the temperature inside the affected tissue to rise. Generally, the dermis layer is in contact with the heating disk. An increased thermal conductivity implies that more heat can be conducted from the heating disk into the skin tissues. If we assume the threshold injury is 318K (45°C) [5] and ignoring the of burn injury (e.g. the degrees of burn etc), we find that a larger dermal thermal conductivity shifts the injury threshold to the right (of that of baseline value). This implies that the injury will spread deeper into the tissue when thermal conductivity is raised. Decreasing the dermis thermal conductivity by half (k = 0.185W/mK) causes the injury threshold to shift towards the left. This means that for lower thermal conductivity, injury will not penetrate as deep as that of a higher thermal conductivity as illustrated in Figures 6 to 8.

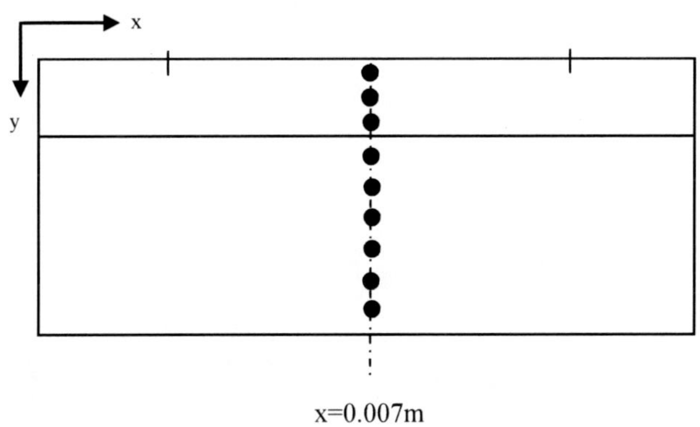

Figure 4. Locations of interior temperatures obtained for parametric study

Table 3. List of parameters values used for parametric study

Parameters	Values
Dermal thermal conductivity	0.185 W/mK 0.37 W/mK 0.74 W/mK
Fat thermal conductivity	0.08 W/mK 0.16 W/mK 0.74 W/mK
Blood perfusion rate	0 $m^3/(sm^3)$ 0.012 $m^3/(sm^3)$ 0.024 $m^3/(sm^3)$
Temperature of disk	333K 363K 393K
Heat transfer coefficient	6250 W/m^2K 12500 W/m^2K 25000 W/m^2K
Ambient Temperature	313K 298K 291K

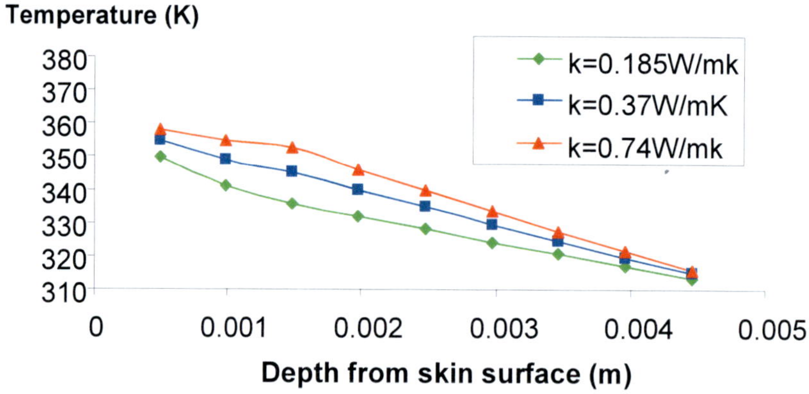

Figure 5. Effects of dermal thermal conductivity on prediction of temperature

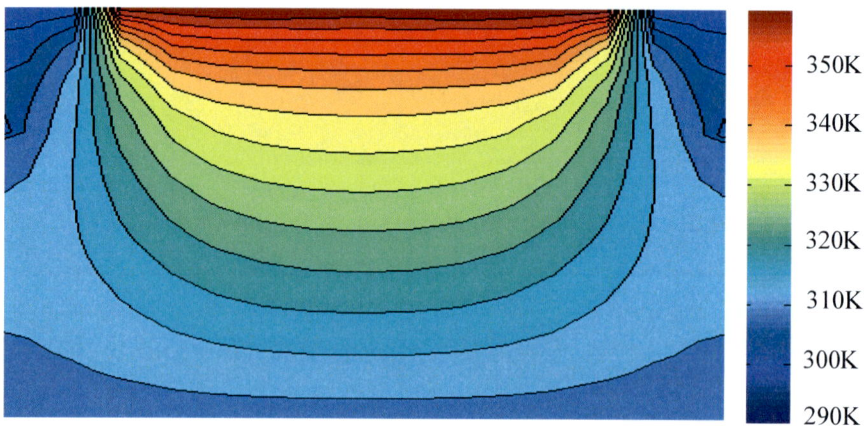

Figure 6. Isotherm plot with lower dermal thermal conductivity

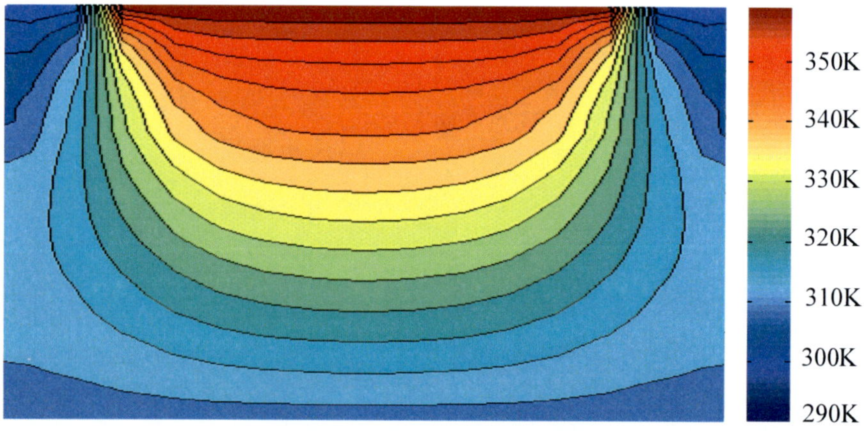

Figure 7. Isotherm plot with baseline dermal conductivity

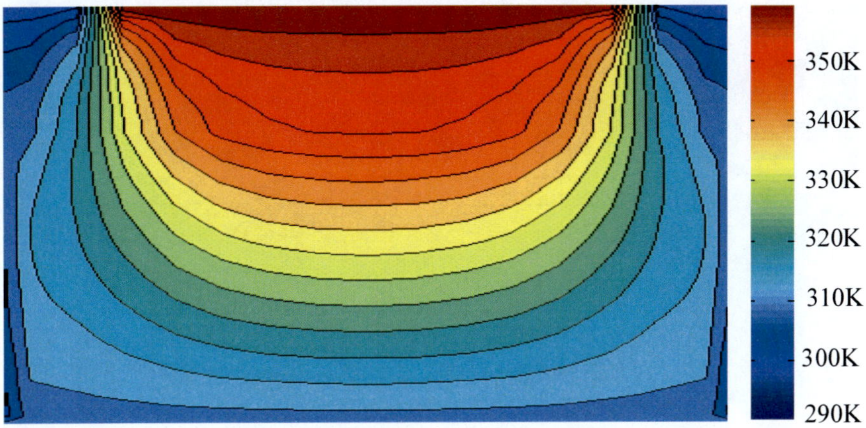

Figure 8. Isotherm plot with higher dermal thermal conductivity

The effect of different values of subcutaneous fat thermal conductivity is shown in Figure 9. The results predicted are contrary to the earlier case of dermal thermal conductivity. By increasing the thermal conductivity of the subcutaneous fat, the temperature in the skin tissue drops. This is likely due to heat being transferred away from the skin surface into the deeper tissue region as thermal conductivity of the subcutaneous fat increases, hence lowering the average temperature of the affected tissue within the dermis layer.

The same rationale may be applied to the threshold injury. When the fat thermal conductivity is increased; the injury threshold shifts to the left of that of baseline value, indicating that the injury penetrates less deep into the tissue. Whereas, when fat thermal conductivity is decreased by half, the injury is inflicted deeper into the affected tissue. This is illustrated in Figure 10 to 12.

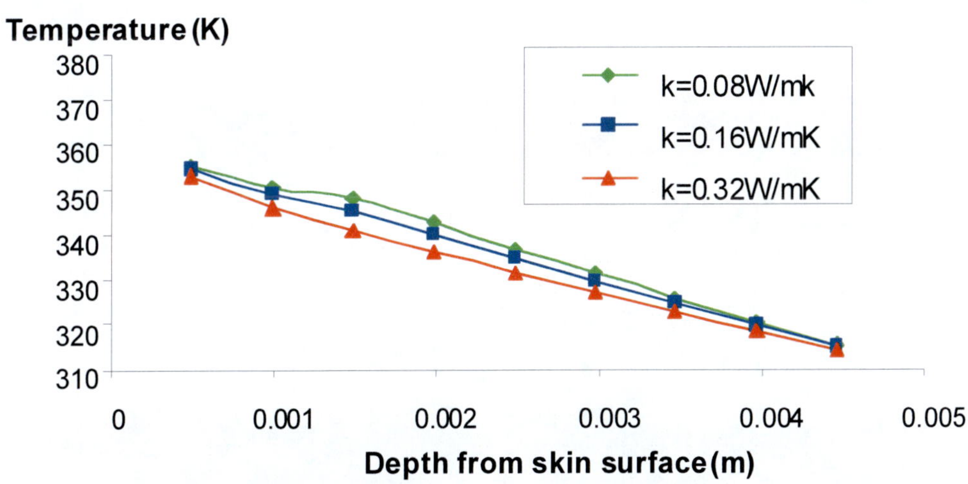

Figure 9. Effects of subcutaneous fat thermal conductivity on prediction of temperature

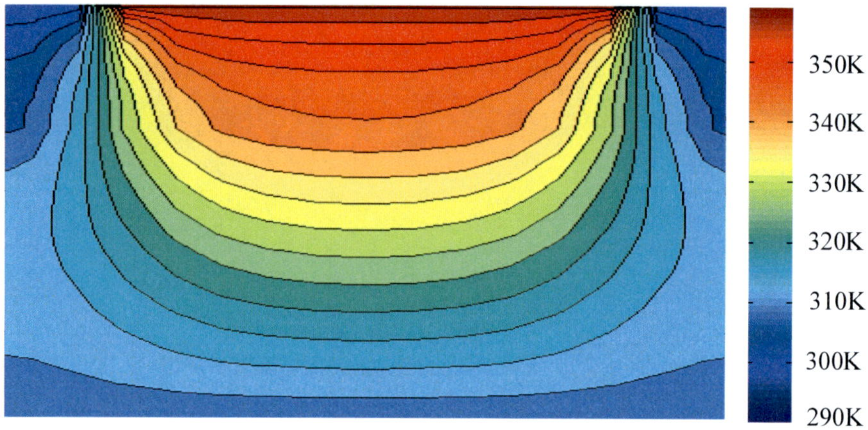

Figure 10. Isotherm plot with lower subcutaneous fat thermal conductivity

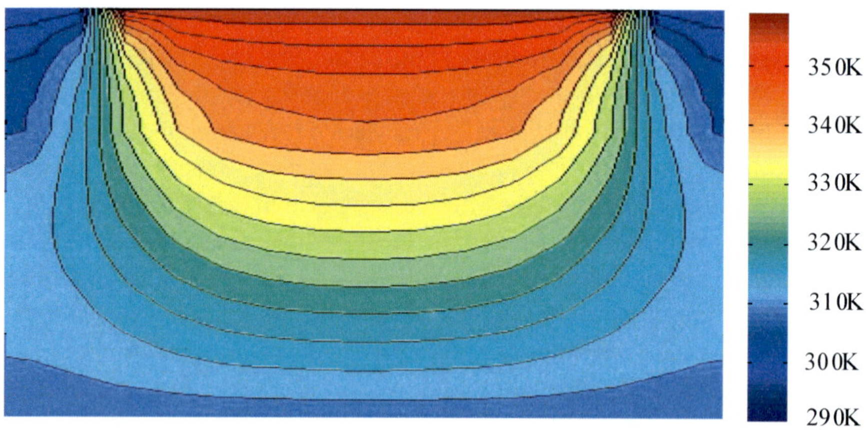

Figure 11. Isotherm plot with baseline subcutaneous fat thermal conductivity

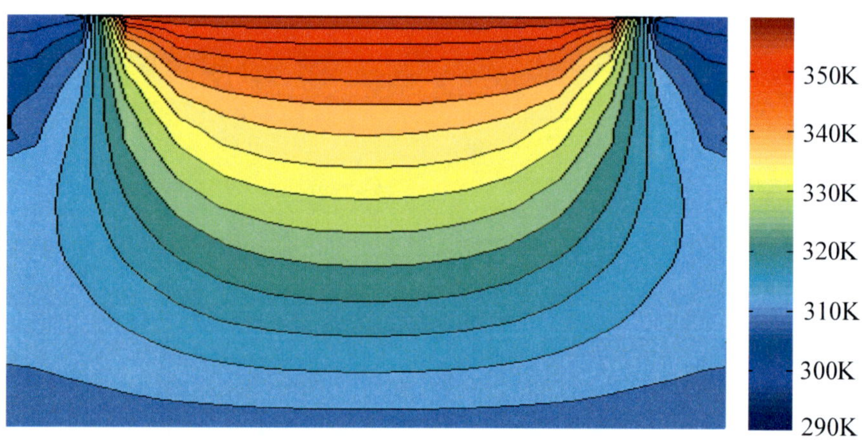

Figure 12. Isotherm plot with higher subcutaneous fat thermal conductivity

Figure 13 shows the temperature distribution inside the skin at x = 0.007m for different values of the blood perfusion rate. By increasing the blood perfusion rate, the temperature of the affected tissue drops. This is evident in the thermoregulatory response of skin tissue. When an increase in temperature is detected, the immediate effect of the body is to dilate the blood vessels inside body (vasodilation). This increases the blood flow, which helps to dissipate the heat accumulated inside the body [13].

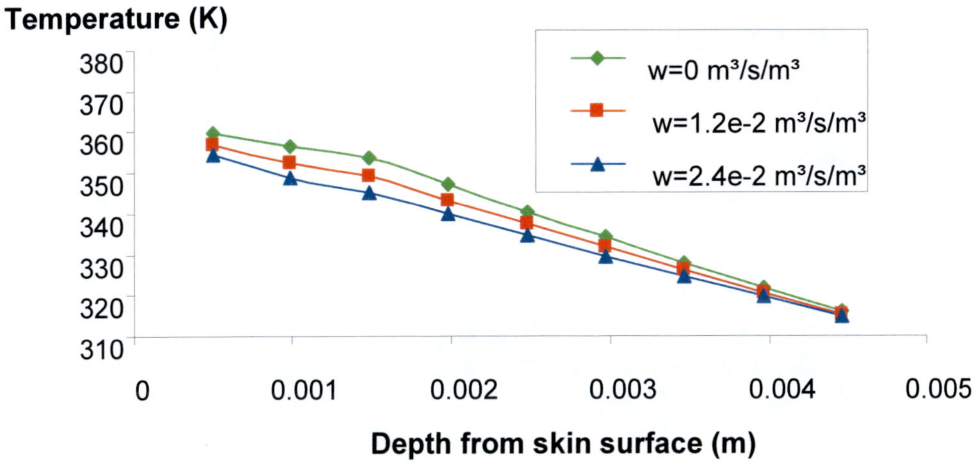

Figure 13. Effects of blood perfusion rate on prediction of temperature

As for the injury threshold, it can be seen from Figure 13 that as blood perfusion rate increases, it shifts to the left, suggesting that the injury does not penetrate into the affected tissue as compared to that of a lower blood perfusion rate (see Figures 14 to 16).

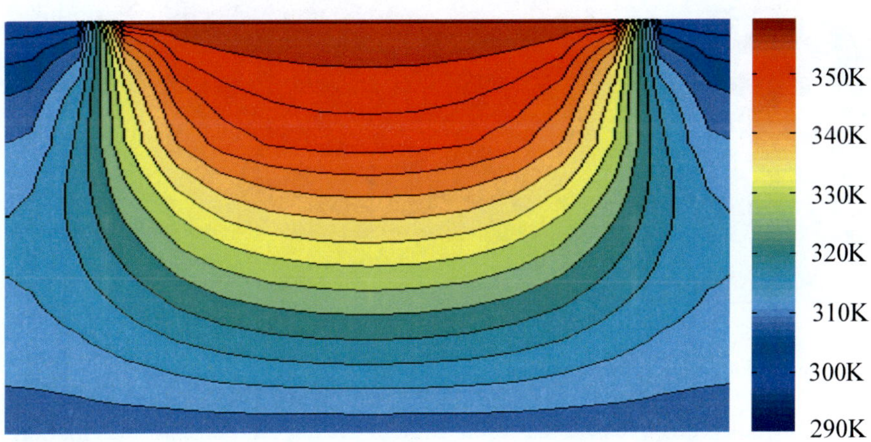

Figure 14. Isotherm plot with no blood perfusion

The temperature distribution inside the skin when heated with different heating disk is shown in Figure 17. The temperature of the affected tissue varies more significantly than the other five factors that are being studied here. Not surprisingly, a heating disk with a higher temperature generally produces warmer skin tissues. Figure 17 suggest that the injury threshold shifts rather significantly to the right when the disk temperature increases, indicating that the burn injury penetrates deeper into the skin tissue. It is also important to note that among the other five factors investigated, by increasing the temperature of disk, it induces the deepest penetration of burn injury into the skin as can be seen from Figure 18 to 20.

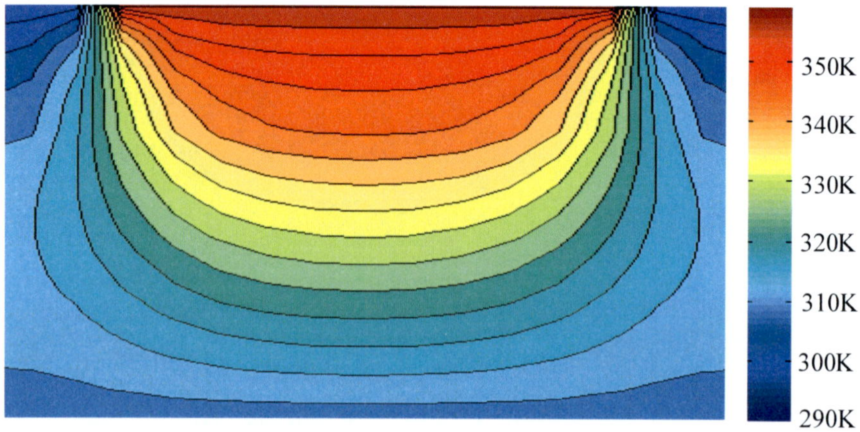

Figure 15. Isotherm plot with half blood perfusion

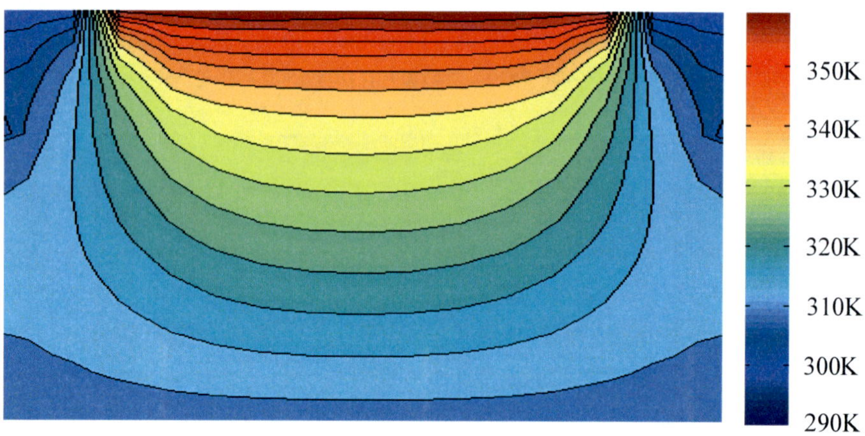

Figure 16. Isotherm plot with full blood perfusion (baseline)

The effect of convective heat transfer coefficient on the temperature distribution inside the skin during burn is displayed in Figure 21. The plot shown in Figure 21 suggests that the convective heat transfer coefficient at the top surfaces does not play a significant part in altering the skin tissue temperature. However, it has to be noted that these values are sampled at the center of skin configuration. From Figures 22 to 24, we find that the tissue temperature at areas where effects of natural convection is significant (surface of dermis exposed to the ambient) drops slightly when the heat transfer coefficient is increased.

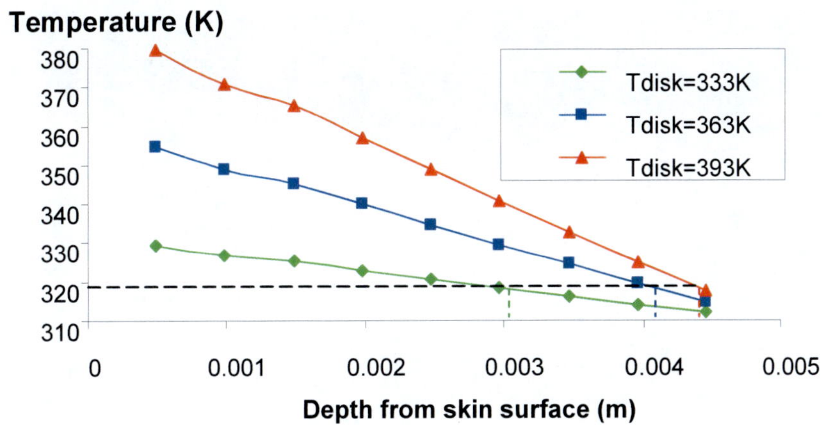

Figure 17. Effects of disk temperature on the prediction of temperature

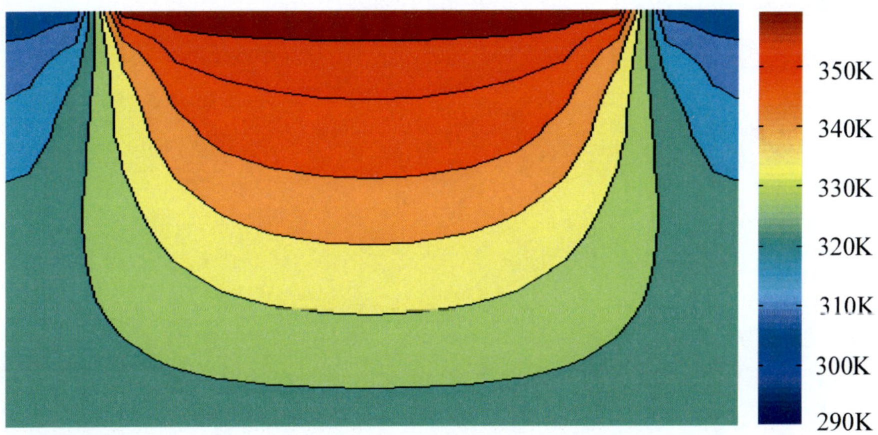

Figure 18. Isotherm plot with cooler disk temperature

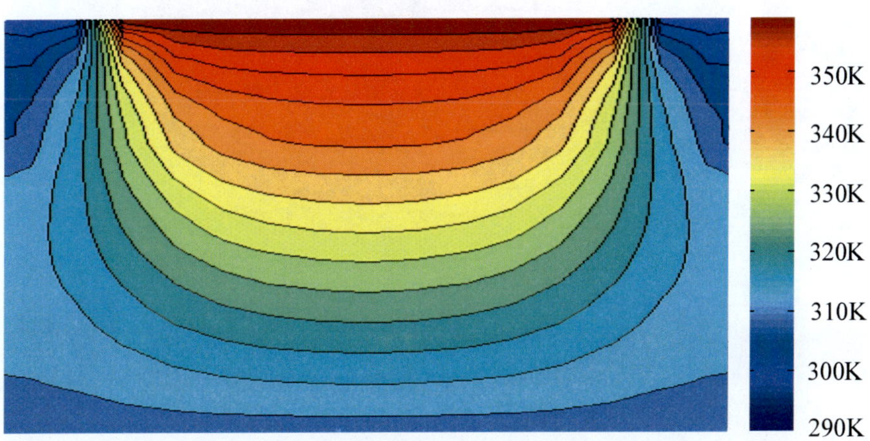

Figure 19. Isotherm plot with baseline disk temperature

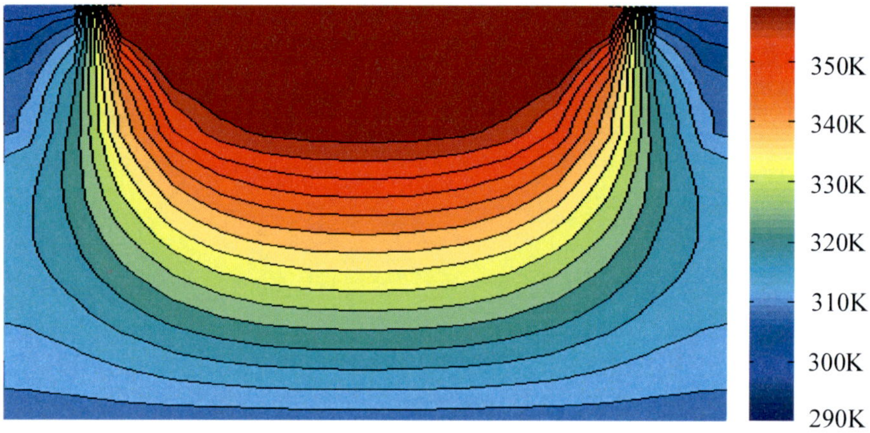

Figure 20. Isotherm plot with hotter disk temperature

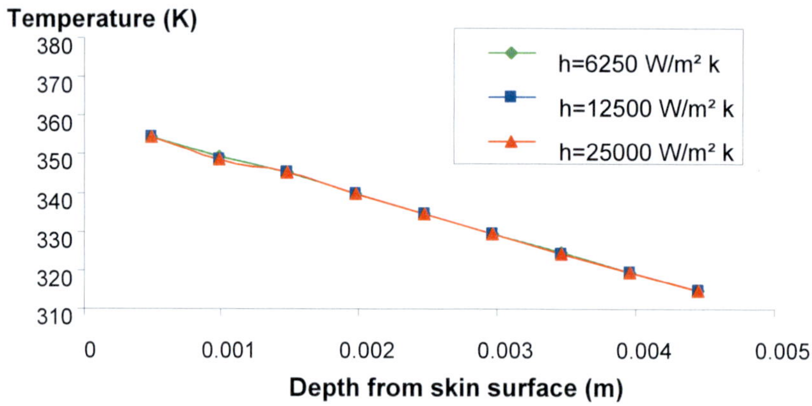

Figure 21. Effects of convective heat transfer coefficient on prediction of temperature

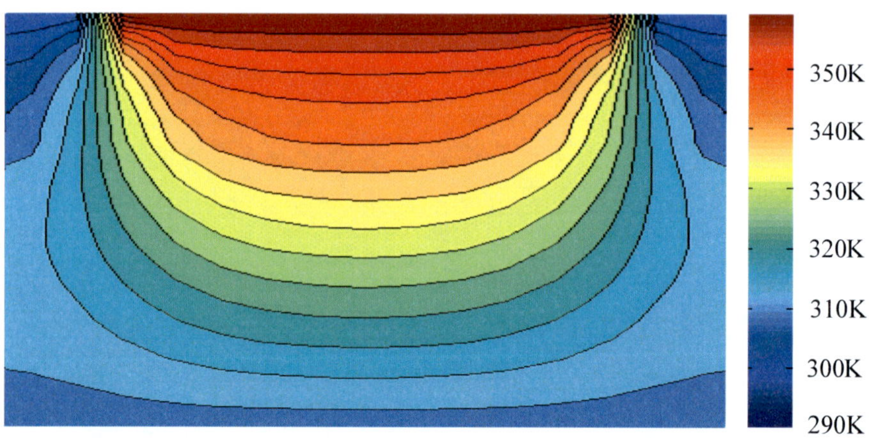

Figure 22. Isotherm plot with lower heat transfer coefficient

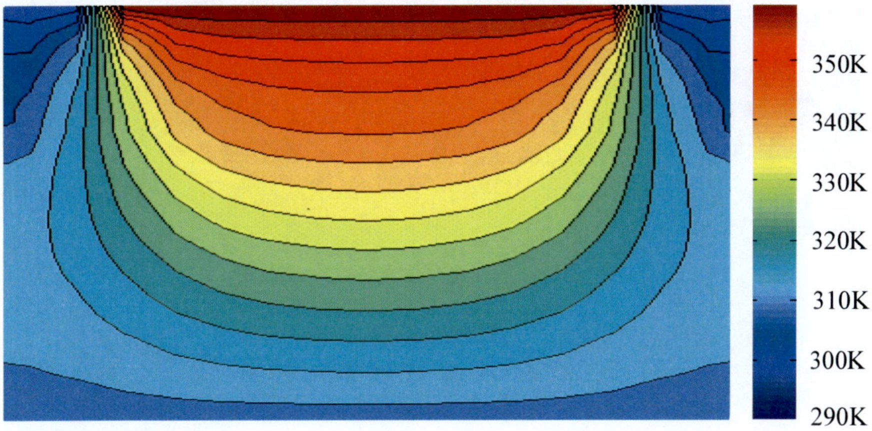

Figure 23. Isotherm plot with baseline heat transfer coefficient

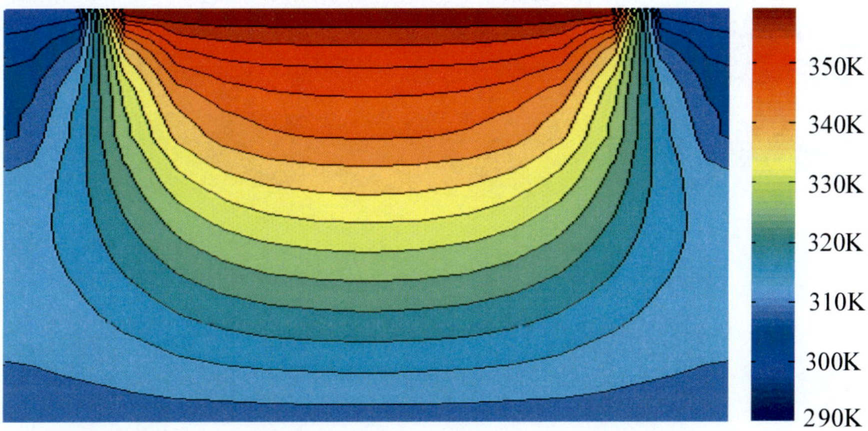

Figure 24. Isotherm plot with higher heat transfer coefficient

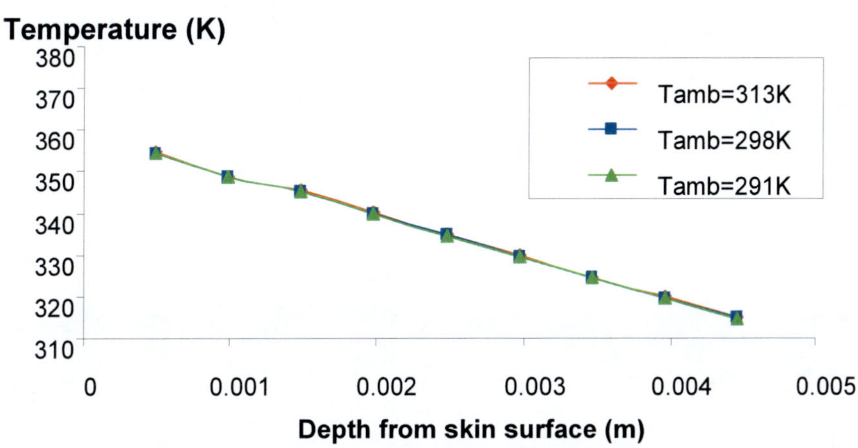

Figure 25. Effects of ambient temperature on the prediction of temperature

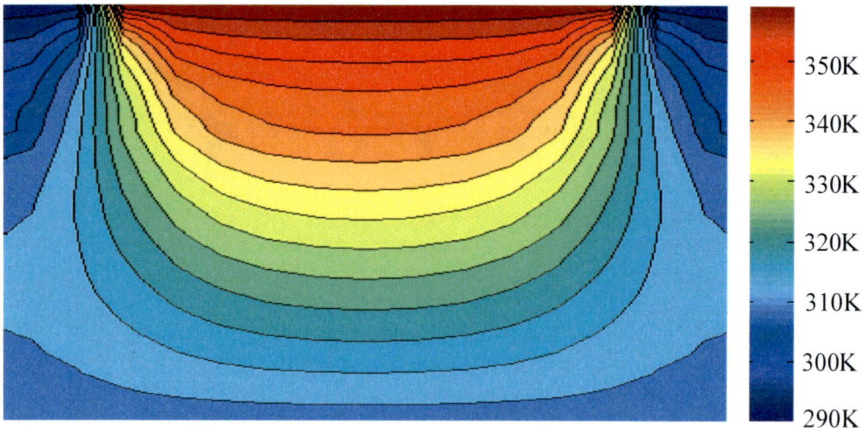

Figure 26. Isotherm plot with lower ambient temperature

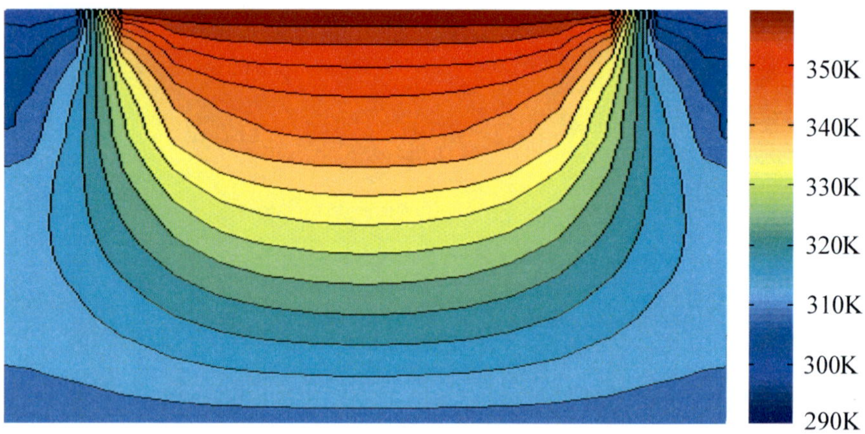

Figure 27. Isotherm plot with baseline ambient temperature

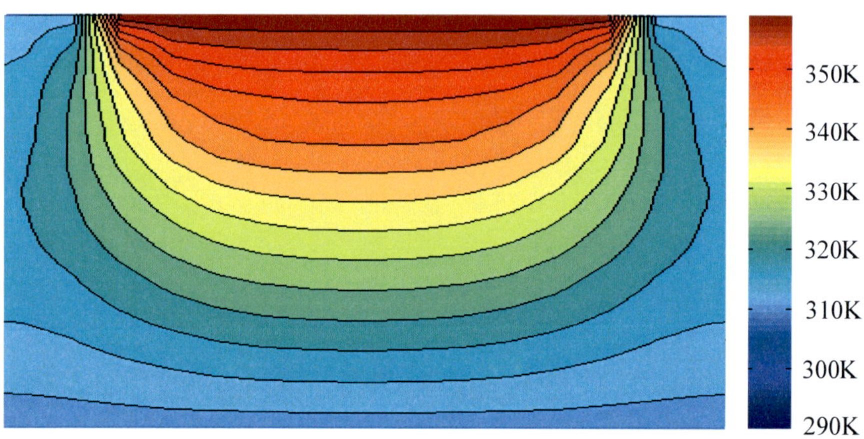

Figure 28. Isotherm plot with higher ambient temperature

The effect of changing the ambient temperature does not have any significant effect on the tissue temperature as indicated in Figure 25. Likewise, the injury threshold does not shift to the right or left. Nevertheless, it is apparent from Figures 26 to 28 that although the temperature at the center of the tissue does not vary much, the temperature at the vicinity do vary significantly. With a lower ambient temperature, the tissue temperature further away from the skin center becomes much cooler and vice versa.

5. Taguchi Method

Taguchi method is carried out in this section and it emphasizes that the control factors must be optimized through the design of experiment rather than by the trial and error approach [14]. A traditional method for improving the quality of an outcome is to adjust one factor at a time to observe the results, such as the sensitivity analysis that has been carried out earlier. The major disadvantage of this method is that it is costly and unreliable due to the interaction between the factors. The Taguchi method is not plagued by these problems. Taguchi method can change many factors simultaneously in a systematic way thus ensuring an independent study of the product factors. Once the factors have been adequately characterized, the quality of an outcome can then be improved.

The location of skin tissue of interest here is limited to the 100 interior points within the dermis layer because greatest burn damage is resulted closer to the skin surface when one is subjected to a heating disk. An average temperature T_{avg} of the 100 interior points is obtained in a single run of the Matlab program.

Table 4 summarizes the six factors used and their parameters in Level 1 and Level 2. L64 (2^6) Taguchi array is selected for the evaluation of these parameters and their interactions.

Table 4. Factors and parameters studied in obtaining the skin temperature

Symbol	Factors	Level 1	Level 2
A	Dermis thermal conductivity, k_1	0.185 W/mK	0.74 W/mK
B	Subcutaneous fat thermal conductivity, k_2	0.08 W/mK	0.32 W/mK
C	Blood perfusion rate, ω_b	0 $m^3/s/m^3$	2.4e-2 $m^3/s/m^3$
D	Temperature of disk, T_{disk}	333K	393K
E	Convective heat transfer coefficient, h	6250W/m^2K	25000W/m^2K
F	Ambient temperature, T_{amb}	291K	313K

Next, the Signal-to-Noise Ratio (SNR), which measures the variation of the observations in a run, is calculated for all the 64 runs. The equation used is given by [14]

$$SNR = -\log\left(\frac{1}{n}\times\frac{1}{y^2}\right) \tag{13}$$

where n is the number of values of each trial conditions (in this case is 2) and y is the observed value (average temperature, T_{avg}).

The average SNR is calculated for each factor at both Level 1 and Level 2. For example, runs involving factor F at level 1, the corresponding values of SNR from runs 1 to 32 are totaled and an average of them is obtained, which is chosen to be SNR_1. Effect is calculated by subtracting SNR of Level 1 from SNR of Level 2 for each factor as tabulated in Table 5.

Table 5. Average SNRs and their effect values

Levels	Average SNR values of the six factors					
	A	B	C	D	E	F
1	53.63331	53.74705	53.76681	**53.21076**	53.71440	53.63331
2	53.78510	53.67136	53.65160	**54.20765**	53.70401	53.78510
Effect	0.15179	-0.07569	-0.11521	**0.99689**	-0.01039	0.15179

Comparing the effect values from Table 5, it can be concluded that factor D, i.e. disk temperature (see bolded numbers) is the single most outstanding factor that affects the skin temperature and is almost nine times greater than the other factors. If it is defined that the higher the skin temperature (resulting in the most damage to the skin for preventive measures) produces the better outcome, then the results in Table 5 suggest that the optimum order of parameters is A2B1C1D2E1F2.

6. Conclusion

A BEM code has been developed to study the temperature distribution inside a two-dimensional skin model during burn. The BEM is used to solve the Pennes bioheat equation. It has been verified with COMSOL Multiphysics (FEM Method) and is useful as an alternative method in determining the temperature within an area of heated skin.

At the middle of the skin configuration (x = 0.007m), interior temperatures of the affected skin are studied and isotherms are produced for the six different factors. From the parametric study, it is concluded that the heating disk temperature affects the skin tissue temperature to the greatest degree when compared to the other five factors. When the disk temperature is increased, it induces the greatest amount of injury depth-wise into the affected skin tissue. The thermal conductivity effects of the dermis and subcutaneous fat, however, produce contrary results. When thermal conductivities of both layers are increased, the dermis conducts more heat from the heating disk, thus increasing the overall average temperature of the affected tissue. On the other hand, the subcutaneous fat conducts heat away from the dermis layer, thus lowering the local temperature at the dermis layer. A higher blood perfusion helps to reduce the skin temperature by transferring away excessive heat. On the contrary, convective heat transfer coefficient and ambient temperature do not play a significant role in changing the temperature at the centre of the tissue (center of burnt area). A significant change in the temperature near the skin surface where convection takes place can be observed however.

From the Taguchi analysis, it is suggested that for a higher skin temperature, the following conditions must be met: the dermis thermal conductivity is set to a higher value, the subcutaneous fat thermal conductivity is set to a lower blood perfusion rate, a high disk temperature, a low convective heat transfer coefficient and, finally, a high ambient temperature set to the higher value.

Several steps may be adopted in the future to improve model and the analysis presented in this chapter. These include:

(a) an inclusion of the epidermal layer,
(b) a time-dependent analysis to investigate the transient temperature changes during burn. This allows the thermal damage induced onto the skin to be predicted using the standard Arrhenius model for damage rate
(c) the use of a three-dimensional or an axisymmetric skin model, and
(d) incorporating the effects (if any) of inhomogeneous and anisotropic conditions of the various tissue layers.

References

[1] Singapore Civil Defense Force Fire and Ambulance Statistics Fire Incident Statistics (Jan-Dec), http://www.nfpc.gov.sg (last accessed: 18/8/2008)

[2] Burn Centre under the Singapore General Hospital Singhealth http://www.sgh.com.sg/MedicalSpecialtiesnServices/SpecialistCentres/Burns/ (last accessed: 18/8/2008)

[3] Pennes H.H., 1948, Analysis of tissue and arterial blood temperatures in the resting forearm. *J. Appl. Physiol.* **1**, 93-122.

[4] Cheng A.H.D. and Cheng D.T., 2005, Heritage and early history of the boundary element method, *Eng Anal Bound Elem*, **29**, 268-302

[5] Henriques, F.C., and Moritz A.R., 1947 Studies of thermal injury: The conduction of heat to and through skin and the temperatures attained therein. A theoretical and an experimental investigation. *American Journal of Pathology*, **23**, 489–502

[6] Diller K.R. and Hayes L.J., 1983, A finite element model of burn injury in blood-perfused skin. *J Biomech Eng*, **105**, 300–307

[7] Torvi D.A. and Dale J.D., 1994, A finite element model of skin subjected to a flash fire. *J Biomech Eng*, 116, 250–255

[8] Ng E.Y.K. and Chua L.T., 2000, Mesh-independent prediction of skin burns injury. *J Med Eng Technol*. 24, 255–261

[9] Ng E.Y.K. and Chua L.T., 2002, Comparison of one- and two-dimensional programs for predicting the state of skin burns. *Burns*, **28**, 27–34

[10] Diller K.R., 1998, Modeling thermal skin burns on a personal computer. *J Burn Care Rehabil*, **19,** 420–429

[11] Diller K.R., 1999, Development and solution of finite difference equations for burn injury with spreadsheet software. *J Burn Care Rehabil*, **20**, 25–32

[12] Ng E.Y.K. and Chua L.T., 2002, Prediction of skin burn injury. Part 2: Parametric and Sensitivity Analysis, *Proc IMech, Part H: J Eng Med*, **216**, 171-183

[13] Gray H., 1969, *Anatomy of the Human Body*, 28th ed, (ed: C.M. Goss) Philadelphia: Lea and Febiger

[14] Fiju A. and Fiju F.A., 2001, Teaching the Taguchi Method to Industrial Engineers, *Work Study*, **50**, 141-149

Index

A

B

D

E

F

G

H

J

K

L

M

P

Q

R

S

T

U

V

W

X

Y

Z